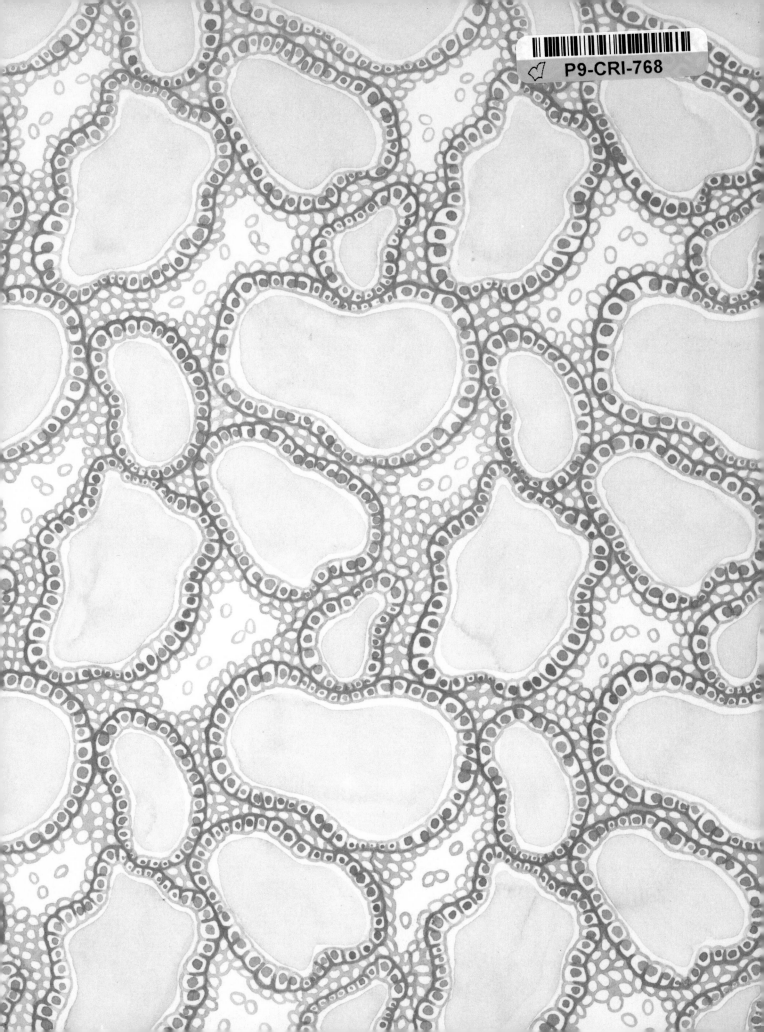

NURSE'S CLINICAL LIBRARY™

ENDOCRINE DISORDERS

NURSING84 BOOKS™
SPRINGHOUSE CORPORATION
Springhouse, Pennsylvania

NURSING84 BOOKS™

Nurse's Clinical Library™

Editorial Director
Helen Klusek Hamilton

Clinical Director
Minnie Bowen Rose, RN, BSN, MEd

Art Director
Sonja E. Douglas

Clinical staff
Clinical Editors
Diane Cochet, RN, BSN; Joanne
Patzek DaCunha, RN; Carole Arlene
Pyle, RN, BSN, MA, CCRN

Drug Information Manager
Larry Neil Gever, RPh, PharmD

Contributing Clinical Editors
Marlene Ciranowicz, RN, MSN; Mary
Gyetvan, RN, BSEd; Sandra Nettina,
RN, BSN; Jo-Ann Olmstead, RN, BS;
Patricia Schull, RN, MSN; Nina Welsh,
RN

Acquisitions
Thomas J. Leibrandt, Susan H.
Brunt, Bernadette M. Glenn

Editorial staff
Managing Editor
Matthew Cahill

Senior Editor
Peter Johnson

Associate Editors
Lisa Z. Cohen, June Norris

Contributing Editors
Laura Albert, Joan Twisdom-Harty,
Marylou Webster, Barbara Hodgson

Copy Supervisor
David R. Moreau

Copy Editors
Dale A. Brueggemann, Diane M.
Labus, Susan L. Baumann, Reni
Fetterolf, Max A. Fogel, Linda
Johnson, Doris Weinstock

Production Coordinator
Sally Johnson

Editorial Assistants
Mary Ann Bowes, Maree DeRosa

Design staff
Senior Designer
Carol Cameron-Sears

Contributing Designers
Jacalyn Bove Facciolo, Donna
Monturo, Mary Wise

Illustrators
Michael Adams, Dimitrios Bastas,
Maryanne Buschini, David
Christiana, David Cook, Design
Management, John Dougherty, Jean
Gardner, William Haney, Tom
Herbert, Robert Jackson, Adam
Mathews, Robert Phillips, George
Retseck, Eileen Rudisill, Eileen
Rudnick, Dennis Schofield

Production staff
Art Production Manager
Robert Perry

Typography Manager
David C. Kosten

Typography Assistants
Ethel Halle, Debra Judy, Diane
Paluba, Nancy Wirs

Senior Production Manager
Deborah C. Meiris

Production Manager
Wilbur D. Davidson

Production Assistant
Tim A. Landis

Special thanks to Regina D. Ford,
RN, BSN, MA.

**Library of Congress Cataloging in
Publication Data**
Main entry under title:
Endocrine disorders.
    (Nurse's clinical library)
    "Nursing84 Books."
    Bibliography: p.
    Includes index.
1. Endocrine glands—Diseases.
2. Endocrine glands—Diseases—
Nursing. I. Series. [DNLM:
1. Endocrinology—nurses' instruction.
WY 155 E563]
RC649.E5137 1984   616.4   84-5509
IBSN 0-916730-71-9

Cover: Color-enhanced thyroid scan.
Photograph by Howard Sochurek.
Inside front and back covers: Thyroid
follicles.

CONTENTS

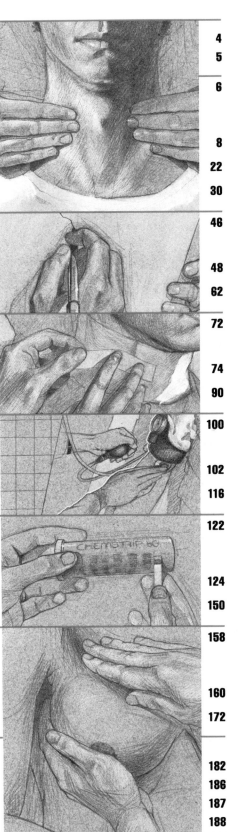

CONTRIBUTORS AND CLINICAL CONSULTANTS

Contributors

At the time of publication, the contributors held the following positions:

Frances Abbruzzo Amorim, RN, MSN, Assistant Professor, Department of Baccalaureate Nursing, Thomas Jefferson University, Philadelphia

Iris Elizabeth Williams Bailey, RNC, MS, Nursing Supervisor, Veterans Administration Medical Center, Memphis

Wendy L. Baker, RN, MS, Staff Nurse, Critical Care Medicine Unit, University of Michigan Hospitals, Ann Arbor

Jo Ann Dorothy Bocchese, RN, MSN, Program Coordinator for Special Child Health Services, Gloucester County Health Department, Woodbury, N.J.

Jeanne Buross-Herlihy, RN, BSN, Assistant Nurse Leader, Clinical Study Unit, New England Medical Center, Boston

Catherine D. Garofano, RN, BS, Clinical Nurse in Endocrinology and Metabolism, Senior Instructor in Medicine, Hahnemann University Medical College and Hospital, Philadelphia

Diana W. Guthrie, RN, EdS, FAAN, C,NCC, Associate Professor and Diabetes Nurse Specialist, Kansas Regional Diabetes Center, University of Kansas School of Medicine, Wichita

Richard A. Guthrie, MD, FAAP, Professor and Director, Kansas Regional Diabetes Center, University of Kansas School of Medicine, Wichita

Sande Jones, RN, BSN, MS, Education Coordinator, Department of Nursing Education, Research, and Standards, Mount Sinai Medical Center of Greater Miami

Joyce L. Kee, RN, MSN, Associate Professor, College of Nursing, University of Delaware, Newark

M. Christene Perkins, RN, MN, Chairperson, Department of Nursing, Kettering (Ohio) College of Medical Arts

Dolores Lake Taylor, RN, MSN, Senior Associate Professor, Bucks County Community College, Newtown, Pa.

Jean Fetzer Walters, RN, MSN, Director, Quality Assurance and Nursing Education, Froedtert Memorial Lutheran Hospital, Milwaukee

Elizabeth Warren-Boulton, RN, MSN, Coordinator for Professional Education, Washington University Diabetes Research and Training Center, St. Louis

Clinical Consultants

At the time of publication, the clinical consultants held the following positions:

Nancy B. Alexander, RN, MSN, Assistant Professor, Duke University School of Nursing, Durham, N.C.

Gregory D. Borowski, MD, Fellow, Division of Endocrinology, Hahnemann University, Philadelphia

James M. Cerletty, MD, Associate Professor of Medicine and Consultant in Endocrinology, Medical College of Wisconsin, Milwaukee

Carol S. Dalglish, RN, MSN, Clinical Specialist in Obstetrics/Gynecology/Infertility, Center for Fertility and Reproductive Research, Vanderbilt University Medical Center, Nashville

Esther Eisenberg, MD, Assistant Professor of Obstetrics and Gynecology, University of Pennsylvania School of Medicine and Pennsylvania Hospital, Philadelphia

Ruth Ann Fitzpatrick, MD, Director, Division of Endocrinology, Crozer-Chester Medical Center, Chester, Pa.

Catherine D. Garofano, RN, BS, Clinical Nurse in Endocrinology and Metabolism, Senior Instructor in Medicine, Hahnemann University Medical College and Hospital, Philadelphia

Gilbert G. Haas, Jr., MD, Associate Professor and Director, Division of Reproductive Endocrinology and Infertility, Department of Obstetrics and Gynecology, University of Oklahoma Health Sciences Center, Oklahoma City

Thad C. Hagen, MD, Chief, Medical Service, Veterans Administration Medical Center; Professor and Co-chairman, Department of Medicine, Medical College of Wisconsin, Milwaukee

Jeanette Taitano Hoffmann, RN, MSN, Assistant Professor, Alverno College, Milwaukee

Anthony S. Jennings, MD, Assistant Professor of Medicine and Pathology, University of Pennsylvania, Philadelphia

John E. Nestler, MD, Fellow in Endocrinology, University of Pennsylvania, Philadelphia

Linda Niedringhaus, RN, MSN, Instructor in Nursing, St. Louis University School of Nursing

Judith M. Roberts, RN, MSN, FNP, Adjunct Faculty, University of North Carolina; Private Nursing Consultant; Family Nurse Practitioner, Wake Teen Medical Services, Chapel Hill, N.C.

Sarah J. Sanford, RN, MA, CCRN, Vice-President, Nursing Services, Overlake Hospital, Bellevue, Wash.

Barbara Solomon, RN, MSN, Clinical Nurse Specialist in Endocrinology, National Institutes of Health, Bethesda, Md.

Ann Gill Taylor, RN, MS, EdD, FAAN, Professor and Director, Medical-Surgical Nursing, School of Nursing, University of Virginia, Charlottesville

Richard W. Tureck, MD, Assistant Professor of Obstetrics and Gynecology, University of Pennsylvania School of Medicine, Philadelphia

Madeline Wake, RN, MSN, Administrator, Continuing Education in Nursing; Assistant Professor of Nursing, Marquette University, Milwaukee

FOREWORD

Endocrine disorders challenge your professional skills in many complex ways. Obviously, they require accurate and continually updated information, as advancing knowledge leads to ever newer and more sophisticated diagnostic tests and treatments. For example, when managing diabetes, you need to be aware of programmable insulin pumps and genetically engineered insulins.

But keeping up with new information is only part of it. Equally important is your ability to recognize and deal with these disorders' profound and wide-ranging physical and psychological effects. Patients with endocrine disorders must often contend with prolonged treatments, emotional distress, social isolation, and, at times, disfigurement caused by hormonal imbalances. To help these patients, you must be prepared to act as educator, counselor, and care coordinator. For example, you must teach and motivate patients with chronic disorders, such as diabetes mellitus, to comply with prescribed treatment and help them understand and correct the underlying reasons for noncompliance. You must provide psychological support and direction for patients with irreversible impairments, such as for some patients with primary hypogonadism. And you must coordinate the efforts of endocrinologists, psychologists, social workers, nutritionists, and exercise therapists to minimize these disorders' debilitating effects.

Meeting these varied responsibilities starts with reliable information. This volume, ENDOCRINE DISORDERS, provides such information, gathered from the clinical specialists who deal with these disorders most often. The introductory chapter reviews endocrine anatomy and physiology, the function and effects of hormones, and the pathophysiology of hormonal imbalance. The second chapter explains endocrine assessment techniques and offers guidelines for developing nursing diagnoses based on the patient history and physical examination. The third chapter provides information on diagnostic tests—blood and urine hormone assays, provocation tests, and the latest forms of radiography—and discusses the implications of test results.

The remaining 10 chapters discuss specific endocrine disorders. Each chapter consists of three major sections. *Pathophysiology* covers the etiology of each disorder, its characteristic signs and symptoms, and its effects on other body systems. *Medical management* summarizes appropriate diagnostic tests and findings, current treatment, and prognosis. *Nursing management,* organized according to the nursing process, offers detailed guidelines for accurate assessment and includes characteristic assessment findings and their implications and the nursing diagnoses that flow from them. Using these diagnoses, this section summarizes nursing goals, appropriate interventions for achieving these goals, and guidelines for evaluation.

To illustrate and amplify the text, this volume contains many anatomic drawings, graphs, charts, and diagrams, including a comprehensive map of endocrine physiology and hormonal pathways. Other graphically highlighted elements emphasize patient-teaching aids, which offer tips for routine care, and emergency care of life-threatening complications, such as thyroid storm. The appendices summarize information on rare endocrine syndromes and frequently used endocrine drugs.

With endocrine disorders affecting more than 10% of the population, all practicing nurses need to keep their knowledge of these disorders current and accurate. This volume will help nurses at all professional levels gain this necessary knowledge and improve their nursing care.

DIANA W. GUTHRIE, RN, EdS, FAAN, C,NCC
Associate Professor and Diabetes Nurse Specialist
Kansas Regional Diabetes Center
University of Kansas School of Medicine at Wichita

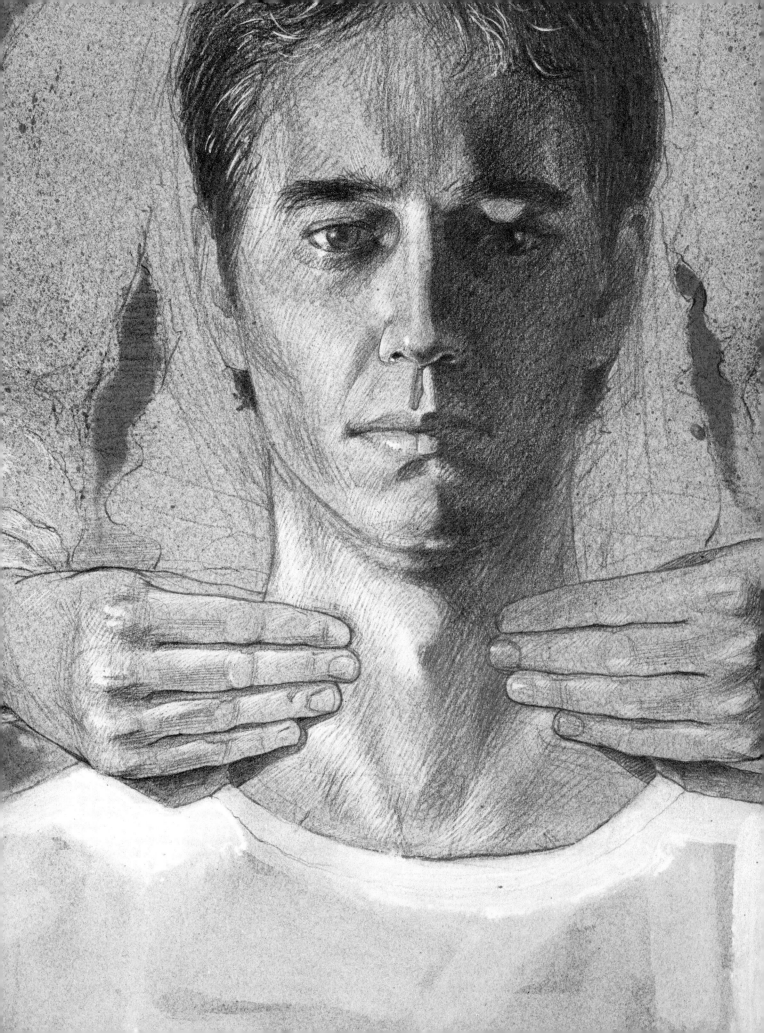

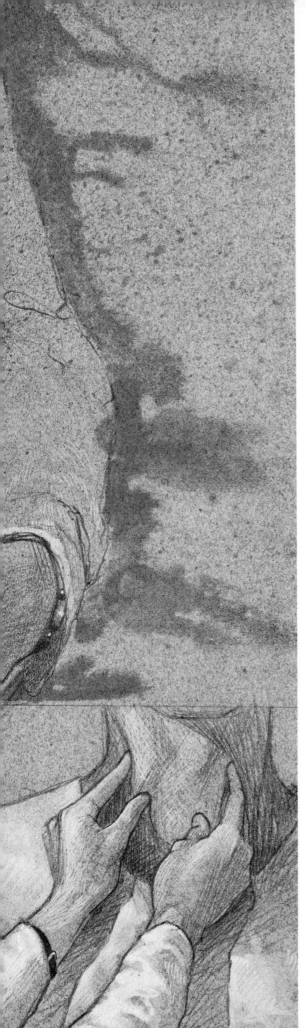

FUNDAMENTAL ENDOCRINE FACTS

1 REVIEWING FUNDAMENTAL PRINCIPLES

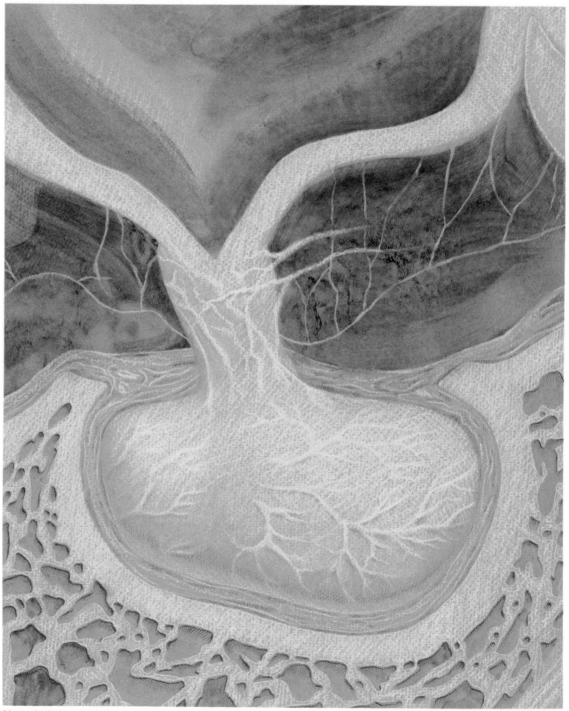

Normal pituitary gland

Endocrine glands are largely responsible for maintaining the homeostasis of some 50 *billion* cells. These glands secrete many hormones into the bloodstream, regulating the hundreds of chemical reactions involved in growth, maturation, reproduction, metabolism, and even behavior. The complexity of endocrine function contributes to the large number and diversity of endocrine disorders, which exact an enormous economic, social, and psychological toll. Diabetes mellitus, the most common endocrine disorder, affects roughly 10 million people in the United States. Thyroid disorders, also relatively common, generate high care costs. Pituitary and gonadal disorders can cause disfigurement, social maladjustment, and emotional stress.

What does this mean to you? Obviously, it means you'll frequently be dealing with endocrine disorders—no matter where you practice nursing. As more sophisticated diagnostic tests and treatments emerge, you'll need expanded assessment and therapeutic management skills. Also, you'll be expected to play an important role in promoting patient self-management skills in chronic diseases and in providing thorough patient education and emotional support.

To successfully meet these nursing challenges, you'll need to be thoroughly familiar with endocrine anatomy and physiology, the function of hormones and their effects on target organs and tissues, and the causes of endocrine pathology.

What is the endocrine system?

The endocrine system works with the nervous system to regulate and integrate the body's metabolic activities. This system consists of ductless glands and other structures that secrete hormones directly into the bloodstream. Hormones are a class of proteins that act as chemical messengers that stimulate target tissues; they're essential for controlling normal growth, development, and reproduction, and for maintaining homeostasis.

The endocrine glands include the pituitary (hypophysis), thyroid, parathyroid, adrenals, islet cells of the pancreas, testes, and ovaries. The pineal and thymus glands also secrete hormones, but their endocrine function isn't well understood. The placenta and the gastrointestinal mucosa also produce hormones. Placental hormones promote embryo growth; gastrointestinal hormones aid digestion. (See *Understanding endocrine anatomy,* page 10.)

UNDERSTANDING HORMONAL MECHANISMS

Hormones are classified into three structural types: peptides, steroids, and amino acid analogues. The peptides include the hormones secreted by the anterior and posterior pituitary and by the parathyroids and the pancreatic hormones insulin and glucagon. The steroids, synthesized from cholesterol, include the sex hormones and the adrenocortical hormones. The amino acid analogues include the thyroid hormones and the catecholamines epinephrine and norepinephrine, secreted by the adrenal medulla. Prostaglandins, a group of hormonelike substances, have wide-ranging somatic effects, and their influence on the endocrine system is being intensively studied.

Hormones controlled by feedback

Hormonal secretion is controlled by feedback mechanisms, which act to stabilize blood hormone levels. For example, elevated thyroid hormone levels inhibit secretion of thyroid-stimulating hormone (TSH) from the pituitary, while reduced thyroid hormone levels stimulate TSH secretion. Metabolite levels may also regulate hormone release. For example, blood glucose levels regulate insulin release from the pancreas, and calcium regulates parathyroid hormone levels. Many of these feedback mechanisms combine to maintain cellular homeostasis. (See *Understanding endocrine dynamics,* pages 12 and 13.)

Mediators and activators

Hormones act on target cells in one of two ways: through a *mediator* or by *gene activation*. The nucleotide cyclic adenosine monophosphate, commonly called cyclic AMP, is an important intracellular mediator for many peptide hormones and the catecholamines. In such cases, a hormone exerts its effect on a target cell by activating cyclic AMP in the cell. Typically, a stimulating hormone combines with a specific hormone receptor at the cell membrane. This hormone-receptor complex stimulates the cyclic AMP mechanism, which generates the appropriate cellular response. For example, TSH acts through cyclic AMP to cause thyroid cells to produce thyroxine (T_4).

Steroid and thyroid hormones act through *gene activation*. A steroid hormone binds to a receptor protein in the cytoplasm, forming a complex that enters the cell nucleus after it's been changed to a form with smaller molecular weight. The new protein-hormone

Understanding endocrine anatomy

The endocrine glands secrete hormones directly into the bloodstream to regulate body function. This illustration shows the location of these glands and that of the placenta and gastrointestinal mucosa, which also secrete hormones.

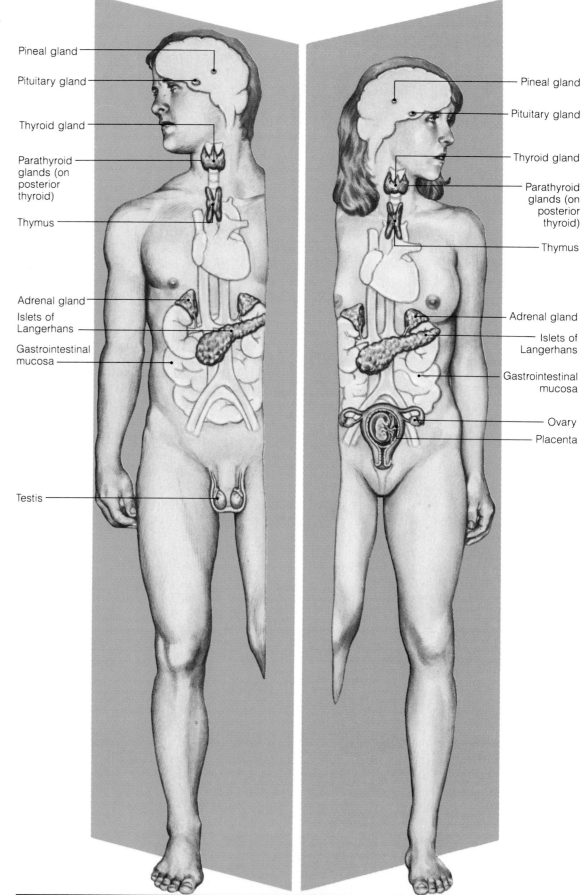

Pineal gland

Pituitary gland

Thyroid gland

Parathyroid glands (on posterior thyroid)

Thymus

Adrenal gland

Islets of Langerhans

Gastrointestinal mucosa

Testis

Pineal gland

Pituitary gland

Thyroid gland

Parathyroid glands (on posterior thyroid)

Thymus

Adrenal gland

Islets of Langerhans

Gastrointestinal mucosa

Ovary

Placenta

complex activates genes in the nucleus to form messenger RNA, which diffuses into the surrounding cytoplasm and stimulates new protein formation in the ribosomes. For example, upon entering a renal tubular cell, aldosterone combines with a receptor protein and causes the cell to manufacture new proteins that promote sodium reabsorption and potassium secretion in the tubules. (See *Steroid and thyroid hormone action,* page 16.)

Hormone levels vary
Levels of circulating hormones reflect the rate of secretion, inactivation, and excretion. (See *Hormone storage and release,* page 15.) These levels may vary with the time of day or the patient's metabolic state, posture, and intrinsic rhythms. Such factors must be considered when evaluating endocrine function during a diagnostic workup.

THE PITUITARY GLAND
Also known as the *hypophysis*, the pituitary gland is about 1 cm in diameter and weighs 0.5 to 0.75 g. It lies in a cavity of bone at the base of the skull (the *sella turcica*) and is connected to the hypothalamus by the *pituitary stalk*. The pituitary has two distinct parts: an anterior lobe (*adenohypophysis*) and a posterior lobe (*neurohypophysis*). The anterior lobe constitutes most of the gland.

Role of the hypothalamus
The endocrine system meets the nervous system at the hypothalamic-pituitary interface. The hypothalamus regulates pituitary activity through two pathways. *Neural* pathways extend from the hypothalamus, where two hormones—antidiuretic hormone (ADH) and oxytocin—are synthesized, to the posterior pituitary lobe, where the hormones are stored and secreted. *Portal venous* pathways, which connect the hypothalamus to the anterior pituitary lobe, carry hypothalamic releasing and inhibiting hormones as well as most of the lobe's blood supply.

Anterior pituitary
Releasing and inhibiting hormones secreted by the hypothalamus into the anterior pituitary control the release of various adenohypophyseal hormones, which, in turn, stimulate their target cells. By binding to specific cell membrane receptors in the anterior pituitary, the hypothalamic hormones stimulate production and release of pituitary hormones into the bloodstream. For example,

thyrotropin-releasing hormone (TRH) from the hypothalamus reaches the anterior pituitary, where it stimulates secretion of TSH, which travels through the bloodstream to the thyroid gland. TSH causes the thyroid to produce T_4, which has wide-ranging effects on cell growth and metabolism.

Besides TRH, other important hypothalamic hormonal secretions include corticotropin-releasing factor (CRF), growth hormone-releasing hormone (GH-RH), growth hormone-inhibitory hormone (GHIH), luteinizing hormone-releasing hormone (LH-RH), and prolactin-inhibitory factor (PIF).

The anterior pituitary itself synthesizes and secretes at least seven important hormones, including growth hormone (GH), prolactin, adrenocorticotropic hormone (ACTH), follicle-stimulating hormone (FSH), luteinizing hormone (LH), thyroid-stimulating hormone (TSH), and melanocyte-stimulating hormone (MSH). Let's look at each of these in turn.

Growth hormone. Although this hormone doesn't affect a specific target organ or tissue, it promotes protein synthesis and tissue growth and induces mobilization of fat from adipose tissue into the bloodstream. It indirectly stimulates cartilage and bone growth by causing formation of small peptides called *somatomedins*, which mediate collagen deposition required for bone and cartilage growth. Necessary for body growth in children, the hormone is thought to maintain normal size and function of adult body organs and to regulate protein synthesis. Growth hormone also depresses carbohydrate metabolism, raising blood glucose levels above normal and causing a diabetogenic effect. This decreased carbohydrate metabolism may result in part from increased fat metabolism.

Secretion of GH occurs in waves and is related to sleep and other neurogenic factors, such as stress and exercise. Plasma GH levels vary with age, and this hormone continues to be secreted even after skeletal growth stops.

Prolactin. Similar in chemical structure to GH, prolactin stimulates milk production in the mammary glands after they have been prepared first by the influence of other hormones, including GH, estrogen, progesterones, T_4, parathyroid hormone, insulin, and corticosteroids. Prolactin synthesis and secretion is reduced by PIF; postpartum decline in PIF levels markedly increases prolactin secretion. The stimulus produced by the infant's suckling and removal of milk from the breast also in-

Understanding endocrine dynamics

The endocrine system works together with the nervous system to maintain bodily functions. Although nerve cells generate electrical impulses that travel rapidly along specialized pathways, they're rapidly fatigued by prolonged and repeated stimulation. Generally slower-acting, the endocrine system uses *hormones,* which travel in the fluid parts of the body, such as the bloodstream, to produce specific effects in target tissues.

Hormones are secreted by endocrine glands and by other structures having endocrine functions, such as the gastrointestinal mucosa and the placenta.

This flow diagram depicts endocrine tissues, hormones, and the interactions that link them in an intricate system of checks and balances. Endocrine glands and tissues are shown as octagons. Hormones appear as solid lines colorcoded from the gland of origin. The thin, lightly shaded lines indicate feedback from target tissues. Triangles show major points of nonhormonal stimulation, and rectangular areas indicate other endocrine effects. The hypothalamus has been given its own shape to indicate its position as an important point of contact between the nervous and endocrine systems.

Key:

ACTH Adrenocortico-
tropic hormone
ADH Antidiuretic
hormone
CCK Cholecystokinin
FSH Follicle-stimulating
hormone
GH Growth hormone
HCG Human chorionic
gonadotropin
HPL Human placental
lactogen
LH Luteinizing hormone
MSH Melanocyte-
stimulating
hormone
TSH Thyroid-stimulating
hormone

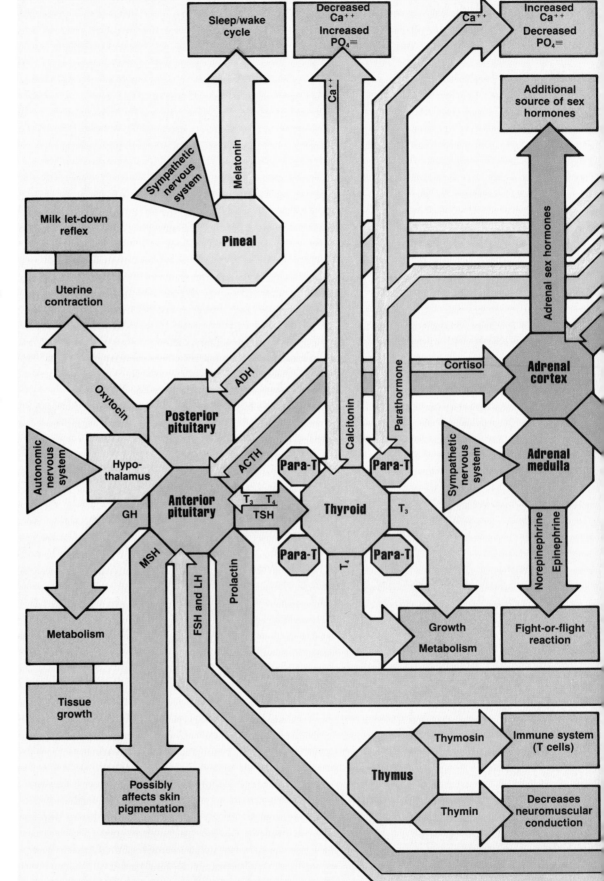

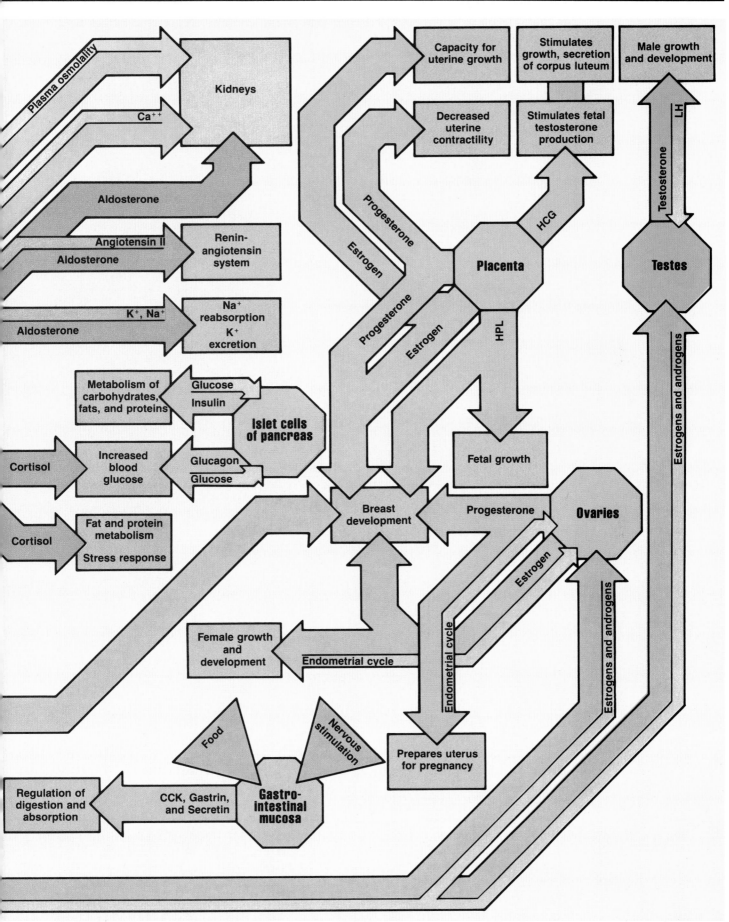

creases prolactin secretion and maintains milk production.

Adrenocorticotropic hormone. Also known as corticotropin, this hormone stimulates production of aldosterone, cortisol, and other glucocorticoids. Plasma cortisol levels largely control ACTH secretion through a negative feedback mechanism. For example, high cortisol levels act directly on the corticotropic cells in the pituitary to suppress ACTH secretion. ACTH also has some melanocyte-stimulating activity and increases amino acid uptake by muscle cells, promotes lipolysis by fat cells, stimulates pancreatic beta cells to secrete insulin, and may contribute to GH release.

Plasma ACTH levels vary diurnally, peaking in the early morning and ebbing in the evening. Physical and emotional stress greatly increases ACTH secretion and can override the negative feedback effect of plasma cortisol levels.

Follicle-stimulating hormone (FSH) and luteinizing hormone (LH). The secretion of these hormones is regulated by LH-RH and by circulating levels of sex hormones. In women, FSH promotes ovarian follicle growth and maturation; secretion fluctuates rhythmically during the menstrual cycle, peaking at ovulation. Both FSH and LH are required to stimulate ovarian estrogen secretion. LH triggers ovulation and maintains the corpus luteum, which, in turn, secretes progesterone. In males, continuous secretion of FSH (and testosterone) stimulates and maintains spermatogenesis. LH stimulates the interstitial (Leydig's) cells in the testes to secrete testosterone, which, with FSH, stimulates and maintains spermatogenesis.

Thyroid-stimulating hormone. Also known as thyrotropin, this hormone is secreted upon stimulation by TRH from the hypothalamus and causes the thyroid gland to release thyroxine (T_4) and triiodothyronine (T_3). Elevated circulating T_4 and T_3 levels exert a negative feedback effect on TSH secretion from the pituitary.

TSH also stimulates increases in size, number, and secretory activity of thyroid cells; and heightens "iodine pump activity" (active transport of iodine across the basal cell membrane), often raising the ratio of intracellular to extracellular iodine as much as 350:1.

Melanocyte-stimulating hormone. This pigment-metabolizing hormone disperses melanocytes containing the dark pigment melanin and is structurally similar to ACTH. In most animals, MSH is produced in the intermediate lobe of the pituitary from the same precursor that gives rise to ACTH. However, in humans this lobe is nearly absent and produces little MSH. Although detected in the fetus, the hormone's presence in the adult is controversial.

Posterior pituitary

Although the posterior pituitary doesn't secrete hormones, it's connected to the hypothalamus by terminal nerve endings. These nerve endings store oxytocin and ADH, which are produced in the hypothalamus.

Oxytocin. Although this hormone is present in the male, it has no known function. In the female, oxytocin exerts its effects primarily during labor and lactation. Although it doesn't initiate labor, it does stimulate uterine contractions and is especially important in the breast's postpartum let-down reflex. The stimulus produced by the newborn's suckling triggers oxytocin release from the posterior pituitary. Reaching the breast via the circulation, the hormone causes the alveoli to contract and express milk into the milk ducts. When released during sexual stimulation, oxytocin promotes fertilization of the ovum by causing contractions in the uterus and fallopian tubes that help propel semen through the fallopian tubes.

Antidiuretic hormone. Also known as vasopressin, ADH regulates fluid balance by making the collecting ducts and distal renal tubules more permeable to water. Osmoreceptor cells in the hypothalamus control the secretion of ADH into the circulation. In a dehydrated patient, the osmolality of extracellular fluid increases, drawing water across an osmotic gradient from body cells. As a result, the cell volume of osmoreceptors decreases, causing them to stimulate release of ADH. Conversely, excessive circulating water reduces extracellular fluid osmolality, and water flows into body cells. This increases receptor cell volume and inhibits ADH release.

THE THYROID GLAND

This important gland consists of two lateral lobes, connected by an isthmus. The lobes partially envelop the anterior and lateral surfaces of the trachea, just below the cricoid cartilage. In the adult, the thyroid weighs about 20 g. It's partially composed of follicular cells containing an iodinated colloidal protein, *thyroglobulin,* which acts as a reservoir for thyroid hormone precursors and for iodide,

Hormone storage and release

Endocrine cells manufacture and release their hormone products in several ways, as shown here.

1. Many endocrine cells possess receptors on their cell membranes that respond to stimuli, such as abnormal extracellular ion levels, hormones from other glands, or impulses from neurons impinging on the membrane. For example, neural stimulation of this pancreatic beta cell synthesizes the hormone precursor *preproinsulin* and converts it to *proinsulin* in beadlike *ribosomes* located on the endoplasmic reticulum. Proinsulin is transferred to the Golgi complex, which collects it into secretory granules. Insulin is formed in the Golgi complex and the secretory granules. These granules move to the cell wall, where they fuse with the plasma membrane and disperse insulin into the bloodstream. Hormonal release by membrane fusion is called *exocytosis*.

2. Thyroid cells store a hormone precursor, colloidal iodinated thyroglobulin, which contains iodine and thyroglobulin. When stimulated by TSH, a follicular cell takes up some of the stored thyroglobulin by *endocytosis*—the reverse of exocytosis. The cell membrane extends fingerlike projections into the colloid, then pulls portions of it back into the cell. Lysosomes in the cell fuse with the colloid, which is then degraded by proteolysis into T_3 and T_4, which are released into the circulation and the lymphatic system by exocytosis.

3. Anterior and posterior pituitary secretions are controlled by hypothalamic signals. On the left of this drawing, the hypothalamic neuron produces ADH, which travels down the axon and is stored in secretory granules in nerve endings in the posterior pituitary. When the axon membrane is depolarized, calcium ions flow into the axon, the hormone granules fuse with the membrane of the terminal bulb, and the hormone is released.

The right side of the drawing shows how the anterior pituitary is stimulated to produce its many hormones. Here, a hypothalamic neuron manufactures *hormone releasing factors* and secretes them into a capillary of the portal system; the factors travel down the pituitary stalk to the anterior pituitary. There, they cause release of many pituitary hormones, including ACTH, TSH, GH, FSH, LH, and prolactin.

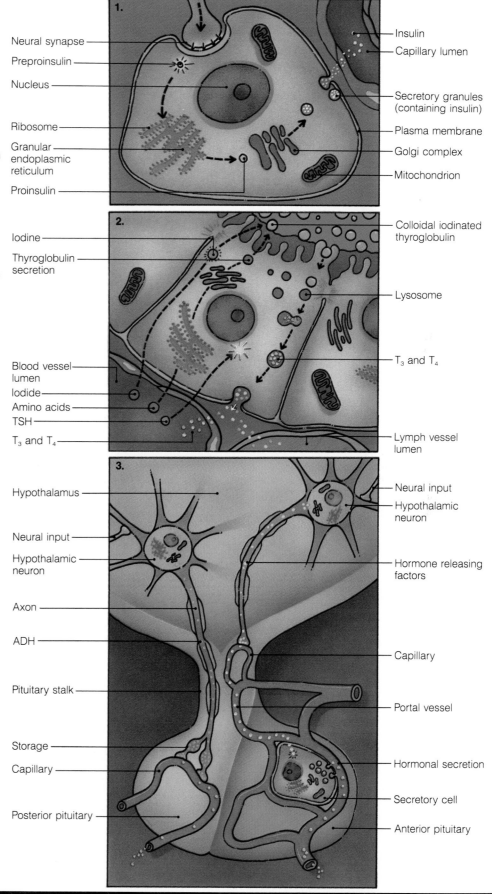

1.
- Neural synapse
- Preproinsulin
- Nucleus
- Ribosome
- Granular endoplasmic reticulum
- Proinsulin
- Insulin
- Capillary lumen
- Secretory granules (containing insulin)
- Plasma membrane
- Golgi complex
- Mitochondrion

2.
- Iodine
- Thyroglobulin secretion
- Blood vessel lumen
- Iodide
- Amino acids
- TSH
- T_3 and T_4
- Colloidal iodinated thyroglobulin
- Lysosome
- T_3 and T_4
- Lymph vessel lumen

3.
- Hypothalamus
- Neural input
- Hypothalamic neuron
- Axon
- ADH
- Pituitary stalk
- Storage
- Capillary
- Posterior pituitary
- Neural input
- Hypothalamic neuron
- Hormone releasing factors
- Capillary
- Portal vessel
- Hormonal secretion
- Secretory cell
- Anterior pituitary

which the gland actively concentrates from ingested food and water. TSH causes the parafollicular cells to synthesize triiodothyronine (T_3) and its suspected precursor, thyroxine (T_4) from thyroglobulin and to release them directly into the bloodstream. From 50% to 90% of T_3 is thought to be derived from T_4. The remaining 10% or more is secreted directly by the thyroid gland.

Most circulating T_3 and T_4 is bound to a serum protein, *thyroxine-binding globulin,* leaving a minute amount of the hormones free to exert their effects. The plasma level of free thyroid hormones mediates a complex negative feedback system based on TSH secretion from the anterior pituitary.

Thyroid hormones increase the metabolic activities of all body tissues. They increase the rate of nutrient use for energy production as well as the rate of protein synthesis and breakdown. These hormones increase oxygen consumption, especially in the heart, kidneys, liver, and skeletal muscle, and also accelerate the rate of growth in children. Many other endocrine glands often increase their activity in the presence of thyroid hormones.

Steroid and thyroid hormone action

Steroid hormones (ST) combine with receptors in the cytoplasm, whereas thyroid hormones (T) enter the nucleus before combining with receptors (R). These activated receptors bind to the DNA in the chromatin, where they modulate transcription of specific genes to form messenger RNA (mRNA). The mRNA enters the cytoplasm and promotes formation of new proteins in the ribosomes, which then mediate the appropriate response to the hormone.

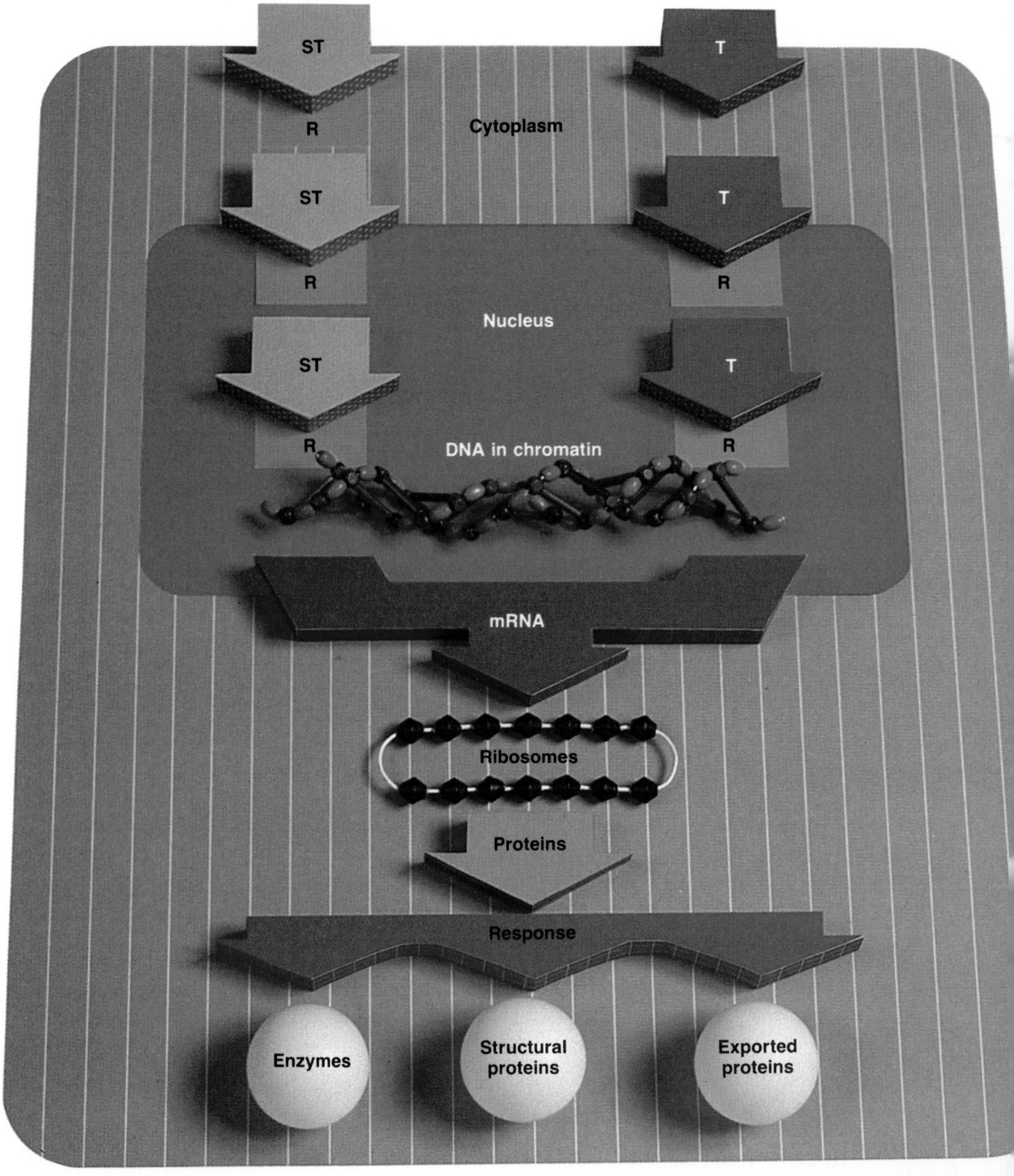

ST

T

R

Cytoplasm

ST

T

R

R

Nucleus

ST

T

R

R

DNA in chromatin

mRNA

Ribosomes

Proteins

Response

Enzymes

Structural proteins

Exported proteins

Calcitonin is a hypocalcemic hormone, secreted predominantly by thyroid parafollicular cells in response to hypercalcemia. The exact role of calcitonin in normal human physiology is not fully defined. Its principal effect is to inhibit bone resorption. Calcitonin is also secreted by the parathyroid glands.

THE PARATHYROID GLANDS

Four small parathyroid glands, each weighing about 30 mg, are normally located beside the thyroid, embedded in the dorsal surface of each upper and lower pole. Composed mainly of agranular *chief cells* and large granular *oxyphil cells*, these glands secrete *parathyroid hormone* (PTH) and calcitonin, which regulate calcium and phosphorus metabolism.

PTH stimulates reabsorption of calcium and phosphate from bone by activating bone-removing *osteoclast* cells and transiently depressing bone-renewing *osteoblast* cells. In the kidneys, this hormone acts on the renal tubules to cause excretion of phosphate and reabsorption of calcium and magnesium. It also increases calcium and phosphate absorption in the intestines. Vitamin D, after it's activated to its most potent metabolite, 1-alpha-dihydroxyvitamin D_3, enhances the absorption of calcium and phosphate from the intestinal tract.

Control of PTH largely depends on extracellular calcium levels. Depressed calcium levels increase PTH secretion, and elevated calcium levels suppress PTH secretion. Calcitonin opposes the effects of PTH, reducing serum calcium levels.

THE ADRENAL GLANDS

The adrenal glands lie at the superior poles of the kidneys and weigh about 4 to 5 g each. They're composed of two morphologically and physiologically distinct parts—an outer *cortex* and an inner *medulla*.

Adrenal cortex

This tissue constitutes almost 90% of the gland. It's divided into three distinct cellular zones: the *zona glomerulosa*, a thin outer layer making up about 15% of the cortex and secreting aldosterone, a mineralocorticoid; the *zona fasciculata*, or middle layer, constituting about 75% of the cortex; and the *zona reticularis*, constituting the rest. The last two zones secrete glucocorticoids and androgen precursors, respectively.

Aldosterone causes the kidneys to retain sodium and excrete potassium, thereby influencing extracellular fluid volume, blood pressure, and electrolyte balance. Many factors influence aldosterone secretion, including potassium, sodium, and ACTH levels and the feedback from the renin-angiotensin system.

The adrenal glucocorticoids include the major hormone *cortisol* (hydrocortisone), corticosterone, and cortisone. Secreted in response to ACTH stimulation, the adrenal glucocorticoids help the body to resist physical and mental stress. They inhibit inflammation and promote normal metabolism of carbohydrates, fats, and proteins, thereby raising blood glucose levels.

Besides mineralocorticoids and glucocorticoids, the adrenal cortex secretes androgen precursors and minute amounts of estrogens and progesterones, but these normally exert minimal effects.

Adrenal medulla

This portion of the adrenal gland is composed mostly of chromaffin cells and acts as a functional extension of the sympathetic nervous system. After sympathetic stimulation, the medulla secretes *catecholamines,* primarily epinephrine and norepinephrine; their effects on target organs persist about 10 times longer than direct nervous stimulation.

Both catecholamines work with the sympathetic nervous system to produce a physiologic response to stress—the fight-or-flight response—that increases heart rate and cardiac output, dilates the pupils, constricts blood vessels in the skin, elevates serum glucose and fatty acid levels, and induces an aroused mental state.

THE PANCREAS

Composed of both endocrine and exocrine tissue, the pancreas lies transversely across the posterior abdominal wall in the epigastric and hypochondriac regions of the body. In adults, the pancreas is about 5″ (13 cm) long and weighs about 2.5 oz (70 g). In its exocrine function, it secretes digestive enzymes via ducts that empty into the duodenum.

The endocrine function of the pancreas is carried out by about 1 million distinct *islets of Langerhans*, which are composed of beta-, alpha-, and delta-secretory cells. (See *Islets of Langerhans,* page 18.) The beta cells secrete insulin, which directly regulates glucose metabolism and the processes necessary for intermediary metabolism of fats, carbohydrates, and proteins. Alpha cells secrete glucagon, which counters the action of insulin.

Islets of Langerhans

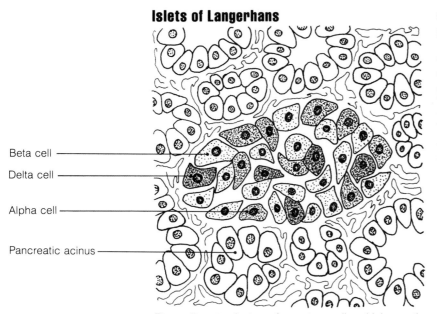

Beta cell

Delta cell

Alpha cell

Pancreatic acinus

These discrete clusters of secretory cells, which constitute the endocrine portion of the pancreas, are made up of three cell types: beta cells, which secrete insulin; alpha cells, which secrete glucagon; and delta cells, which secrete somatostatin.

Delta cells secrete the hormone *somatostatin,* the function of which isn't clearly understood.

The role of insulin

Insulin primarily controls glucose homeostasis, maintaining serum glucose levels within a narrow range whether the individual is eating or fasting. During eating, insulin promotes the transfer of glucose across cell membranes of insulin-sensitive tissues, such as muscle and fat. Some important cells, such as neurons, brain cells, erythrocytes, and liver cells, can metabolize glucose without insulin. During eating, insulin also stimulates storage of glucose as glycogen in the liver, and it suppresses gluconeogenesis.

In the fasting state, insulin levels drop, decreasing glucose utilization and increasing glucose production by gluconeogenesis and glycogenolysis.

Glucagon, secreted by the pancreas when blood glucose is low, stimulates liver glycolysis and glycogenolysis, thereby increasing the blood glucose level. It can reverse insulin-induced hypoglycemia in patients with adequate liver glycogen stores. Glucagon resembles epinephrine in its effects on the liver, heart, and intestines. Blood glucose concentration is the major determinant of both insulin and glucagon secretion. An increase in blood glucose triggers insulin secretion and suppresses glucagon secretion. When blood glucose falls below about 100 mg/ml, insulin secretion drops to a low level and triggers glucagon release.

THE TESTES

The testes produce spermatozoa and male sex hormones (androgens), of which testosterone is the most important. The two testes each weigh about 21 g and are held in the scrotum, a pouchlike sac suspended outside the abdominal cavity. Each testis is divided into compartments (lobules) by fibrous septa. The lobules contain seminiferous tubules in which sperm are formed and loose connective tissue with clusters of interstitial cells, called *Leydig's cells,* which secrete testosterone.

During fetal life, testosterone mediates the development of male sex organs and the descent of the testes into the scrotum. After infancy, little testosterone is secreted until puberty, when, stimulated by LH, it promotes growth of the penis, scrotum, and testes as well as development of secondary sex characteristics, such as increased hair distribution, deepened voice, and increased musculature. FSH from the anterior pituitary stimulates spermatogenesis; final sperm maturation requires FSH, LH, and testosterone.

THE OVARIES

Almond-shaped and weighing about 14 g each, the ovaries are suspended on either side of the uterus by ligaments and lie close to the fimbriated end of the fallopian tubes. Each ovary consists of an outer *cortex* and an inner *medulla* and is enclosed in an outer layer of germinal epithelium with a layer of connective tissue beneath it.

The ovaries release gametes (eggs) for fertilization and secrete female sex hormones that affect growth and function of the reproductive tract and other target tissues.

Estradiol, the major estrogen, and *progesterone* are the two principal ovarian sex hormones. Estrogens promote development of genitalia, growth of other body cells, and development of secondary sex characteristics, such as fat distribution and breast growth. Progesterone prepares the uterus for pregnancy and the breasts for lactation.

The female gonads secrete only slight amounts of estrogens and progesterone until puberty, when the hypothalamus stimulates the anterior pituitary to secrete FSH and LH, which regulate the menstrual cycle. These hormones stimulate follicular development and estrogen secretion, leading to ovulation. After ovulation, the secretory cells of the follicle form the *corpus luteum*, which secretes mostly progesterone and some estrogens for about 14 days. If fertilization does not occur during this period, the corpus luteum atrophies and stops secreting its hormones; menstruation begins, to start the cycle anew.

THE THYMUS

The thymus is the central gland of the lymphatic system. Enclosed in a capsule of connective tissue, it's located beneath the sternum and comprises two lateral lobes of lymphatic tissue. The lobes divide further into numerous lobules, each containing an outer cellular cortex and an inner medulla. The size of the thymus varies with age: up to age 2, it's large in relation to the body; by puberty it shrinks to the size of a chestnut. After puberty it atrophies gradually and weighs about 10 g in an adult.

The thymus produces the hormones *thymosin* and *thymin* (thymopoietin). The gland's endocrine activity probably depends on the activity of thymosin, which is composed of biologically active peptides critical to maturation and development of the immune system. The T cells of the cell-mediated immune response develop in the thymus before migrating to the lymph nodes and the spleen. Although researchers have shown that thymin blocks neuromuscular transmission, this effect may not be clinically significant.

THE PINEAL GLAND

Still poorly understood after decades of research, the pineal gland is about the size of a pea, weighs about 0.1 to 0.18 g, and is divided into anterior and posterior lobes. It's attached by a small stalk to the posterior part of the third ventricle of the brain. The pineal serves a neuroendocrine function since it responds to neural stimulation rather than to hormones secreted by other glands. In this respect, it's similar to the adrenal medulla.

The pineal gland is not considered essential to life, and most information regarding its function has been derived from animal experiments. However, the gland may possibly be involved in regulating growth and function of the pituitary, adrenal, and thyroid glands, and the gonads.

THE PLACENTA

During pregnancy the placenta secretes several hormones, including *human chorionic gonadotropin* (HCG), *human placental lactogen* (HPL), estrogens, and progesterone.

HCG is thought to act on the corpus luteum to prolong and increase its secretions of progesterone and estrogen beyond its usual 14-day life span. However, after about 11 weeks of gestation, the placenta can secrete enough progesterone and estrogen to support the pregnancy to term. HCG is also thought to stimulate the fetal testes to secrete testosterone before the fetal pituitary secretes LH.

HPL was first thought to influence breast development and lactation, but this has not been proved. Apparently, the primary function of HPL is maternal glucose and fat metabolism. By decreasing insulin sensitivity and glucose metabolism in the mother, HPL diverts more glucose to the fetus. By promoting release of free fatty acids from maternal fat stores, it releases this alternate source of energy for her metabolic needs. HPL also has some slight somatotropic properties.

Estrogen and progesterone secretion increase markedly toward the end of pregnancy. Estrogens cause enlargement of the uterus, breasts, and external genitalia. Progesterone prepares the endometrium for ovum implantation and development of the placenta, aids lactation, and depresses uterine contractility.

THE GASTROINTESTINAL MUCOSA

Gastrointestinal hormones are secreted into the bloodstream by endocrine cells that are scattered throughout the walls of the stomach and intestines rather than clustered into discrete structures or glands. These endocrine cells contain secretory granules that respond to stimuli, such as ingested food, blood factors, or neural stimulation.

The known gastrointestinal hormones are *gastrin*, *secretin*, and *cholecystokinin*. Gastrin, found in the antrum and first part of the duodenum, stimulates the release of gastric acid and pepsin and promotes growth of acid-secreting mucosa. Secretin, with cholecystokinin, is distributed throughout the small bowel. Both hormones act on pancreatic acinar cells, promoting secretion of bicarbonate and water. Cholecystokinin also stimulates pancreatic enzyme secretion and gallbladder contraction.

The role of prostaglandins

Found in tiny quantities in most body tissues, prostaglandins are extremely potent substances derived from fatty acids. Unlike hormones, which often act on distant target tissues, prostaglandins act in the immediate vicinity of their origin. Apparently, they play a part in cellular metabolism and the mediation

Endocrine function: Too little or too much?

Endocrine disorders are usually classified as hyperfunctional or hypofunctional. The dysfunction may originate in the hypothalamic-pituitary unit, the hormone-producing gland, the target organ, or possibly a tumor.

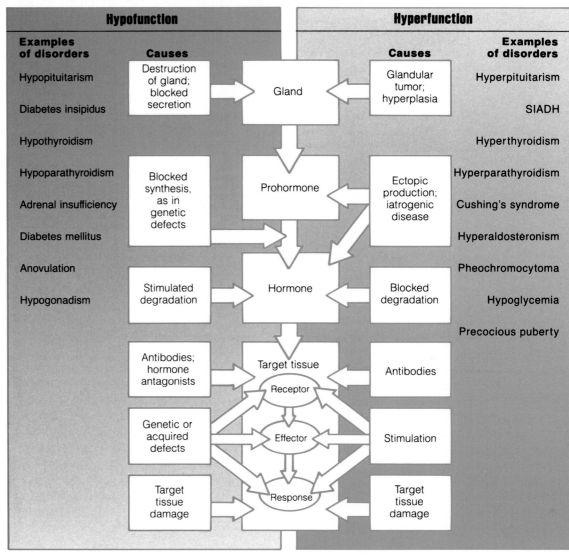

Hypofunction				Hyperfunction	
Examples of disorders	**Causes**			**Causes**	**Examples of disorders**
Hypopituitarism	Destruction of gland; blocked secretion	Gland		Glandular tumor; hyperplasia	Hyperpituitarism
Diabetes insipidus					SIADH
Hypothyroidism					Hyperthyroidism
Hypoparathyroidism	Blocked synthesis, as in genetic defects	Prohormone		Ectopic production; iatrogenic disease	Hyperparathyroidism
Adrenal insufficiency					Cushing's syndrome
Diabetes mellitus					Hyperaldosteronism
Anovulation	Stimulated degradation	Hormone		Blocked degradation	Pheochromocytoma
Hypogonadism					Hypoglycemia
					Precocious puberty
	Antibodies; hormone antagonists	Target tissue / Receptor		Antibodies	
	Genetic or acquired defects	Effector		Stimulation	
	Target tissue damage	Response		Target tissue damage	

of hormone-cellular reactions by cyclic AMP.

Research into the function of prostaglandins will provide further insights into basic biological processes as well as engender new types of medical treatment. Certain prostaglandins are used clinically to induce labor and terminate pregnancies; others that reduce gastric secretions may be potentially useful against gastrointestinal ulcers. Still others may help to treat asthma or reduce blood pressure.

ENDOCRINE PATHOPHYSIOLOGY

Endocrine disorders result from hormonal imbalances. These disorders can be classified as primary or secondary hyperfunction and hypofunction; functional disorders caused by nonendocrine disease; failed end-organ response; abnormal or ectopic hormone production; or iatrogenic disorders. (See *Endocrine function: Too little or too much?*, above.)

Primary hyperfunction

Excessive hormone production by a gland may be caused by a tumor or other abnormal stimulus and usually causes disease. *Tumors* may arise from neoplastic changes occurring during cell division within the gland. Abnormal cell proliferation (hyperplasia) causes excessive secretion without prior stimulation. Such tumors usually are benign. *Tissue hyperplasia* may arise in response to a hormone-secreting tumor or to antibodies that mimic hormonal stimulators. Other causes of hyperplasia have been harder to identify.

Primary hypofunction

Endocrine hypofunction can result from congenital abnormalities, neoplasms, infarctions, infections, and autoimmune disorders affecting the gland itself. Frequently, hypofunction develops slowly, without influencing the gland's basal hormone production until a late stage. By the time secretion levels decrease, the gland's reserve capacity is usually compromised, preventing it from responding to increased demand. This can lead to intermittent clinical manifestations that are difficult to diagnose.

Secondary dysfunction
When an abnormal stimulus causes excessive or inadequate hormone production by a target gland, it's called secondary hyper- or hypofunction. For example, an abnormally low stimulus at the hypothalamic-pituitary level causes hyposecretion by target glands, such as the gonads, thyroid, or adrenals.

Measurement of pituitary and target gland hormones helps distinguish between primary and secondary endocrine failure. For example, inadequate ovarian estrogen secretion occurring with normal LH and FSH levels indicates hypothalamic-pituitary disease, while a low to normal estrogen level with elevated FSH and LH implies an ovarian disorder.

Functional disorders
Nonendocrine disease may affect synthesis and secretion of hormones from endocrine glands. In chronic renal failure, for example, secondary hyperparathyroidism may result from abnormal levels of phosphate and calcium. Hyperaldosteronism secondary to liver disease, renal disease, or heart failure can aggravate the edematous tendencies of these disorders. Chronic liver disease affects both the pituitary gland and testes, leading to decreased testosterone production and increased estrogen levels. Estrogens are increased because of peripheral conversion of androgens to estrogens in liver disease. Testicular atrophy and gynecomastia are present in about 50% of patients with cirrhosis of the liver.

Failure of end-organ response
Since the target organ often fails to respond to hormonal stimulation, hormone levels must be interpreted with regulatory feedback-system factors in mind. The presence of normal or elevated hormone levels without normal hormonal action indicates hormone resistance. This can also be illustrated by diminished or absent response to administration of exogenous hormone. Mechanisms of hormone resistance may be genetic or acquired and include defects at receptor sites, antibody reaction to hormone receptors, and defective postreceptor hormone action.

Abnormal hormone production
Frequently resulting from an inborn error of metabolism, such defects include excessive production of hormone precursors due to a block in synthesis and enzyme deficiencies that impair hormone synthesis. If such defects are not complete, increased stimuli may compensate by causing glandular hyperplasia, resulting in normal hormone levels.

Ectopic hormone production
Hormone production by nonendocrine tissue is usually caused by a malignant tumor. Since peptides are more easily synthesized than steroids, most ectopic hormones are peptides. Although different tumors can produce hormones, some cell types are more commonly associated with specific tumors. For example, certain cells of endodermal origin, called *amine precursor uptake and decarboxylation cells,* are found in oat cell carcinomas of the lung and tumors of the thymus and pancreas; they are often associated with ectopic hormone production.

Iatrogenic disorders. Some endocrine disorders may be induced by medical treatments, such as therapy for a nonendocrine disorder or excessive therapy for an endocrine disorder.

Iatrogenic Cushing's syndrome has become more common than endogenous hypercortisolism due to widespread use of large doses of corticosteroids. Exogenous corticosteroids can suppress the hypothalamic-pituitary-adrenal axis and cause adrenal atrophy; if corticosteroid dosage is then abruptly terminated or rapidly decreased, or if the patient is stressed by acute illness or surgery, the adrenal gland will be unable to respond with the extra corticosteroids required. Iatrogenic disorders can also be caused by the effects of chemotherapy, radiation, and surgical removal of glands. Hypofunction can occur with destruction or removal of the gland or if the gland's blood supply is compromised.

A complex and challenging field
Understanding advances in endocrinology provides a continuing nursing challenge. A basic understanding of endocrine anatomy and physiology enables you to most effectively care for patients with endocrine disorders. Such knowledge will improve your assessment skills and allow you to set realistic care goals and develop appropriate nursing interventions. Also, you'll be better able to help the patient understand, accept, and manage his disease, thereby helping him maintain his well-being.

Points to remember

- The endocrine system acts together with the nervous system to maintain homeostasis.
- The endocrine glands or structures include the pituitary, thyroid, parathyroid, adrenals, islet cells of the pancreas, testes, ovaries, pineal, thymus, placenta, and gastrointestinal mucosa.
- Endocrine glands release hormones directly into the bloodstream.
- A hormone is a potent chemical messenger that exerts a physiologic effect on specific target cells and tissues.
- Excessive or diminished hormone secretion causes most endocrine disorders.

2 ASSESSING ENDOCRINE FUNCTION

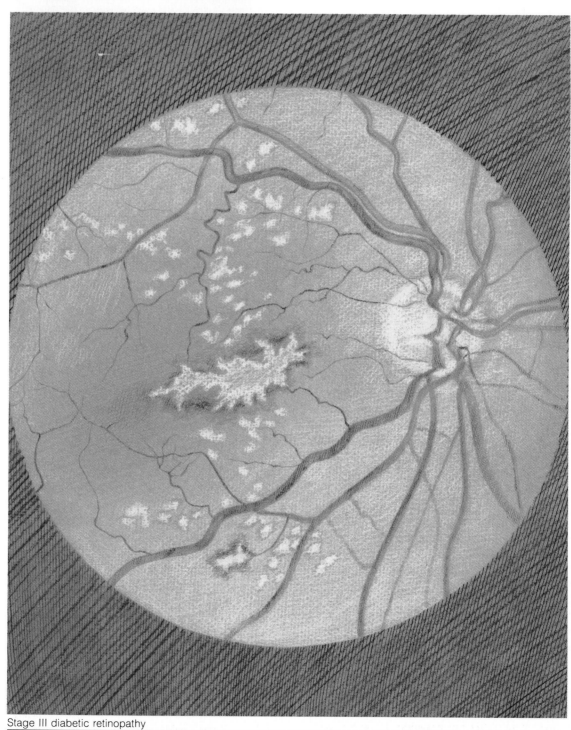

Stage III diabetic retinopathy

The pervasive effects of endocrine disorders make assessment of this complex system a formidable nursing challenge. For example, cardiac dysrhythmia may actually result from calcium imbalance caused by parathyroid dysfunction. Or an acute psychotic episode may stem from Cushing's syndrome.

Endocrine assessment is especially difficult because you can't directly examine the endocrine glands, except for the thyroid. Instead, you'll need to understand the delicate balance between endocrine and other body functions to achieve accurate assessment findings. This chapter will help you achieve this understanding—beginning with the patient's complaints and symptoms, progressing through all stages of assessment, and ending with the nursing diagnosis.

Prepare the equipment

Begin the endocrine assessment by gathering equipment: a thermometer, blood pressure cuff, gloves, tongue depressor, ophthalmoscope, cotton balls, reflex hammer, tuning fork, nasal speculum, and, of course, an interview form and pen. Then, make sure the examining room is well lit and offers privacy. This is especially important for eliciting information about puberty or emotional distress and for examining the breasts and genitalia.

Prepare the patient

Introduce yourself to the patient and be sure he understands the purpose of the assessment. Let him fully express his feelings about the assessment. Stress the privacy of the interview, especially if the patient is young or apprehensive. If the patient is a child, decide at what points in the examination he needs the comfort of a parent or trusted adult, and at what points you should question each alone.

Try to understand the patient's feelings about his illness and its impact on his life. Because endocrine disorders often alter appearance and cause emotional distress, the patient may experience depression. Accept the patient's feelings and offer comfort.

If the patient has difficulty discussing excretion, sexuality, or other bodily functions, postpone this part of the interview until he feels more comfortable.

HISTORY AND OBSERVATION

During the patient interview, form an overall impression of his appearance. Look for obvious signs of endocrine disorders, such as abnormal body size or proportions, or unusual facial features. Note the distribution of body fat, which should be evenly spread on a man and concentrated in the shoulders, breasts, buttocks, inner thighs, and pubic symphysis on a woman.

Pay attention not only to what the patient says, but to how he says it. Is his speech abnormally slow or fast? Is it coherent? Does it reflect anxiety or the need for reassurance?

Record information as the patient presents it, but also note your impressions as you go along. Ask questions slowly, and allow the patient time to respond fully.

Discuss the chief complaint

Help the patient focus on his major problem by asking the reason for his visit. Then, encourage him to elaborate on his chief complaint. Ask about its onset, quality, quantity, location, duration, and any aggravating or alleviating factors. Find out if symptoms have changed over time. Ask about comfort measures, prescribed drugs, and previous treatments. List previous hospitalizations, medical visits, or surgical procedures relating to the chief complaint in chronological order.

Collect background information

Once you've explored the chief complaint, ask the patient to supply background information. First, find out if the patient has noticed any change in weight, body size, or proportions. Ask if his appetite or nutritional habits have changed recently; persistent loss of appetite may suggest an organic rather than a psychological cause. Is he thirstier than usual or urinating more frequently? Does he urinate in small or large amounts? Does he awaken at night to urinate? The patient's responses to these questions will help you distinguish urinary tract infection from diabetes.

Ask about any gastrointestinal disturbances. Nausea, vomiting, constipation, or diarrhea can result from thyroid or adrenal disorders. Abdominal pain can signal diabetes.

Ask about energy level changes. Are such changes continuous or intermittent? Is he sleeping enough? Weakness and fatigue from endocrine disorders usually worsen at day's end and after exercise, and are generalized.

Ask about muscle tremors, palpitations, headaches, or visual disturbances, since these symptoms may signal a thyroid disorder. Also find out about skin changes, such as drying, scaling, or excessive bruising—and about hair-growth or fingernail changes. Excessive hair growth occurs in Cushing's syndrome; fingernail changes suggest a thyroid or parathyroid disorder. Ask about the patient's response to sudden, extreme temperature changes. Intolerance to heat indicates hyperthyroidism; intolerance to cold indicates hypothyroidism or Addison's disease.

Ask about sexual and reproductive problems that may reflect endocrine dysfunction. Has he noticed a loss of libido or impotence? A change in the size or color of genitalia? Ask a woman about any change in the menstrual cycle or an inability to conceive.

Complete the health history
Ask about the patient's general health, including his normal activity level, strength, and average weight. Explore dietary habits and sleeping patterns. Ask about any recent or long-term illnesses and food or drug allergies. Ask about previous hospitalizations, noting the reasons, admission dates, and treatment.

If the patient is a child, find out about immunizations, communicable diseases, and physical development. Ask the mother about her prenatal care, labor, and the child's habits.

Ask about use of prescribed, over-the-counter, or street drugs. Drug abuse can produce symptoms that mimic hyperthyroidism and adrenal imbalance. Also ask about smoking or use of alcohol.

Ask the patient about his life-style. For instance, does he jog? Jogging decreases pulse rate. Has he experienced any recent emotional loss or trauma?

Because certain endocrine disorders may be inherited or have familial tendencies, ask about and list any family history of diabetes, thyroid disorders, heart or kidney disease, hypertension, cancer, or any hereditary or congenital disorders.

At the end of the interview, allow the patient time to express his fears and concerns before performing the physical exam.

THE PHYSICAL EXAMINATION
After collecting subjective data from the interview, you're ready to begin a physical examination, using either the major systems or head-to-toe approach. As you know, the physical exam requires skillful use of inspection, palpation, percussion, and auscultation.

Check vital signs first
Begin the exam by positioning the patient comfortably and taking vital signs. Some en-

docrine disorders, such as hyperthyroidism, raise temperature. Ask the female patient the date of her last period, so you can estimate time of ovulation. Remember that body temperature rises immediately after ovulation.

Next, palpate the radial pulse for at least 30 seconds, noting and recording its rate, quality, and rhythm. Keep in mind that cardiovascular and thyroid drugs can affect pulse rate, as can cardiovascular, thyroid, parathyroid, and adrenal disorders.

Count the patient's respirations for at least 15 seconds and record their rate and quality. In diabetic ketosis, you'll detect Kussmaul's respirations. Also check for a sweetish breath odor, which can indicate ketosis.

Take blood pressure in both arms. Adrenal tumors, especially pheochromocytoma, and Cushing's syndrome elevate blood pressure. In Addison's disease, abnormal aldosterone secretion decreases sodium, decreasing blood pressure. Insufficient antidiuretic hormone (ADH) secretion may also decrease blood pressure; excessive secretion of ADH may elevate blood pressure.

Inspect the skin
First, check skin color on exposed areas and at pressure points. Remember that pigmentation reflects racial and ethnic variations and is greater on the face, the back of the hands, the areolae, and genitals, especially during pregnancy. Pregnancy may also darken pigmentation along the midline of the abdomen.

Hyperpigmentation ranges from tan to brown and may indicate Addison's disease, diabetes mellitus, or thyroid disorders. Yellow skin can indicate jaundice or myxedema; however, yellow sclerae result from jaundice, not myxedema.

Examine the skin for hydration, temperature, texture, and turgor. Dry, rough skin can indicate dehydration or hypothyroidism, while smooth, flushed, sweaty skin suggests hyperthyroidism. Also check for lesions and note their location, size, shape, color, and distribution. Note excessive bruising or petechiae, found in Cushing's syndrome. Check for edema (pitting and non-pitting, peripheral and central) and document its location and severity. Peripheral or central edema can accompany myxedema, Cushing's syndrome, and acromegaly.

Assess the hair and nails
Check for abnormal hair distribution or loss. Hirsutism—the presence of excessive facial,

chest, or abdominal hair in women—can indicate adrenal dysfunction. Unusual hair loss can indicate pituitary, thyroid, and parathyroid disorders. Also check hair texture. Fine, silky hair occurs in hyperthyroidism; coarse, dry hair in hypothyroidism.

Observe the patient's fingernails. Thick, brittle nails suggest hypothyroidism; malformed, pitted nails suggest hypoparathyroidism; pigmented nails, Addison's disease. Check for separation of the nails from the nailbed (onycholysis), a sign of hyperthyroidism.

Examine the head
Study the patient's facial features. Are they fine or coarse? Is his expression alert, dull, anxious, or flat? A prominent forehead and a large jaw can indicate acromegaly, whereas facial adiposity (moon face) can indicate Cushing's syndrome. A dull face with coarse, puffy, dry features can characterize myxedema in an adult or cretinism in a child.

Observe the eyes. Protruding eyeballs and retracted upper eyelids characterize exophthalmos, a sign of hyperthyroidism. Infrequent blinking, excessive tearing, tremor of closed lids, and conjunctival edema often accompany hyperthyroidism. Typically, patients with this disorder complain of a sandy, full feeling in the eye and, at times, blurred or double vision.

Assess cranial nerves III (oculomotor), IV (trochlear), and VI (abducens), to detect pituitary tumor. First, check pupillary reactions and extraocular movements, noting any ptosis or nystagmus. Then ask the patient to assume these expressions in succession: to raise the eyebrows, to frown, to close his eyes tightly, to puff his cheeks, to show his teeth, and to smile. Observe for asymmetry in each posture. Also, ask the patient to clench his teeth, and note the strength of bilateral muscle contraction.

Check for visual field defects, which can indicate pituitary tumor. First, instruct the patient to cover his right eye with his right hand. Then, stand about 2′ from him and cover your left eye with your left hand. Tell him to stare at your right eye while you move two waving fingers into his visual field from each quadrant. Ask the patient to tell you when he first sees your fingers. Assuming your visual fields are normal, the patient should see your fingers at the same time you do. Next, repeat these steps for the other eye.

Now, perform the funduscopic examination (this exam is usually not performed by the staff nurse), following these steps:

Signs of Cushing's syndrome

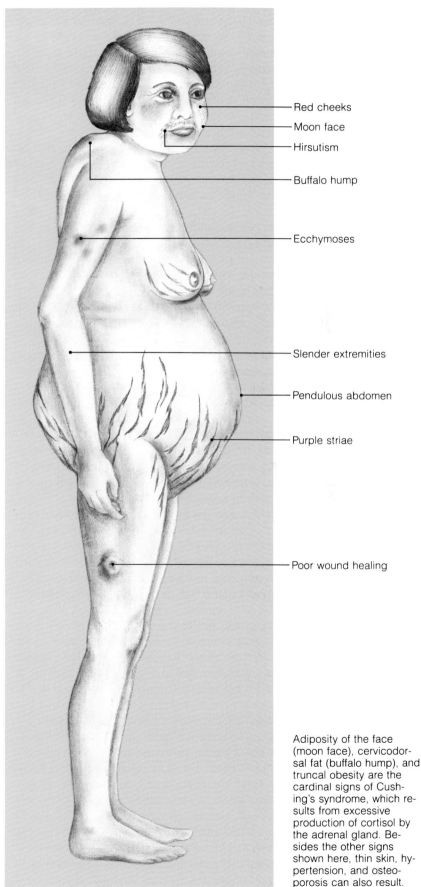

- Red cheeks
- Moon face
- Hirsutism
- Buffalo hump
- Ecchymoses
- Slender extremities
- Pendulous abdomen
- Purple striae
- Poor wound healing

Adiposity of the face (moon face), cervicodorsal fat (buffalo hump), and truncal obesity are the cardinal signs of Cushing's syndrome, which results from excessive production of cortisol by the adrenal gland. Besides the other signs shown here, thin skin, hypertension, and osteoporosis can also result.

• In a darkened room, stand about 12″ to 15″ from the patient, holding an ophthalmoscope in your right hand. Look with your right eye into the patient's right eye.

• Turn on the ophthalmoscope. (If you wear glasses, keep them on.) Direct the light into the patient's pupil at a 25° angle to his right side. You should see a red retinal reflex transparent through the anterior and posterior chambers.

• Move the ophthalmoscope closer to the pupil. Inspect the cornea and lens, which should be transparent; the retina, which should be free from hemorrhagic spots or pigmented areas; the optic disk, which should be circular, yellowish-pink, and smooth; the macular area, which surrounds the fovea and should be avascular; and blood vessels, which should be well-defined and move outward from the disk in all areas but the macula.

Abnormal funduscopic findings can indicate neurologic disorders, diabetes, pituitary tumors, or hyperthyroidism.

Use a nasal speculum to check the patency of the nares. Note the color of mucous membranes, and any discharge, odor, obstruction, or excessive hair growth. Reddened mucous membranes, discharge, obstruction, and odor can result from infection secondary to Cushing's syndrome. Highly inflamed nares do not always result from an endocrine disorder. Sometimes inflammation may result from chronic inhalation of glue, paint, or cocaine.

Observe the lips, noting their symmetry, color, edema, abnormalities, and lesions. Inspect the tongue for size, color, coating, and ulceration. An enlarged tongue can indicate myxedema; tooth malformation and moniliasis commonly occur in hypoparathyroidism.

Examine the thyroid gland
To examine this gland, use techniques of observation, palpation, and auscultation. Stand facing the patient and observe the lower half of his neck, first in normal position and then with the neck slightly extended. Observe for thyroid enlargement (goiter) or asymmetry. Then, ask the patient to swallow. (Provide a glass of water, if necessary.) The thyroid should move up as he swallows. Ask if he has noticed any difficulty swallowing, hoarseness, or a choked feeling in his throat.

Next, palpate the thyroid from both the front and the back. (See *Palpating the thyroid,* page 27.) Note the thyroid's size, shape, location, and tone. Check for the presence of nodules, which feel like knots or swellings. A firm, fixed nodule may be a tumor.

If you palpate a suspected tumor, determine if it's compressing the trachea by applying slight pressure to the lobes as the patient inhales deeply. If the trachea is compressed, he'll feel stridor and dyspnea.

Auscultate an enlarged thyroid for systolic bruits. Place the stethoscope's diaphragm over one lateral lobe of the gland and listen carefully for a bruit—a soft, rushing sound. Bruits occur in hyperthyroidism, as accelerated blood flow through the arteries of the gland produces vibrations. Because breath sounds can interfere with auscultation of bruits, you may want to ask the patient to hold his breath as you listen.

To tell a bruit from a venous hum, press the jugular vein on the side you're auscultating. The venous hum should disappear.

Examine the chest
Inspect the size, shape, and symmetry of the chest and note any deformities. Then listen for the apical pulse at the fifth left intercostal space, about 7 to 9 cm to the left of the midsternal line. Assess heart rate and rhythm, since dysrhythmia can indicate hyperthyroidism, hypoparathyroidism, and electrolyte imbalance as well as other endocrine and cardiovascular disorders.

Examine the female breasts for size, shape, symmetry, and pigmentation. Pendulous breasts with red-purple striae indicate Cushing's syndrome. Check the areolae for cracks, crusts, infection, or drainage. Galactorrhea can occur in both males and females with pituitary dysfunction or hypothyroidism. If you suspect galactorrhea, milk the breast or ask the patient to do so. Then, describe any drainage. Also, examine the male breasts for swelling or discharge, since gynecomastia may occur in Graves' disease.

Examine the abdomen
With the patient in the supine position, inspect the abdomen for surgical scars, rashes, striae, bulges, and discolorations. A discolored, striated, protruding abdomen suggests Cushing's syndrome; an obese, hypotonic abdomen suggests hypothyroidism.

Auscultate the abdomen for bowel sounds, which should occur 5 to 35 times a minute and sound like stomach grumblings. Note their frequency, pitch, duration, and location, and ask the patient if pain or cramping accompanies these sounds. Decreased or absent bowel sounds occur in electrolyte disturbances and

Palpating the thyroid

To palpate the thyroid *from the front,* stand in front of the patient and place your index and middle fingers below the cricoid cartilage on both sides of the trachea. Palpate for the thyroid isthmus as he swallows. Then, ask the patient to flex the neck to the side being examined as you gently palpate each lobe. Typically, you'll feel only the isthmus connecting the two lobes. However, if the patient has a thin neck, you may feel the whole gland. If he has a short, stocky neck, you may have trouble palpating even an enlarged thyroid.

To locate the right lobe, use your right hand to displace the thyroid cartilage slightly to your left. Hook your left index and middle fingers around the sternocleidomastoid muscle to palpate for thyroid enlargement. Then, examine the left lobe, using your left hand to displace the thyroid cartilage and your right hand to palpate the lobe.

To palpate the thyroid *from the back,* stand behind the patient and ask him to lower the chin to relax the neck muscles. Curve your fingers and place them on either side of the trachea. Feel for the isthmus with your index and middle fingers as the patient swallows. To palpate the left lobe, turn the patient's head slightly to the left, displace the trachea to the left side with the fingers of your right hand, and examine the left lobe with your left hand. To palpate the right lobe, turn the head slightly to the right, displace the trachea to the right with your left hand, and examine the lobe with your right hand.

Palpating the right lobe, from the front.

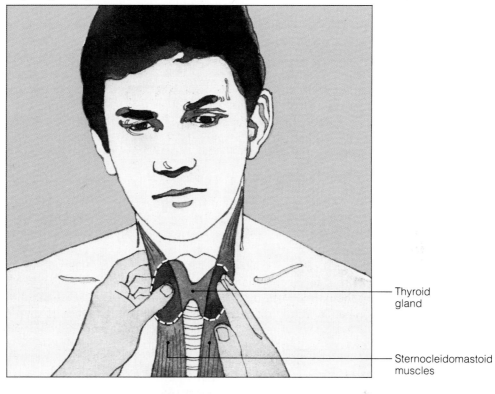

Thyroid gland

Sternocleidomastoid muscles

Palpating the left lobe, from the back.

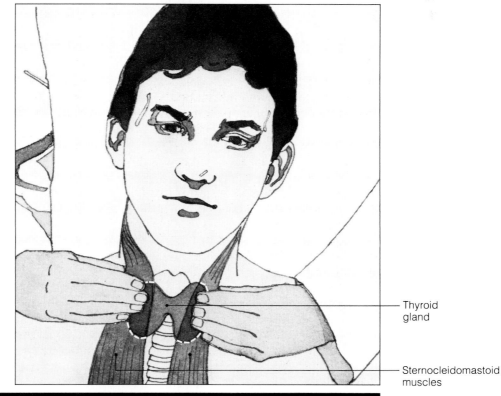

Thyroid gland

Sternocleidomastoid muscles

hypothyroidism. Hyperactive bowel motility accompanies hyperthyroidism.

Percuss the abdomen, starting at the right midclavicular line below the umbilical level. Mark the spot in the upper right quadrant where tympany changes to dullness. This is the lower border of the liver. Move up to the lower thorax and percuss downward, noting the point where resonance over the lung changes to dullness in the upper right quadrant. This is the upper border of the liver. Estimate the size of the liver. In uncontrolled or poorly regulated diabetes, the liver may be enlarged from fatty infiltration.

Continue to percuss the abdomen for ascites. (See *Percussing the abdomen for ascitic fluid.*) Dullness in the bulging flanks can indicate ascitic fluid from myxedema or certain ovarian disorders. Watch for shifting fluid when the patient moves from his back to his side.

Lightly palpate all four quadrants of the abdomen. Then, use deep palpation to detect any tenderness, masses, or enlarged organs. Note the patient's response and facial expression. Remember that severe tenderness of the upper abdomen is characteristic in acute pancreatitis and may mark the onset of acute, severe diabetes.

Palpate the liver—it should feel firm and smooth. (See *Palpating the liver,* page 29.) Enlargement can indicate uncontrolled diabetes.

Examine the genitalia

Inspect pubic hair for quantity and distribution, keeping in mind normal standards for the patient's age. Note the location of the meatus. Also observe any lesions, such as vesicles, and any discharge. Note the size and color of the scrotum and penis or the labia. With a gloved hand separate the labia and note the location and size of the clitoris. An enlarged clitoris in a woman can indicate virilization. In congenital adrenocortical hyperplasia, a female infant has an enlarged clitoris closely resembling a penis. With a gloved hand, palpate the testicles and note their location and size. Asymmetrical testes in a man may indicate a tumor; undescended testes, adrenal dysfunction or delayed maturity; small testes can indicate hypogonadism. Assess for precocious puberty in preadolescents of both sexes.

Assess the musculoskeletal system

Evaluate the patient's body proportions. Abnormally short height suggests dwarfism. Disproportionately large hands and feet occur in acromegaly and other growth hormone disorders. Check for bone deformities and joint enlargements common in acromegaly, Cushing's syndrome, and hyperparathyroidism.

Examine the patient's arms and legs for size, appearance, symmetry, and muscle tone. Note any masses, signs of wasting, hypertonia, or hypotonia.

Check for postural tremors, which can accompany hypothyroidism. Ask the patient to close his eyes and hold both hands out in front of him with fingers extended. Describe any tremors in the arms or legs. Check for head movements or facial twitching.

Check for muscle atrophy. Describe its location and type (unilateral or bilateral).

Percussing the abdomen for ascitic fluid

Tympany

Dullness

Bulging flank

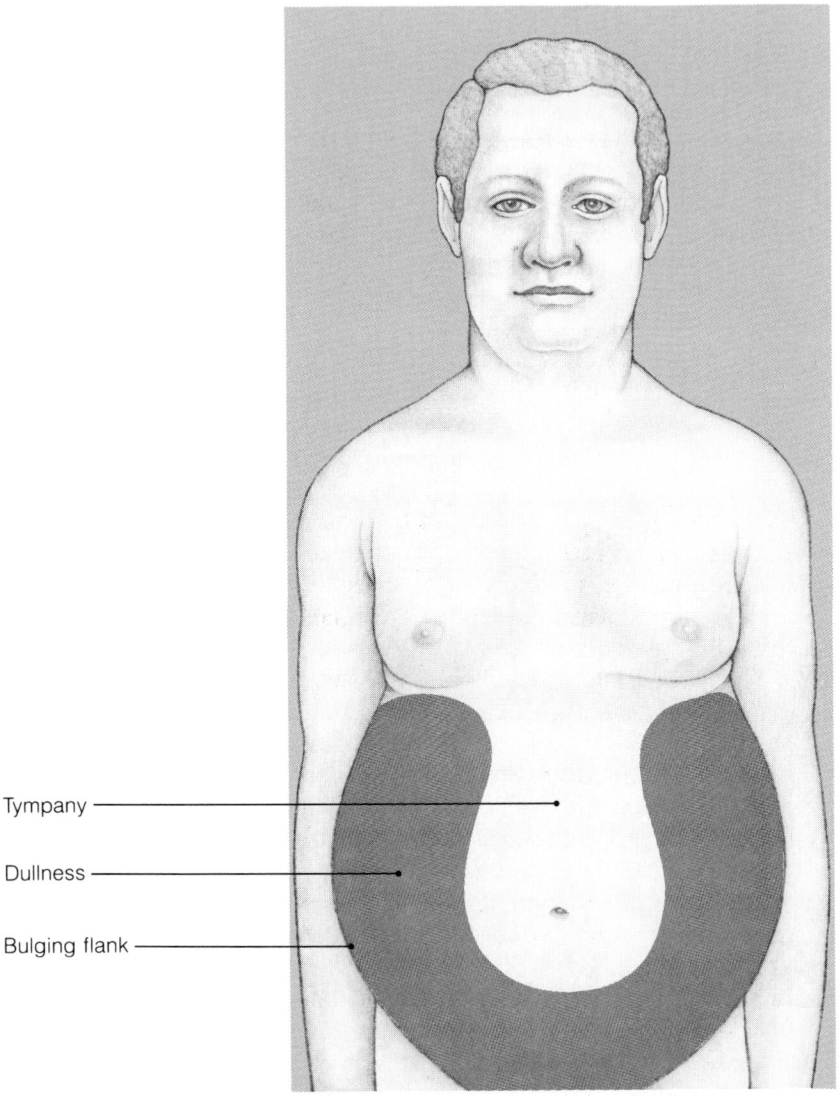

In myxedema, ascitic fluid accumulates in the lower abdomen, producing bulging flanks. Typically, percussion of these flanks reveals dullness. Also, percussion of the area around the umbilicus reveals tympany.

Palpating the liver

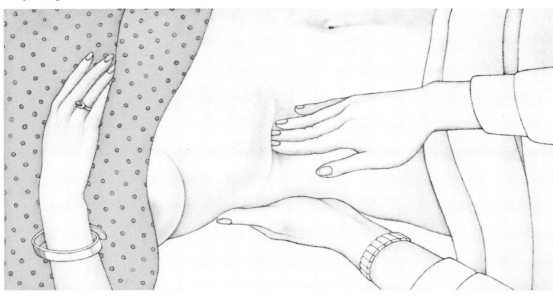

With the patient supine, place your left hand under the right 10th to 12th ribs and lift slightly. Using your right hand, point your fingers toward the rib cage and press beneath the costal margin as the patient inhales deeply. Normally, the liver feels firm and smooth. But you won't be able to palpate the liver in every patient.

Remember, tremor, muscle fatigue, and muscle wasting accompany various endocrine disorders, such as diabetes, Cushing's syndrome, Addison's disease, hyperthyroidism, and hyperparathyroidism. However, these signs can also indicate a degenerative neurologic disorder, such as Huntington's chorea.

Check sensory responses

Ask the patient to close his eyes. Then touch him lightly with a cotton ball at several places along the inner and outer arms and legs. Squeeze or pinch the same spots to test pain response. Place a vibrating tuning fork over bony prominences to test vibrating sense. Paresthesia, hyperalgesia, and hyperesthesia characterize diabetic neuropathy. Now, ask the patient to close his eyes and check sensory response on his other side.

If the patient reports tingling and numbness in his hands, feet, and around the mouth, and experiences tetany with muscle cramps, he may have hypocalcemic tetany from hypoparathyroidism or parathyroid gland removal. Check for hypocalcemic tetany by testing for Trousseau's sign and Chvostek's sign.

To elicit Trousseau's sign, apply a blood pressure cuff to the arm and inflate it to occlude blood flow. If occlusion causes carpal spasms, contractions of the fingers into a claw-like position, and inability to open the hand, Trousseau's sign is positive.

To test for Chvostek's sign, place one finger in front of the patient's ear at the angle of the lower jaw, just over the facial nerve. If this causes spasms or contracture of the lateral facial muscles, Chvostek's sign is positive. But remember, Chvostek's sign may occur in normal patients.

Interpret your findings

After finishing the assessment, remember that signs and symptoms of endocrine disorders also characterize other body system disorders. For example, muscle fatigue and tremors also accompany neurologic disorders. Consequently, try to view your assessment findings with objectivity and suspicion. Identify those areas that require further, more definitive study and, if necessary, discuss appropriate diagnostic tests with the doctor.

Once you're satisfied with the assessment, you're ready to form nursing diagnoses. As you know, a nursing diagnosis describes a set of signs and symptoms that indicate an actual or potential health problem requiring nursing intervention. When writing a nursing diagnosis, keep it simple. First, establish a baseline assessment using a nursing data base, and then write your diagnostic statement—reflecting a problem related to etiology. If you've identified the cause of the problem, your nursing diagnosis should clearly describe it.

Mastering the steps from assessment to nursing diagnosis can help you detect and interpret the sometimes subtle signs of endocrine disorders—and allow timely, appropriate interventions.

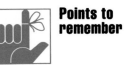

Points to remember

- A comprehensive endocrine assessment includes patient history taking and physical examination, which enable you to formulate nursing diagnoses. It can help detect subtle endocrine disorders that may initially appear to result from other body system dysfunctions.
- The patient interview provides important subjective information to help you interpret your examination results. Carefully conducted, it can help distinguish endocrine from psychological disorders.
- The thyroid is the only endocrine gland that you can palpate. Skillful palpation can reveal enlargement, nodules, or tumors.
- Before forming a nursing diagnosis, carefully consider your assessment findings.

3 IMPLEMENTING THE DIAGNOSTIC WORKUP

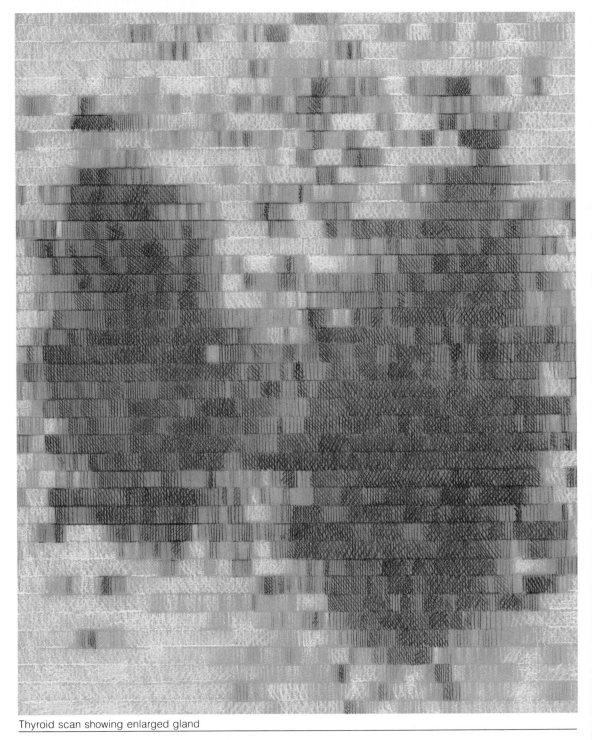

Thyroid scan showing enlarged gland

Tremendous strides have been made in the past decade in developing more sophisticated diagnostic tests of endocrine function. Radioimmunoassay (RIA), for example, allows direct measurement of serum thyroxine (T_4) and has largely replaced the often unreliable protein-bound iodine and butanol-extractable iodine tests, which merely provided indirect estimates of T_4. The thyroid scan, a nuclear medicine test, reveals hyperfunctioning or hypofunctioning nodules and can indicate the need for further diagnostic tests. Thyroid ultrasonography, a safe, noninvasive test, can accurately differentiate between a cyst and a tumor. However, the accuracy of these and other endocrine tests depends greatly on thorough patient preparation and teaching. For serum and urine studies, it also depends on timely collection and transport of samples for laboratory analyses.

FOUR TYPES OF ENDOCRINE TESTS
Tests of endocrine function fall into four major categories: measurement of serum or plasma hormone levels; measurement of urine levels of a hormone or its metabolite; measurement of hormonal reserve and regulation by stimulation and suppression studies; and radiographic and nuclear imaging tests.

The diagnostic workup in suspected endocrine disorders begins with standard screening tests, which can provide clues to endocrine function. For example, routine urinalysis helps detect endocrine disorders that change urine specific gravity or cause glucosuria. Electrolyte studies may reveal abnormal calcium and phosphate levels, suggesting a parathyroid disorder. (See *Laboratory findings in endocrine disorders,* page 32.)

However, the results of such screening tests require careful interpretation. Urine free cortisol levels, for example, commonly rise in Cushing's syndrome resulting from adrenal hyperplasia, adrenal or pituitary tumors, or ectopic adrenocorticotropic hormone (ACTH) production. They may also rise in the presence of many drugs, such as steroids, amphetamines, reserpine, phenothiazines, or morphine. Thus, the patient's drug history must be checked, and drug restrictions enforced to avoid misleading results.

Serum and plasma tests
These tests are commonly performed to evaluate hormonal balance. Circulating blood hormone levels have great diagnostic significance because a change in the blood level of one hormone eventually affects the secretion of other hormones. Many tests based on RIA techniques have been devised to detect and evaluate these changes. (See *Principle of radioimmunoassay,* page 43.) Blood tests are subject to such variables as drug effects, stress, nutritional status, or diurnal rhythms in hormone secretions, which necessitate careful collection scheduling.

Urine tests
Although many hormones are commonly measured in the blood, some hormones and their metabolites can easily be measured in the urine. Urine hormone and metabolite levels closely reflect the serum levels of circulating hormones. Hormone metabolites also serve as valuable diagnostic indicators when the hormones themselves aren't excreted in detectable quantities. Urine tests are especially useful in diagnosing or confirming adrenal and gonadal disorders. Usually, a 24-hour urine specimen is collected. This reflects total daily secretion, offsets diurnal variations (an advantage over blood tests), and masks temporary fluctuations.

Provocative tests
Through stimulation or suppression of glandular secretion, these tests assess the gland's ability to respond to stimuli as an index of its reserve capacity and to confirm glandular hyper- or hypofunction, especially if blood and urine testing gives borderline results. The tests may also help locate endocrine defects.

Radiography and nuclear imaging tests
Including such diverse approaches as X-rays, computerized tomography (CT) scans, scintiscans, or arteriography, radiographic and nuclear tests may accompany or follow other laboratory tests. These tests usually are ordered to identify or confirm suspected glandular neoplasms, cysts, or hyperplasias.

SPECIFIC TESTS OF GLANDULAR FUNCTION
To help pinpoint specific endocrine dysfunction, multiple tests of blood, urine, or glandular function are often required. The following tests are the most commonly performed for evaluating specific endocrine glands.

Tests of pituitary function
The pituitary gland is composed of an anterior lobe and a posterior lobe. The anterior pitu-

Laboratory findings in endocrine disorders

Category	Increased levels	Test	Decreased levels
Electrolytes	Adrenal hypofunction Hyperparathyroidism Hyperthyroidism	Calcium	Hypoparathyroidism Cushing's syndrome
	Hyperparathyroidism	Chloride	Primary hyperaldosteronism Adrenal hypofunction
	Adrenal hypofunction Early-stage diabetic acidosis	Magnesium	Hyperparathyroidism Hyperthyroidism Primary hyperaldosteronism
	Acromegaly Hypoparathyroidism	Phosphate	Hyperparathyroidism
	Adrenal hypofunction	Potassium	Cushing's syndrome Primary hyperaldosteronism
	Cushing's syndrome Diabetes insipidus Hyperosmolar hyperglycemic nonketotic coma (HHNC) Primary hyperaldosteronism	Sodium	Adrenal hypofunction Chronic primary adrenocortical insufficiency
Blood chemistry	Diabetic acidosis Hypothyroidism	Albumin	Hyperthyroidism
	Acromegaly Hyperparathyroidism Hyperthyroidism	Alkaline phosphatase	Hypothyroidism
	Cushing's syndrome	Bicarbonate	Adrenal hypofunction
	Adrenal hypofunction Uncontrolled diabetes mellitus	Blood urea nitrogen (BUN)	Acromegaly
	Hypothyroidism	Cholesterol	Hyperthyroidism
	Adrenal hypofunction Uncontrolled diabetes mellitus	Creatinine	
	Acromegaly Cushing's syndrome Diabetes mellitus Hyperpituitarism (GH, ACTH) Hyperthyroidism Pheochromocytoma	Glucose	Adrenal hypofunction Hypopituitarism (GH, ACTH) Hypothyroidism Insulinoma
	Hypothyroidism Severe diabetic acidosis	Lactic dehydrogenase	
	Hypothyroidism Diabetic acidosis	SGOT	
	Diabetic acidosis Hypothyroidism	Total protein	Chronic uncontrolled diabetes mellitus Hyperthyroidism
Hematology	Adrenal hypofunction Cushing's syndrome Diabetic acidosis Pheochromocytoma	Hematocrit	
	Cushing's syndrome Pheochromocytoma	Hemoglobin	Ectopic ACTH syndrome Hypopituitarism Hypothyroidism
	Pituitary tumors	Red blood cells	Adrenal hypofunction
	Cushing's syndrome Diabetic acidosis	White blood cells Neutrophils	Adrenal hypofunction
	Adrenal hypofunction Hyperthyroidism Anterior pituitary hypofunction	Eosinophils	Cushing's syndrome Diabetic acidosis
	Hypothyroidism Anterior pituitary hypofunction	Basophils	Hyperthyroidism
	Adrenal hypofunction Hyperthyroidism	Lymphocytes	Cushing's syndrome Diabetic acidosis

Testing pituitary function

Test	Normal values/findings	Clinical significance of abnormal findings
Anterior		
Growth hormone (GH), serum	Adult: male, 0 to 5 ng/ml; female, 0 to 10 ng/ml Child: 0 to 16 ng/ml	*Increased levels:* acromegaly (in adults), gigantism (in children), bronchogenic or gastric cancer, psychosocial deprivation syndrome (in infants), hypoglycemia *Decreased levels:* pituitary dwarfism (in children), psychosocial deprivation syndrome (in older children), ingestion of glucose-load hyperglycemia, pharmacologic doses of glucocorticoids
Growth hormone stimulation (arginine stimulation)	Rise in GH to more than 10 ng/ml in men, 15 ng/ml in women, and 48 ng/ml in children	*Increased levels:* acromegaly, gigantism, tumors *Decreased levels:* dwarfism
Growth hormone suppression (glucose loading)	GH suppressed to < 3 ng/ml at some time during test	*Increased levels:* gigantism, acromegaly, tumors
CT scan of pituitary	Pituitary appears normal in size and structure.	Pituitary tumors
Posterior		
Antidiuretic hormone, serum	1 to 5 pg/ml	*Increased levels:* syndrome of inappropriate secretion of antidiuretic hormone (SIADH), hyperthyroidism, adrenal insufficiency, severe hemorrhage, circulatory shock, stress, pain *Decreased levels:* diabetes insipidus, metastatic disease, viral infection, head trauma
Osmolality, serum	275 to 295 mOsm/kg water	*Increased levels:* hypernatremia, hyperosmolar nonketotic hyperglycemia, hyperglycemia, diabetes insipidus, hypercalcemia *Decreased levels:* excessive fluid intake, SIADH
Water loading test	> 80% of water excreted over 5 hr. Urine osmolality falls to < 100 mOsm/kg	*< 40% excretion:* SIADH
Water deprivation test	Decreased urine flow to < 0.5 ml/min. Urine osmolality > 800 mOsm/liter	*Increased urine volumes and decreased urine concentration:* possible diabetes insipidus
Skull X-ray	Normal size, shape, thickness, and position of cranial bones	Pituitary lesion
Anterior and posterior		
X-ray of sella turcica	Normal-volume area	Erosion and destruction of the sella turcica suggest pituitary tumor

itary lobe secretes growth hormone (GH), prolactin, thyroid-stimulating hormone (TSH), ACTH, luteinizing hormone (LH), and follicle-stimulating hormone (FSH). The posterior pituitary lobe secretes antidiuretic hormone (ADH) and oxytocin. Most tests for evaluating pituitary function are based on plasma levels of pituitary hormones. These are measured in a basal state, after stimulation of hypothalamic releasing hormones, or after suppression of hormones produced by pituitary hormone target tissues.

Anterior pituitary studies. These tests include measurement of serum GH by RIA and GH stimulation and suppression tests. (See *Testing pituitary function.*)

The *GH stimulation test* measures plasma GH levels after I.V. administration of arginine, an amino acid that normally stimulates GH secretion. At times, this test is performed with an insulin tolerance test (because insulin-induced hypoglycemia stimulates GH secretion) or after administration of other GH stimulants, such as glucagon, vasopressin, and L-dopa.

The *GH suppression test* assesses elevated baseline GH levels by measuring the secretory response to a loading dose of glucose. GH

Scanning the pituitary

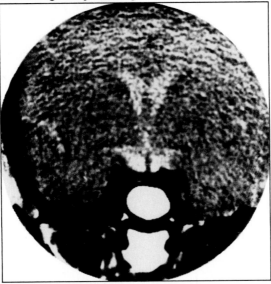

This CT scan shows the normal size and structure of the pituitary gland.

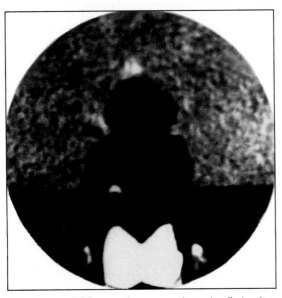

This abnormal CT scan shows an enlarged sella turcica with a lesion, indicating a pituitary tumor.

normally exerts an anti-insulin effect by raising plasma glucose and fatty acid concentrations; increased insulin secretion counteracts these effects. Therefore, a glucose load should suppress GH secretion. Failure to suppress indicates anterior pituitary hypersecretion of GH, resulting in acromegaly and gigantism.

Because the anterior pituitary strongly influences the gonads, serum FSH, plasma LH, serum estrogens, and plasma progesterone are commonly measured to detect ovarian failure or gonadal dysfunction. (See also *Testing gonadal function,* page 44.)

Posterior pituitary studies. These tests include measurements of serum and urine os-molality, water deprivation tests (Mosenthal's test, Fishberg concentration test, renal function test, or 8-hour or 14-hour deprivation test), and water loading tests (saline challenge, water load, or Hickey-Hare osmolality test). Direct measurements of serum and urine ADH levels are rare.

The pituitary may be X-rayed to assess glandular volume and to detect erosion or enlargement within the sella turcica. (See *Scanning the pituitary.*)

Tests of thyroid function

The thyroid gland is a primary regulator of body metabolism and secretes two vital hormones—T_4 and triiodothyronine (T_3)—to maintain a normal cellular metabolic rate. Thyroid tests include RIAs, provocative tests, isotope studies, scanning, and ultrasonography. (See *Testing thyroid function,* page 35.)

Serum thyroxine. T_4 is secreted by the thyroid in response to TSH from the pituitary and, indirectly, in response to thyrotropin-releasing hormone (TRH) from the hypothalamus. Only a fraction of the T_4 circulates freely; most of it binds strongly to thyroxin-binding globulin (TBG). However, the free T_4 is responsible for the clinical effects of thyroid hormone on body cells and tissues.

The serum T_4 RIA, one of the most common indicators of thyroid function, measures the total circulating T_4 level when TBG is normal.

Serum triiodothyronine. T_3 is derived primarily from T_4 and, like it, is secreted in response to TSH and TRH. It's more potent than T_4 and binds less firmly to TBG. The T_3 RIA is highly specific and measures the total (bound and free) serum contents of T_3 to investigate thyroid dysfunction. This assay is the most sensitive test for thyrotoxicosis.

Generally, T_3 levels are more reliable than T_4 in thyrotoxicosis, because thyrotoxicosis increases T_3 levels disproportionately, even though it raises both T_3 and T_4 levels in most patients. In hypothyroidism, T_3 levels are less reliable; they may fall within the normal range and may not be diagnostically significant.

Serum free T_4 and T_3. Often performed simultaneously, these tests measure serum levels of free T_4 and T_3, which are not bound to TBG. Since levels of circulating free T_4 and free T_3 are regulated by a feedback mechanism that compensates for changes in binding protein concentrations by adjusting total hormone levels, measurement of free hormone levels is the best indicator of thyroid function. This test may be useful in the 5% of patients in whom the standard T_3 or T_4 tests are not diagnostic.

T_3 resin uptake. This test indirectly measures free T_4 levels by demonstrating the availability of serum protein-binding sites for T_4. Results of this test are frequently combined with a T_4 RIA to determine the free T_4 index, a mathematical calculation that is thought to reflect free T_4 levels by correcting for TBG abnormalities.

Radioactive iodine uptake. Measuring thyroid uptake of radioactive iodine (^{131}I) permits direct evaluation of thyroid function and is especially significant in thyroid hyperfunction, assessment of thyrotoxicosis factitia, and subacute thyroiditis. This test measures the amount of orally ingested ^{131}I accumulating in the thyroid after 2, 6, and 24 hours. An external detector measures radioactivity in the thyroid as a percentage of the original dose, indicating the gland's ability to retain iodine. When performed concurrently with a thyroid scan and T_3 resin uptake test, the ^{131}I uptake test helps differentiate thyrotoxicosis from

Testing thyroid function

Test	Normal values/findings	Clinical significance of abnormal findings
Thyroxine (T_4), serum	RIA: 5 to 13.5 mcg/dl	*Increased levels:* thyrotoxicosis, acute thyroiditis, pregnancy *Decreased levels:* hypothyroidism, anterior pituitary hypofunction, chronic debilitating illness
Triiodothyronine (T_3), serum	Adult: 90 to 230 ng/dl Neonate: 134 to 146 ng/dl Ages 1 to 2: 116 to 132 ng/dl Ages 3 to 10: 131 to 141 ng/dl Adolescent: 129 ng/dl	*Increased levels:* thyrotoxicosis, T_3 toxicosis, Hashimoto's thyroiditis *Decreased levels:* severe acute illness, trauma, malnutrition
T_3 resin uptake	Normally, 25% to 35% of radioactive T_3 binds to the resin.	*Increased levels:* thyrotoxicosis, protein malnutrition *Decreased levels:* hypothyroidism, pregnancy
Thyroid-stimulating hormone (TSH), serum	0 to 10 μIU/ml	*Increased levels:* primary hypothyroidism *Decreased levels:* secondary hypothyroidism, anterior pituitary hypofunction, thyrotoxicosis

Thyroid circulating antibody
  Antimicrosomal antibody (microsomal antibody, antithyroid microsomal antibody)
  Antithyroglobin antibody titer (thyroid autoantibody)
	Titer: < 1:100
	
	Titer: < 1:20
		High titers: Hashimoto's thyroiditis, thyrotoxicosis
		
		Low titers: thyroid disorders, pernicious anemia, myasthenia gravis, primary myxedema, juvenile-onset diabetes

Thyroid suppression (T_3 suppression)	TSH levels fall below baseline value; T_4 levels fall to < 50% of baseline value.	*Failure to suppress:* primary hyperthyroidism (multinodular goiter)
TSH stimulation (thyrotropin-releasing factor)	Prompt rise in TSH, peaking in 15 to 30 min Women: peak value 16 to 26 μIU/ml from base of 6 μIU/ml Men: slightly lower	*No response:* hypothyroidism from pituitary failure; hyperthyroidism from functional autonomy of the thyroid, as in toxic goiter *Subnormal response:* euthyroidism therapy for Graves' disease, multinodular goiter *Normal response:* primary hyperthyroidism, hypothyroidism from deficiency but not absence of pituitary or hypothalamic function
Radioactive iodine uptake (^{131}I uptake)	After 2 hr, 1% to 13% of radioactive iodine accumulates in thyroid; after 6 hr, 2% to 25%; and after 24 hr, 15% to 45%.	*Increased levels:* thyrotoxicosis, thyroiditis *Decreased levels:* hypothyroidism
Thyroid scan	Thyroid gland about 2″ (5 cm) long and 1½″ (3.8 cm) wide, with uniform uptake of radioisotope and without tumors	*Hot spots* (gray-black regions): hyperfunctioning thyroid gland *Cold spots* (white regions): hypofunctioning thyroid gland, thyroid tumor (malignant)
Ultrasonography	Uniform echo pattern throughout gland	Variation in echo pattern distinguishes cyst from tumor.

hypofunctioning toxic adenoma. The test is accurate for thyrotoxicosis but less accurate for hypothyroidism, due to increased use of iodinized food, which suppresses ^{131}I uptake.

Serum thyroid-stimulating hormone. This RIA is a reliable test for primary hypothyroidism and helps determine whether it results from thyroid gland failure or from pituitary or hypothalamic dysfunction. Normal serum TSH levels rule out primary hypothyroidism because an absence of thyroid hormone in the serum stimulates pituitary hypersecretion of TSH through negative feedback.

TRH challenge. This test evaluates thyroid function and directly tests pituitary reserve. After a baseline TSH level is obtained, synthetic TRH is injected intravenously. As many as five samples are then drawn at 5-, 10-, 15-, 20-, and 60-minute intervals to assess thyroid response. A sudden spike above the baseline TSH reading indicates a normally functioning pituitary but suggests hypothalamic dysfunction. A normal rise but a delayed peak in the TSH level suggests hypothalamic hypothyroidism. If the TSH level fails to rise or remains undetectable, pituitary failure is likely. In thyrotoxicosis or thyroiditis, high concentrations of thyroid hormones inhibit TSH secretion. Consequently, TSH levels fail to rise when challenged by TRH.

Thyroid suppression. When serum T_3 and T_4 values are borderline, a thyroid (T_3) suppression test may confirm or rule out a case of borderline thyrotoxicosis. If TSH secretion is suppressed after oral administration of T_3, thyrotoxicosis can be ruled out.

Antithyroid antibodies. Two tests to detect circulating antithyroid antibodies—antithyroglobulin antibody and long-acting thyroid stimulator—are performed when evidence indicates Hashimoto's thyroiditis, Graves' disease, or other autoimmune disorders.

Scintiscanning and ultrasonography. These tests are used to assess thyroid anatomy. A *thyroid scan* visualizes the gland after administration of ^{131}I. The scan indicates the gland's size and shape and defines areas of hyperfunction (hot spots) and hypofunction (cold spots). This test is commonly used to assess a palpable mass, gland enlargement, or asymmetrical goiter. It's generally performed with thyroid ultrasonography, serum T_3 and T_4 measurements, and thyroid uptake tests.

In *thyroid ultrasonography,* the gland is visualized by variable reflectance of high frequency sound waves. Mainly used to distinguish cysts from tumors, it's also useful in evaluating thyroid nodules during pregnancy, because it doesn't expose the fetus to ^{131}I.

Tests of parathyroid function

The four small parathyroid glands, located close to the posterior surface of the thyroid gland, secrete parathyroid hormone (PTH), which is essential for serum calcium and phosphorus homeostasis. Abnormalities in serum calcium and phosphorus levels are often the first clue to parathyroid dysfunction. (See *Testing parathyroid function,* page 37.)

Serum parathyroid hormone. Normally, PTH release is regulated by a negative feedback mechanism involving serum calcium. Normal or elevated circulating calcium inhibits PTH release, while decreased calcium stimulates PTH release. PTH raises plasma levels of calcium while lowering phosphorus levels. An excess or deficiency of PTH is directly related to the effects of PTH on the renal tubules and on bone and to its interaction with ionized calcium and biologically active vitamin D. Consequently, measuring serum calcium, phosphorus, and creatinine levels with a serum PTH radioimmunoassay is useful in identifying parathyroid dysfunction.

In the urine, PTH can be measured directly by determining its effect on phosphate reabsorption. Because this hormone inhibits renal tubular reabsorption of phosphorus, its serum level can be estimated by comparing creatinine clearance with phosphate clearance and calculating the amount per minute of phosphate reabsorbed by the tubules. The urine PTH test detects hyperparathyroidism in patients with clinical signs of the disorder and borderline or normal serum levels of calcium, phosphate, and alkaline phosphatase.

Other blood and urine tests. Sulkowitch's test monitors urine calcium levels by using a reagent to precipitate calcium out of the urine. A heavy, milky precipitate indicates hypercalcemia; absence of a precipitate, hypocalcemia.

Magnesium, an electrolyte vital to neuromuscular function, also influences intracellular calcium levels through its effect on secretion of PTH. Serum and urine magnesium tests may be used along with other parathyroid tests to determine the etiology of tetany, an acute manifestation of hypoparathyroidism.

Provocative testing for parathyroid disorders. Such tests include measuring urinary cyclic adenosine monophosphate (cyclic AMP) excretion after I.V. infusion of a standard dose of PTH (in suspected hypoparathyroidism), and phosphate loading and calcium

Testing parathyroid function

Test	Normal values/findings	Clinical significance of abnormal findings
Parathyroid hormone C-terminal PTH: Intact PTH:	< 150 to 375 pg/Eq/ml 163 to 347 pg/Eq/ml (depends on serum calcium level)	*Increased levels:* hyperparathyroidism, parathyroid tumors *Decreased levels:* parathyroid trauma, postparathyroidectomy
Calcium, serum	Adults: 8.9 to 10.1 mg/dl (atomic absorption) or from 4.5 to 5.5 mEq/liter Children: up to 12 mg/dl (atomic absorption)	*Increased levels:* hyperparathyroidism, metastatic bone tumors, nonparathyroid PTH-producing tumors (lung, breast, kidney), milk-alkali syndrome *Decreased levels:* hypoparathyroidism, alcoholism, chronic renal disease, malabsorption syndrome
Phosphates, serum	Adult levels range from 2.5 to 4.5 mg/dl (atomic absorption) or from 1.8 to 2.6 mEq/liter. Levels are higher in children and can rise to 7 mg/dl or 4.1 mEq/liter during periods of increased bone growth.	*Increased levels:* hypoparathyroidism, hypocalcemia, renal insufficiency or failure *Decreased levels:* hyperparathyroidism, hypercalcemia
Calcium, urine (Sulkowitch's qualitative urine test)	1+ to 2+ (also reported as negative, moderately positive, and strongly positive)	*Increased levels:* concentrated urine, hyperparathyroidism, osteoporosis, renal tubular acidosis, hyperthyroidism, vitamin D intoxication *Decreased levels:* dilute urine, hypoparathyroidism, malabsorption disorders, vitamin D deficiency
Tubular reabsorption of phosphate (TRP)	Renal tubules reabsorb 80% or more of phosphate.	*Low TRP:* primary hyperparathyroidism, hypercalcemia from PTH-secreting malignancy, renal defects
Cyclic AMP	After I.V. infusion of parathyroid hormone: 10- to 20-fold increase in cyclic AMP	*Increased levels:* primary hyperparathyroidism *Decreased levels:* hypoparathyroidism
Ultrasonography	Glands appear as solid masses, 5 mm or smaller, with echo pattern of less amplitude than thyroid tissue.	Glandular enlargement usually characteristic of tumor growth or of hyperplasia

infusion tests, which are unreliable. The glucocorticoid suppression (dexamethasone suppression) test may help diagnose hyperparathyroidism because, although glucocorticoids generally don't affect calcium levels in hyperparathyroidism, they do suppress hypercalcemia from other disorders.

Ultrasonography and other studies. Examining the neck with ultrasound helps identify small parathyroid lesions except in the mediastinal area. Mediastinal parathyroid lesions may be detected by CT scan. If a lesion is found, thyroid arteriography may confirm the diagnosis.

Tests of adrenal function

The adrenal glands consist of two portions, the outer *cortex* and the inner *medulla*. The cortex secretes the mineralocorticoids and glucocorticoids essential to life. The medulla secretes catecholamines (mainly epinephrine, norepinephrine, and dopamine) as part of the body's fight-or-flight reaction. A wide range of tests evaluates cortical and medullary function (see *Testing adrenal function,* pages 38 and 39).

Cortex studies

ACTH, which is secreted by the anterior pituitary gland, stimulates the adrenal cortex to secrete cortisol, aldosterone (mainly controlled by the renin-angiotensin system), and androgens. Tests to determine adrenocortical hypofunction or hyperfunction can be divided into two major groups: absolute determination of individual blood and urine hormone values and provocative tests that investigate hormonal interdependency and feedback mechanisms.

Serum and plasma tests. The *serum aldosterone* RIA identifies aldosteronism and, when supported by plasma renin levels, distinguishes between the primary and secondary forms of that disorder. *Plasma ACTH,* also an RIA, may be ordered for patients with signs of adrenal hypofunction (insufficiency) or hyperfunction (Cushing's syndrome). ACTH suppression or stimulation testing is usually needed to confirm the diagnosis of these disorders.

Plasma cortisol is usually ordered for suspected adrenal dysfunction, but provocative tests—suppression tests for hyperfunction and

Testing adrenal function

Test	Normal values/findings	Clinical significance of abnormal findings
Cortex		
Cortisol, plasma	8 a.m.: 7 to 28 mcg/dl 4 p.m.: 2 to 18 mcg/dl	*Increased levels:* adrenocortical hyperfunction, obesity, stress, pregnancy, renal disease, diabetes mellitus *Decreased levels:* adrenal hypofunction, hypopituitarism
ACTH, plasma	8 a.m., fasting: 20 to 100 pg/ml 4 p.m., nonfasting: 10 to 50 pg/ml	*Increased levels:* primary adrenal insufficiency, stress, pituitary neoplasm *Decreased levels:* adrenal hypofunction, hypopituitarism
Aldosterone, serum	7 a.m., recumbent: normal sodium intake—3 to 10 ng/dl 9 a.m., upright: normal sodium intake—4 to 30 ng/dl On low sodium diet, normal values increase twofold to fivefold.	*Increased levels:* primary aldosteronism, secondary aldosteronism, hypertension, nephrotic syndrome *Decreased levels:* hypotension, adrenal hypofunction, toxemia of pregnancy, hypothyroidism
Cortisol, urine (free cortisol)	24 to 108 mcg/24 hr	*Increased levels:* adrenal hyperplasia, adrenal or pituitary tumor, emotional stress *Decreased levels:* clinically insignificant
17-OHCS, urine	Female: 2 to 10 mg/24 hr Male: 3 to 12 mg/24 hr	*Increased levels:* adrenal hyperfunction, adrenal cancer, hyperpituitarism, hyperthyroidism *Decreased levels:* adrenal hypofunction, hypopituitarism, hypothyroidism
17-ketosteroids (17-KS), urine	Marked daily variations in 17-KS secretion Adult: female, 4 to 17 mg/24 hr; male, 6 to 21 mg/24 hr; levels progressively decline after age 60 Pediatric: under age 11, 0.1 mg to 3 mg/24 hr; ages 11 to 14: 2 to 12 mg/24 hr	*Increased levels:* adrenocortical hyperfunction, adrenogenital syndrome, adrenocortical carcinoma, testicular neoplasm, ovarian neoplasm, hirsutism *Decreased levels:* adrenal hypofunction, hypogonadism, hypopituitarism
17-ketogenic steroids, urine	Adult: female, 2 to 15 mg/24 hr; male, 4 to 22 mg/24 hr Pediatric: under age 11, 0.1 to 4 mg/24 hr; ages 11 to 14: 2 to 9 mg/24 hr	*Increased levels:* adrenal hyperfunction, adrenogenital syndrome, adrenal carcinoma *Decreased levels:* adrenal hypofunction, panhypopituitarism
Aldosterone, urine	2 to 16 mcg/24 hr	*Increased levels:* primary aldosteronism, secondary aldosteronism, stress *Decreased levels:* adrenal hypofunction, toxemia
ACTH stimulation (modified Thorn, ACTH infusion, provocative ACTH)	8-hr infusion test (modified Thorn): twofold to fourfold increase in plasma cortisol, 17-KS, or 17-OHCS levels over baseline Screening test: 30-, 60-, or 120-min plasma cortisol should double over baseline or increase 10 mcg/dl within 60 min (if ACTH given I.M., peak effect delayed) 5-day test: plasma cortisol more than double baseline	*Increased levels:* pituitary insufficiency (secondary adrenal insufficiency), some adrenal adenomas, adrenocortical hyperplasia *Decreased levels:* adrenal insufficiency *Delayed response:* long-term suppression of adrenal activity secondary to substantial steroid therapy
Metyrapone response (when plasma cortisol and urinary metabolites are used to evaluate results, it may be called cortisol/compound S, metyrapone combination; compound S metyrapone/cortisol combination; cortisol/11-deoxycortisol)	Compound S baseline: < 1 mcg/dl Postmetyrapone: > 7 mcg/dl (or twofold to fourfold increase in urinary 17-OHCS) Cortisol: a.m., 7 to 18 mcg/dl; p.m., 2 to 9 mcg/dl	*Exaggerated increase in compound S, decreased cortisol:* Cushing's disease, pituitary-dependent adrenal hyperplasia *No increase in compound S, normal cortisol:* Cushing's disease owing to adrenal carcinoma, autonomous adrenal function, or androgenital syndrome *No increase in compound S with low baseline plasma cortisol:* pituitary failure, hypothalamic failure
Dexamethasone suppression	Overnight screening test: plasma cortisol, measured at 8 a.m., is less than 5 mcg/dl	*Increased levels:* Cushing's syndrome
Aldosterone stimulation (furosemide)	Urine aldosterone increases twofold to threefold; plasma aldosterone increases twofold to fivefold.	*Increased levels:* primary aldosteronism *Decreased levels:* hypoaldosteronism
Aldosterone suppression (deoxycorticosterone, fludrocortisone, saline infusion, spironolactone)	> 50% decrease in secretion or excretion of aldosterone	*Little or no suppression:* primary aldosteronism

Testing adrenal function (continued)

Test	Normal values/findings	Clinical significance of abnormal findings
Medulla		
Catecholamine fractionation, plasma	Supine: epinephrine—0 to 150 ng/liter; norepinephrine—103 to 193 ng/liter Standing: epinephrine—0 to 150 ng/liter; norepineph-rine—293 to 489 ng/liter	*Increased levels:* pheochromocytoma (> 1,000 ng/ml), neuroblastoma, ganglioneuroblastoma
Vanillylmandelic acid, urine	Adult: 0.7 to 6.8 mg/24 hr Pediatric: ages 1 to 2, < 2 mg/24 hr; ages 12 to 14, < 5 mg/24 hr	*Increased levels:* pheochromocytoma, neuroblastoma, ganglioblastoma, physical and mental stress, myocardial infarction, muscle disorders
Cortex and medulla		
Adrenal arteriography	Adrenal artery vasculature appears normal.	Abnormal vasculature may suggest neoplasms of the adrenals (pheochromocytomas, adrenal adenomas, carcinomas) or bilateral adrenal hyperplasia.
Adrenal vein catheterization	Plasma cortisol levels of blood drawn through catheter in adrenals are normal.	*Plasma cortisol markedly elevated on one side:* unilateral adrenal tumor causing Cushing's syndrome *Plasma cortisol bilaterally elevated:* possibly bilateral adrenal hyperplasia *Plasma catecholamine markedly elevated on one side:* possibly unilateral pheochromocytoma *Plasma catecholamine bilaterally elevated:* possibly bilateral pheochromocytomas, most likely familial
CT scan	Adrenals appear normal in size and structure.	Small tumors of the adrenal glands (adenomas, carcinomas, and pheochromocytomas)

stimulation tests for hypofunction—are generally required to confirm a diagnosis.

Serum potassium determination is an indirect evaluation of adrenal function. Normally, the adrenocortical hormones cortisol and aldosterone promote urinary excretion of potassium and urinary retention of sodium. Adrenal hyperfunction produces serum potassium deficit; adrenal hypofunction produces serum potassium excess.

Urine tests. Serum aldosterone concentration is normally low and thus more difficult to measure than urine aldosterone. To measure *urine aldosterone,* a 24-hour specimen is ordered to compensate for short-term variations owing to diurnal rhythms and other factors, such as ACTH; for changes in sodium or potassium levels; and to reduce overlap between normal and abnormal ranges. Other 24-hour urine studies used to determine hormone values include *17-hydroxycorticosteroids (17-OHCS), 17-ketogenic steroids (17-KGS),* and *17-ketosteroids (17-KS).* The 17-OHCS test measures the metabolites of the hormones that regulate glycogenesis and some small amounts of aldosterone. Because more than 80% of all urinary 17-OHCS is metabolized from cortisol, the primary adrenocortical steroid, test findings reflect cortisol secretion and, indirectly, adrenocortical function. The 17-KGS test is similar to 17-OHCS but also measures urine levels of other adrenocorticoids, such as pregnanetriol, that can be oxidized to 17-KS in the laboratory. Because 17-KGS represents so many steroids, it provides an excellent overall assessment of adrenocortical function.

The 17-KS test also measures the metabolites of testosterone and other androgens. However, because this test does not include all the androgens (for example, testosterone, the most potent androgen, is not a 17-KS), these levels provide only a rough estimate of androgenic activity. For additional information about androgen secretion, plasma testosterone levels may be measured concurrently; 17-KS fractionation may also be appropriate.

The adrenal cortex also secretes sex steroids—estrogens and androgens. Urine estrogens, FSH, and pregnanediol (progesterone metabolite) analyses are obtained to detect ovarian disorders. Urine levels of estriol, the predominant estrogen excreted in urine during pregnancy, are checked closely in high-risk

Understanding glycosylation

Glucose molecules gradually attach to hemoglobin A in the red blood cells—a process called glycosylation. The glycosylated hemoglobin level reflects an average of glucose fluctuations that occurred in the blood during the past 2 to 3 months.

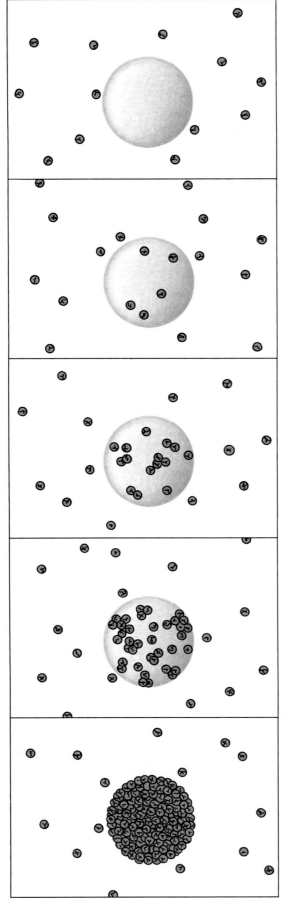

pregnancy to monitor fetal well-being.

Provocative tests. These tests may help to evaluate adrenal function but are seldom used because plasma ACTH can now be measured directly. The ACTH stimulation tests now being used are modified versions of the original Thorn test, in which the eosinophil count is measured after I.M. administration of ACTH. By measuring urinary metabolites of cortisone and cortisol as well as plasma cortisol after administration of measured amounts of ACTH, these tests reveal the adrenal gland's capacity for steroid secretion. If plasma cortisol levels rise after ACTH infusion, significant primary adrenal hypofunction is ruled out.

A *metyrapone suppression test* identifies pituitary-dependent bilateral adrenal hyperplasia (Cushing's disease) and differentiates it from Cushing's syndrome, which is caused by ectopic ACTH syndrome. The *dexamethasone suppression test* suppresses ACTH production and is used to evaluate the pituitary feedback mechanism. Both the *aldosterone stimulation test* (using furosemide) and *suppression test* (using deoxycorticosterone) may be ordered to differentiate between an adrenal disorder and essential hypertension.

Medulla studies

Measurement of plasma and urine catecholamines (epinephrine, norepinephrine, dopamine) is important in assessing adrenal medulla function. Urine vanillylmandelic acid (VMA), a catecholamine metabolite, is also used in such an assessment; however, certain drugs, strenuous exercise, and stress can raise VMA levels, causing false-positive results.

Radiographic studies

Radiographic visualization of the adrenal glands helps detect calcification, which can occur in either adrenal carcinoma or tuberculosis associated with Addison's disease. Intravenous pyelography and CT scans provide additional information about the gland's size and shape and may also reveal displacement of other organs resulting from adrenal gland abnormality. Other radiographic tests used to identify structural abnormalities include venography, angiography, and ultrasonography.

Tests of pancreatic function

In the pancreas, the islets of Langerhans secrete insulin (from beta cells) and glucagon (from alpha cells). Both hormones are vitally important for carbohydrate metabolism. Insulin, a simple protein, acts as a hypoglycemic by stimulating cellular absorption of glucose and promoting its conversion to storage forms. Glucagon, another small protein, acts as a hyperglycemic. When blood glucose concentration is low (during periods of fasting) and insulin secretion falls, the alpha cells secrete glucagon to maintain body glucose levels (insulin's hypoglycemic role suppresses glucagon secretion). Glucagon breaks down stored liver glycogen and combats hypoglycemia. Since glucose is the brain's only nutrient, adequate glucose levels are essential.

Most tests of pancreatic function measure glucose levels, directly or indirectly, in blood and urine. Glucagon is rarely measured be-cause the RIA for this hormone is difficult to perform. Radiographic studies are also of little value in assessing pancreatic function. (See *Testing pancreatic function*.)

Blood glucose tests. These tests measure the capacity for conversion of carbohydrates by insulin. Blood tests used to identify hypo- or hyperglycemic states include fasting plasma glucose, 2-hour plasma postprandial glucose, and glycosylated hemoglobin.

The *fasting plasma glucose test* measures plasma glucose levels after a 12- to 14-hour fast. In the fasting state, plasma glucose levels decrease, stimulating release of glucagon. Glucagon then acts to raise plasma glucose levels by accelerating glycogenolysis, stimulat-

Testing pancreatic function

Test	Normal values/findings	Clinical significance of abnormal findings
Glucose, plasma	Fasting blood sugar: 70 to 100 mg/dl 2-hour postprandial glucose: < 145 mg/dl Random: depends on time of last meal	*Increased levels:* diabetes mellitus, adrenal hyperfunction, acromegaly, stress *Decreased levels:* hypoglycemia, hyperinsulinism, adrenal hypofunction, malnutrition, alcoholism
Glucose tolerance	After 30 min, blood sugar < 160 mg/dl; returns to normal by 2 hr. No urine sugar.	*Prolonged elevated blood glucose, sugar in urine:* possibly diabetes mellitus (Diet, drugs, and many diseases can influence results.)
Insulin, serum	4 to 24 μIU/ml	*Increased levels:* insulinoma, conditions causing reactive hypoglycemia, insulin resistance *Decreased levels:* diabetes mellitus (Type I or Type II), obesity
Glycosylated hemoglobin	< 7.5%	*Increased levels:* hyperglycemia *Decreased levels:* hemolytic states resulting from hemoglobin loss rather than from decreased production
Tolbutamide tolerance (insulin tolerance, Orinase diagnostic, insulin stimulation)	Insulin level usually peaks within 5 min. Plasma glucose peaks within 15 to 30 min (or 50% of basal level). Usually, insulin and glucose return to normal levels in 1½ to 3 hr.	*Diminished response:* possibly diabetes mellitus *Excessive release of insulin:* possibly insulinoma (hypoglycemia)
Copper reduction, urine (Clinitest)	Negative	Tablet indicates color changes in glycosuria, which occurs in diabetes mellitus; adrenal and thyroid dysfunction; hepatic, renal, and central nervous system diseases.
Glucose oxidase, urine (Tes-Tape, Clinistix, etc.) commonly used for self-testing of blood glucose	Negative	Reagent strips show color changes in glycosuria, indicating diabetes mellitus and other disorders, as in copper reduction test.
Ketones, urine	Negative	Reagent strips or tablets indicate color changes in ketonuria and reliably reflect serum ketone levels. Ketonuria occurs in uncontrolled diabetes mellitus, starvation, and as a metabolic complication of total parenteral nutrition.
CT scan	Uniform density; gland normally thickens from tail to head and has a smooth surface.	Changes in size and shape may indicate inflammation, cysts, or tumor.
Ultrasonography	Echo pattern is coarse and uniform; gland appears more echogenic than adjacent liver.	Alterations in size, contour, and parenchymal texture may indicate pancreatic tumors, pseudocysts, or pancreatitis.

ing glyconeogenesis, and inhibiting glycogen synthesis. In a nondiabetic person, insulin secretion checks this rise in glucose levels. In a diabetic patient, absence or deficiency of insulin allows persistently high glucose levels.

The *2-hour postprandial plasma glucose test* is used to screen for diabetes mellitus or to verify results of the fasting plasma glucose test. This test is based on the fact that the greatest difference between normal and diabetic insulin responses, and thus in plasma glucose concentration, occurs about 2 hours after a challenge dose of glucose. A blood sample taken at 2 hours reliably indicates the body's insulin response to carbohydrate ingestion. In borderline test results, the oral glucose tolerance test confirms diagnosis.

The *glycosylated hemoglobin test* is a relatively new diagnostic tool for monitoring hypoglycemic therapy. This test measures glucose levels that were chemically incorporated within three minor hemoglobins (all variants of hemoglobin A) over the preceding 120 days. Since the glycosylated hemoglobin test, unlike other test measures, represents a 120-day span—the life span of the erythrocytes containing glucose—this test provides stable values that may help assess average daily glucose levels over long periods of therapy in patients with diabetes. (See *Understanding glycosylation,* page 40.)

In the *serum insulin RIA,* insulin levels are always measured along with glucose levels because glucose is the primary stimulus for the release of insulin from the islet cells. Results are interpreted in light of the prevailing glucose concentration and can aid differential diagnosis of hypoglycemia resulting from a tumor or hyperplasia of the islet cells, glucocorticoid deficiency, or severe hepatic disease.

Tolerance tests. In these tests, challenge doses of glucose are administered after the patient has followed a high-carbohydrate diet for 3 days and then fasted overnight.

The *oral glucose tolerance test* (OGTT) is the most sensitive test for evaluating borderline diabetes mellitus. Normally, the body absorbs the challenge dose rapidly, causing plasma glucose levels to rise and peak within 30 minutes to 1 hour. The pancreas responds by secreting more insulin, which causes glucose levels to return to normal after 2 to 3 hours. During this period, plasma and urine glucose levels are monitored to assess insulin secretion and capacity to metabolize glucose.

In the *tolbutamide tolerance test,* tolbutamide is given I.V. to stimulate insulin secretion

by beta cells. Plasma glucose levels normally drop rapidly after infusion to about half the fasting level, remain low for 30 minutes, then return to pre-test levels in 1½ to 3 hours.

Other tolerance tests. Although the OGTT is the most effective test for detecting diabetes, two other glucose tolerance tests are sometimes used to confirm OGTT findings.

The *I.V. glucose tolerance test* measures blood glucose after an I.V. infusion of 50% glucose over 3 to 4 minutes. Blood samples are then drawn at ½-, 1-, 2-, and 3-hour intervals. After an immediate glucose peak of 300 to 400 mg/dl (accompanied by glycosuria), the normal glucose curve falls steadily, reaching fasting levels within 1 to 1¼ hours. Failure to achieve fasting glucose levels within 2 to 3 hours generally confirms diabetes.

The *cortisone glucose tolerance test* is occasionally used for evaluating patients with borderline carbohydrate-tolerance deficiencies and for those who produce a normal OGTT curve but have a strong familial predisposition to diabetes. After a 3-day high-carbohydrate diet, oral cortisone acetate is given 8½ and 2 hours before the standard OGTT. (Cortisone promotes glyconeogenesis and may accentuate carbohydrate intolerance in latent or mild diabetes.) Values rising about 20 mg/dl above those of standard OGTT after 2 hours demonstrate probable diabetes in some persons with only minimally decreased carbohydrate intolerance. This test is now used primarily for research.

Urine glucose and ketone tests. Methods for detecting glucose in the urine include copper reduction tests (Clinitest) and glucose oxidase tests (dip-and-read reagent strips). These tests produce standardized color reactions by reduction of copper in a hot alkaline solution with formation of a chromatic precipitate or by sequential enzymatic oxidation of glucose. Both reactions indicate the presence of glucose or other reducing substances.

In the *test tablet procedure* (Clinitest), a commercially prepared tablet containing cupric sulfate, citric acid, sodium carbonate, and sodium hydroxide is added to a test tube of water and urine. The chemical reaction of water and sodium hydroxide releases sufficient heat to activate reduction of cupric ions in the presence of glucose. This test may react to substances other than glucose.

Reagent test strips (Clinistix, Diastix, Chemstrip bG strips, and Tes-Tape) are specific for glucose and are impregnated with a mixture of enzymes and a chromogen. They un-

Principle of radioimmunoassay

Radioimmunoassay (RIA) is an umbrella term for a collection of laboratory procedures based on antigen/antibody displacement reactions. It allows highly sensitive and specific measurement of certain hormones, previously measured with great difficulty or not at all.

RIA involves incubation of the hormone or antigen (Ag) being measured with a fixed amount of radiolabeled hormone or antigen (Ag*) and its specific antibody (Ab). The labeled and unlabeled antigens then compete for binding sites on the antibody, forming Ag*-Ab and Ag-Ab complexes. As the concentration of unlabeled antigen increases, it displaces the labeled antigen. Comparing the amount of displacement of labeled hormone to a standard curve indicates the concentration of the unlabeled hormone.

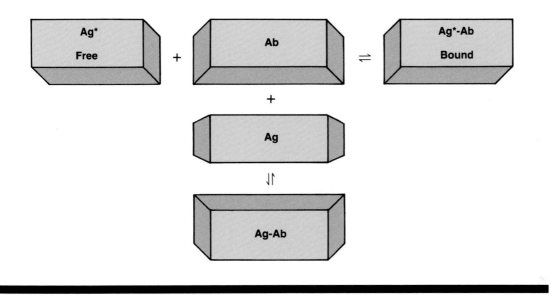

dergo a reaction that, in the presence of glucose, produces an oxidized form of the chromogen.

A similar reagent strip (Ketostix) tests for ketones in urine. The reagent strip is impregnated with sodium nitroprusside and is specific for acetoacetic acid and sensitive to 10 mg/dl. When the strip is dipped into a urine specimen, the presence of acetoacetic acid produces a color change that can be compared with a standard color block to determine approximate concentrations.

Tests of gonadal function

Diagnostic testing of the reproductive system may assess the organs and related structures for abnormalities, detect malignancies, or determine the cause of infertility or sexual dysfunction. Some tests are notably useful in pregnancy. (See *Testing gonadal function,* page 44.)

The gonads are the testes and ovaries. The testes produce the germ cells known as spermatozoa and the hormone testosterone, which induces and maintains secondary sexual characteristics; the ovaries produce ova and the hormones estrogen, progesterone, and androgens, which also promote and maintain secondary sexual characteristics. During pregnancy the placenta serves as a temporary endocrine organ, secreting the hormones human chorionic gonadotropin (HCG) and human placental lactogen (HPL).

The anterior lobe of the pituitary influences gonadal function by secreting prolactin, which stimulates breast development and milk production; and FSH and LH, which allow the gonads to function normally. Blood and urine tests allow evaluation of gonadal function.

Blood tests. The *serum estrogen* test measures levels of estradiol, estrone, and estriol— the only estrogens that are measurable in serum—and helps evaluate female gonadal dysfunction. Tests of hypothalamic-pituitary function may be required to confirm diagnosis.

Serum progesterone. This RIA provides information about corpus luteum function in

Testing gonadal function

Test	Normal values/findings	Clinical significance of abnormal findings
Estrogens, serum Estradiol (E₂) Estriol (E₃)	Female: follicular phase, 3 to 10 ng/dl; luteal phase, 7 to 10 ng/dl 6 to 34 ng/ml	*Increased levels:* female precocity *Decreased levels:* ovarian dysfunction *Decreased levels:* fetal distress, fetal adrenal hyperplasia, hydatidiform mole, placental dysfunction
Progesterone, serum	Female: follicular phase, < 100 ng/dl; luteal phase, > 400 ng/dl; pregnancy, > 800 ng/dl Male: < 20 ng/dl	*Increased levels:* adrenal, testicular, or ovarian tumors; pregnancy, adrenogenital syndrome *Decreased levels:* impending abortion
Testosterone, serum	Female: 30 to 95 ng/dl Male: 300 to 1,200 ng/dl	*Increased levels:* female virilization, adrenogenital syndrome, male precocity *Decreased levels:* delayed male puberty, male hypogonadism
Follicle-stimulating hormone, serum	Female: follicular phase, 5 to 20 mIU/ml; ovulatory, 4 to 35 mIU/ml; luteal phase, 2 to 11 mIU/ml; postmenopausal, 40 to 200 mIU/ml Male: 5 to 20 mIU/ml Pediatric: up to 12 mIU/ml	*Increased levels:* primary gonadal failure *Decreased levels:* hypothalamic or pituitary failure, anovulation, aspermatogenesis
Luteinizing hormone, serum	Female: follicular phase, 5 to 30 mIU/ml; ovulatory, 75 to 150 mIU/ml; luteal phase, 3 to 40 mIU/ml; postmenopausal, 30 to 200 mIU/ml Male: 6 to 30 mIU/ml Pediatric: 4 to 20 mIU/ml	*Increased levels:* primary gonadal failure *Decreased levels:* hypothalamic or pituitary failure
Prolactin, serum (8:00 a.m. fasting)	Female: 6 to 30 ng/ml Male: 5 to 18 ng/ml	*Increased levels:* amenorrhea, galactorrhea, prolactin-secreting tumors, primary hypothyroidism, physical stress *Decreased levels:* pituitary necrosis or infarction
Human chorionic gonadotropin, serum	Male and fertile female: < 5 mIU/liter Postmenopausal female: < 9 mIU/liter Pregnancy: > 40 mIU/liter	*Increased levels:* pregnancy, trophoblastic tumors, HCG-secreting tumors *Decreased levels:* threatened abortion
Human placental lactogen, serum	Male and nonpregnant female: < 0.5 mcg/ml Pregnant female: 5 to 27 weeks, < 4.6 mcg/ml; 28 to 31 weeks, 2.4 to 6.1 mcg/ml; 32 to 35 weeks, 3.7 to 7.7 mcg/ml; 36 weeks to term, 5 to 8.6 mcg/ml	*Increased levels:* > 6.0 mcg/ml after 30 weeks' gestation may suggest an enlarged placenta, (e.g., diabetes mellitus, multiple pregnancy, or Rh disorder). May be found in malignancies. *Decreased levels:* < 4 mcg/ml after 30 weeks' gestation may indicate placental dysfunction.
Human chorionic gonadotropin, urine	Varies according to type of test and trimester of pregnancy	*Increased levels:* threatened abortion, multiple fetuses, trophoblastic tumors; near term, possible Rh disorder, diabetes *Decreased levels:* ectopic pregnancy, threatened abortion
Estrogens, urine Total and fractionation Estrone Estradiol (E₂) Estriol (E₃)	Female: 5 to 100 mcg/24 hr Male: 4 to 25 mcg/24 hr Female: premenopausal, 4 to 31 mcg/24 hr; postmenopausal, 1 to 7 mcg/24 hr Male and prepubertal female: 3 to 8 mcg/24 hr Female: premenopausal, 0 to 14 mcg/24 hr; postmenopausal, 0 to 4 mcg/24 hr Male and prepubertal female: 0 to 5 mcg/24 hr Female: premenopausal, 2 to 30 mcg/24 hr; postmenopausal, 2.2 to 7.5 mcg/24 hr Male and prepubertal female: 0 to 10 mcg/24 hr	*Increased levels:* adrenocortical hyperplasia, adrenocortical tumor, ovarian tumor, testicular tumor, pregnancy *Decreased levels:* ovarian dysfunction, intrauterine death, postmenopausal symptoms
Pregnanediol, urine	Female: follicular phase, 0.5 to 1.5 mg/24 hr; luteal phase, 2 to 7 mg/24 hr; postmenopausal, 0.2 to 1 mg/24 hr Male: 1.5 mg/24 hr	*Increased levels:* pregnancy, ovarian cyst, adrenal hyperplasia *Decreased levels:* ovarian hypofunction, threatened abortion, intrauterine death, neoplasms of ovary or breast
Follicle-stimulating hormone, urine	Adult: 6 to 50 mIU/24 hr Postmenopausal female: > 50 mIU/24 hr Prepuberty: < 6 mIU/24 hr	*Increased levels:* gonadal failure, hyperpituitarism, FSH-producing tumor, Klinefelter's syndrome *Decreased levels:* neoplasms of ovary, adrenal gland or testis; anorexia nervosa
Placental estriol, urine	Varies with week of gestation	*Increased levels:* urinary tract infection *Decreased levels:* fetal distress

fertility studies or placental function in pregnancy.

Testosterone. Using a competitive protein-binding technique, this test measures serum or plasma testosterone levels and, when combined with gonadotropin levels (FSH and LH), reliably aids evaluation of gonadal dysfunction in males and females.

Follicle-stimulating hormone. Performed more often on females than on males, this test measures FSH levels by RIA and may be used in infertility studies. Its overall diagnostic significance often depends on the results of related hormone tests (such as LH, estrogen, or progesterone). Because plasma levels fluctuate widely in females, a true baseline level may require daily testing for 3 to 5 days or multiple blood samples on the same day.

Luteinizing hormone. This test is usually ordered for anovulation and infertility studies and is performed most often on females. For accurate diagnosis, results must be evaluated in light of results from related hormone tests (such as FSH, estrogen, and testosterone).

Prolactin. This RIA test measures serum levels of prolactin, which is similar in molecular structure and biologic activity to GH. This test is considered useful to detect suspected pituitary tumors, which are known to secrete prolactin in excessive amounts.

Human chorionic gonadotropin. This test is more sensitive than the routine pregnancy test, which checks for HCG in urine. If conception occurs, the beta-subunit assay for HCG may detect this hormone in the blood 9 days after ovulation. Elevated HCG beta-subunit levels indicate pregnancy; significantly higher concentrations may suggest a multiple pregnancy or trophoblastic disease.

Human placental lactogen. This RIA measures plasma HPL levels, which are roughly proportional to placental mass, as evidenced by higher levels in a multiple pregnancy. Such assays may be required in high-risk pregnancies (such as those complicated by hypertension or toxemia) or in suspected placental tissue dysfunction. When combined with measurement of estriol levels, this test reliably indicates placental function as well as fetal well-being. It may also be useful as a tumor marker in certain malignancies, such as ectopic tumors that secrete HPL.

Urine tests. *Estrogens.* Total urine levels of the major estrogens—estriol, estradiol, and estrone—are commonly obtained by gel filtration and spectrophotofluorometry. Clinical indications for these tests include tumors of ovarian, adrenocortical, or testicular origin. They are also used to evaluate ovarian activity to help determine the cause of amenorrhea and female hyperestrogenism.

Pregnanediol. Using gas chromatography, this test measures urine levels of the chief urine metabolite of progesterone. Although biologically inert, pregnanediol has diagnostic significance because it reflects about 10% of the endogenous production of its parent hormone. Normally, urine levels of pregnanediol reflect variations in progesterone secretion during the menstrual cycle and pregnancy.

Placental estriol. This test monitors fetal viability by measuring urine levels of placental estriol, the predominant estrogen excreted in urine during pregnancy. Normal levels reflect a properly functioning placenta. The indication for this RIA test is high-risk pregnancy.

Follicle-stimulating hormone. The urine FSH test, which requires a 24-hour urine collection, is seldom used because the serum FSH test is considered more reliable.

Human chorionic gonadotropin. Commonly used to detect pregnancy, this test detects levels of HCG in the urine by immunoassay. The patient's urine is incubated with an antibody to HCG; if the hormone is present in the specimen, it reacts with the antibody to form a complex. The urine-antibody mixture is then added to an indicator system (red blood cells or latex particles coated with HCG). If HCG is present in the urine sample, it has bound to the antibody and cannot react with the indicator; therefore, it does not cause agglutination. Consequently, agglutination of the sample means it does not contain HCG.

Review diagnostic methods
A good way to deepen your understanding of endocrine disorders and their effects and, at the same time, help improve your nursing management skills, is to review the whole range of tests available to detect these disorders. Correctly identifying an endocrine disorder depends very much on laboratory test results. More than ever before, your professional responsibility for patient care includes many aspects of preparing for a test, assisting during its course, and monitoring its effects. To meet these responsibilities effectively, you need much more than a superficial familiarity with any given test. Knowing what test is important for evaluating endocrine function and understanding its implications will help you care for your patients more knowledgeably and efficiently.

Points to remember

- Diagnostic studies are essential in determining endocrine dysfunction.
- RIA techniques have made direct measurement of most hormones possible.
- Provocative tests assess glandular responsiveness to stimuli.
- Knowledge of the test, the ability to explain the test, and understanding of abnormal results are the nurse's responsibility.

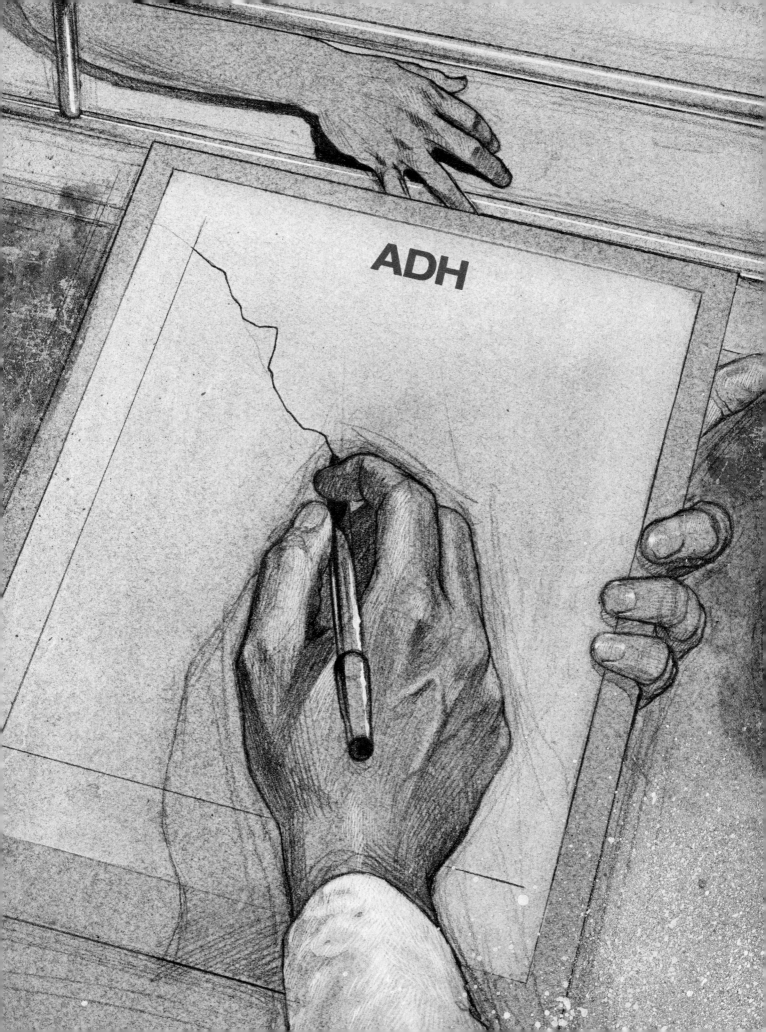

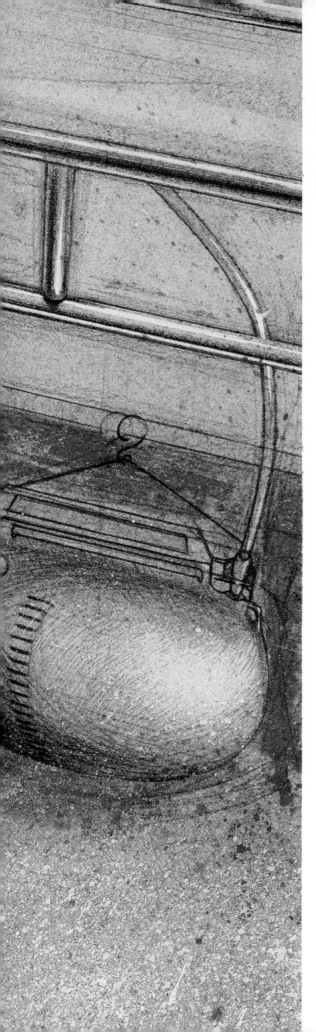

DISORDERS OF
THE PITUITARY
GLAND

4 PINPOINTING ANTERIOR LOBE DYSFUNCTION

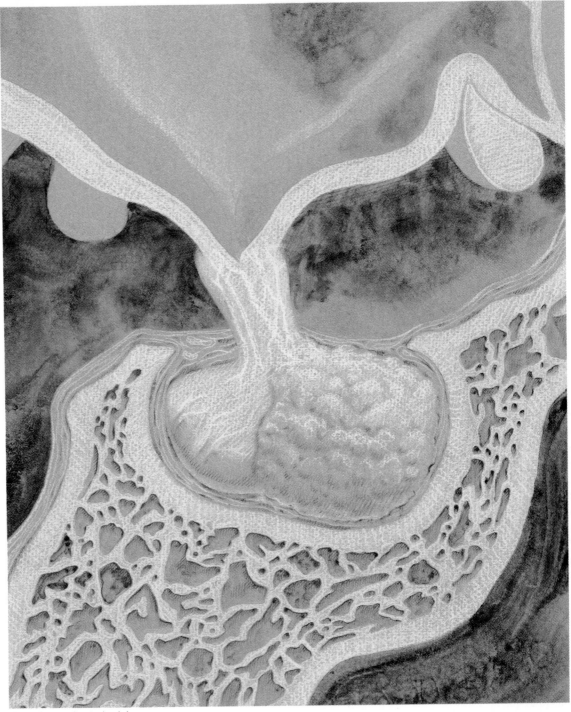

Granuloma of anterior lobe

The anterior pituitary regulates growth, sexual development, and many metabolic activities through the effects of its hormones: growth hormone (GH), prolactin (PRL), adrenocorticotropic hormone (ACTH), follicle-stimulating hormone (FSH), luteinizing hormone (LH), and thyroid-stimulating hormone (TSH). Consequently, anterior pituitary disorders, which interfere with normal secretion of these hormones, cause wide-ranging physical and psychological effects. These disorders respond well to early diagnosis and effective treatment, which can provide a good long-term prognosis. Unfortunately, early diagnosis is often difficult. Anterior pituitary disorders often produce nonspecific symptoms and signs, such as visual field defects and headaches, that tend to obscure the diagnosis. Understanding how these disorders develop and how they produce their systemic effects can prepare you to recognize these sometimes elusive disorders at early, most treatable stages, and to manage them more effectively.

Hyperpituitarism and hypopituitarism

Hyperpituitarism reflects excessive secretion of one or more of the anterior pituitary hormones—usually PRL or GH, occasionally ACTH, and very rarely TSH, FSH, or LH. Its clinical effects depend on which hormone is being overproduced. Hyperpituitarism marked by excessive secretion of PRL causes galactorrhea and amenorrhea in women and gynecomastia in men. Hyperpituitarism marked by excessive secretion of GH is a chronic, progressive disorder marked by hormonal dysfunction and startling skeletal overgrowth. It occurs in two forms, depending on age at onset. Acromegaly, the more common form, occurs after epiphyseal closure, usually in the third or fourth decade, causing bone thickening and transverse growth and visceromegaly. It affects equal numbers of men and women, with about 300 new cases reported annually in the United States. Gigantism, its less common form, begins before epiphyseal closure and causes proportional overgrowth of all body tissue.

Hypopituitarism most commonly reflects GH deficiency or FSH-LH deficiency; less often deficiency of TSH, PRL, or ACTH. Panhypopituitarism, a generalized form of hypopituitarism, reflects deficiency of all anterior pituitary hormones. When unitropic GH deficiency occurs during childhood, it causes pituitary dwarfism. This condition affects up to 15,000 children in the United States.

Both hypopituitarism and hyperpituitarism are rare. However, because initial signs and symptoms of these disorders are often subtle, eluding early diagnosis, reported incidence may be much lower than actual incidence.

PATHOPHYSIOLOGY

Anterior pituitary disorders may be classified as primary or secondary. Both types change the cellular structure of the pituitary—either mechanically or functionally. Mechanical changes result from the impingement of space-occupying lesions within the sella or invasion of the sella from adjacent areas. Functional changes result from deficient or excessive secretion of one or more anterior pituitary hormones.

Primary hyperpituitarism, the most common form, usually results from a tumor. Secondary hyperpituitarism results from hypothalamic disease or from failure of a target organ, such as the thyroid. In primary hypothyroidism, for example, the anterior pituitary perceives decreased thyroid hormone levels as a signal to secrete more TSH. In response to this excessive stimulation, the number of thyrotropic cells increases, sometimes causing hyperplasia.

Primary hypopituitarism results from absence or destruction of hormone-secreting cells caused by a pituitary tumor, ischemia, granuloma formation, radiation treatment for malignant head or neck diseases, and, rarely, syphilis or tuberculosis.

Secondary hypopituitarism results from hypothalamic failure to stimulate secretion of tropic hormones. Its causes include vascular disorders, head trauma, parasellar tumor, inflammatory and infiltrative disease, sarcoidosis, and emotional disturbances that affect hypothalamic function. Panhypopituitarism results from surgical excision of the pituitary, which may occur during excision of a tumor or treatment for breast cancer; or it occasionally follows radiation therapy or occurs as an idiopathic disorder. It may also result from any of the causes of primary hypopituitarism.

Varying tumors; varying effects

Pituitary tumors can be functioning (secretory) or nonfunctioning (nonsecretory). These tumors may be confined to the pituitary (adenoma) or may extend to the parasella. Parasellar tumors (craniopharyngioma, meningioma, optic glioma) and metastatic tumors may invade the sella. Usually, an ade-

The hypothalamic-pituitary axis

Hypothalamic stimulation triggers a complex feedback mechanism that controls the blood levels of many hormones. First, the hypothalamus sends releasing and inhibiting factors or hormones to the anterior pituitary. In response, the anterior pituitary secretes hormones, such as GH, PRL, ACTH, TSH, FSH and LH, and sends them to an appropriate target organ. When these hormones reach normal levels in body tissue, a feedback mechanism inhibits further hypothalamic and pituitary secretion.

For example, reduced cortisol levels stimulate the hypothalamus to send corticotropin-releasing factor to the anterior pituitary, which then secretes ACTH. In turn, ACTH stimulates the adrenal cortex to secrete cortisol. When cortisol levels reach normal, they inhibit the hypothalamic secretion of corticotropin-releasing factor, which in turn prevents the pituitary from secreting ACTH.

Key

Excitatory response

Inhibitory response

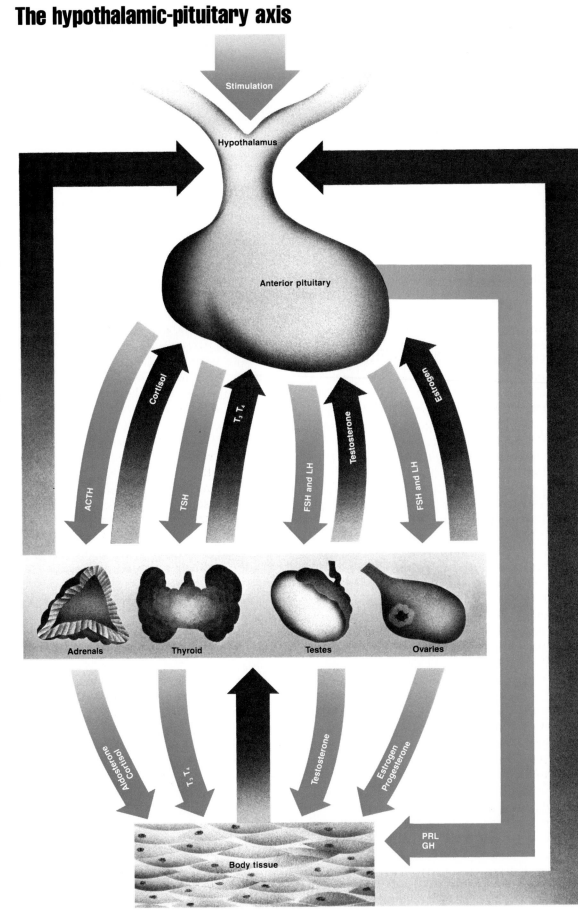

noma autonomously synthesizes and secretes hormones according to its cell type. For example, an adenoma of the somatotroph cells secretes excessive amounts of GH, causing acromegaly in adults and gigantism in children. An adenoma of the lactotroph cells, the most common pituitary tumor, secretes excessive amounts of prolactin.

Tumors may cause hypopituitarism by compressing and obliterating normal cells, thus impairing hormone synthesis and release. When they impinge on and damage the hypothalamus, such tumors may alter the synthesis of hormonal releasing and inhibitory factors, contributing to altered anterior pituitary hormone levels.

Tumors produce multiple signs and symptoms that vary with the extent of decreased hormone secretion, the hormone affected, the patient's age, and speed of onset. (See *Clinical findings in hyperpituitarism and hypopituitarism,* page 59.) For example, when a tumor compresses pituitary tissue and exerts pressure on the overlying dura, headache results. Upward expansion through the sella usually compresses the optic chiasm, leading to bitemporal hemianopia. Continued expansion leads to optic atrophy and, eventually, to complete blindness. Hypothalamic compression may cause temperature fluctuations, hyperphagia, altered sleep patterns, and emotional disturbances. Lateral expansion of the tumor may compress cranial nerves III, IV, and VI and cause paralysis of ocular muscles and diplopia. Downward growth may rupture the sellar floor and cause cerebrospinal fluid (CSF) rhinorrhea.

Space-occupying tumors can cause hypopituitarism by destroying cells that secrete other pituitary hormones. Tumors can also obstruct the pituitary's blood supply, causing ischemic necrosis and pituitary apoplexy—the sudden enlargement or infarction of a pituitary tumor or hemorrhage into a tumor. (See *Pituitary apoplexy,* page 55.) Signs and symptoms of pituitary apoplexy may vary greatly. Slow bleeding causes signs and symptoms of hypopituitarism. Rapid bleeding causes sudden, excruciating headache, loss of vision, and decreased level of consciousness.

Causes of infarction and ischemia
Pituitary infarction is usually associated with Sheehan's syndrome—pituitary necrosis resulting from severe postpartum hemorrhage and shock. Fortunately, with improved medical care, Sheehan's syndrome and other causes

of pituitary infarction, such as diabetic microvascular disease, sickle cell anemia, cavernous sinus thrombosis, temporal arteritis, internal carotid aneurysm, and trauma, occur infrequently.

In Sheehan's syndrome, postpartum hemorrhage, peripheral vascular collapse, and arteriolar spasm (of arterioles that supply the hypothalamic-pituitary portal vessels) or thrombosis of pituitary vessels cause pituitary ischemia. (Thrombosis may occur as part of the generalized intravascular coagulation that accompanies shock.) When circulation is restored, the already enlarged pituitary becomes severely edematous. In this edematous pituitary, confined to the sella turcica, impaired circulation eventually causes necrosis of the anterior lobe. In this situation, the posterior pituitary usually survives because it depends less on portal vessels for nutrition. Unfortunately, destruction of the anterior pituitary usually doesn't produce recognizable clinical signs until years after the initial incident has occurred. When recognizable clinical signs do occur, they include failure to lactate and menstrual irregularities.

Granulomas and other causes
Hypopituitarism can result from granuloma formation in the anterior pituitary caused by tuberculosis, meningitis, syphilis, or sarcoidosis. It can also result from formation of a multifocal eosinophilic granuloma (Hand-Schüller-Christian disease) in the hypothalamus. In both sites, the granuloma damages tissue by replacing or eliminating parenchymal elements and sometimes by causing pronounced fibrosis.

Actually, hypopituitarism can result from any of the disorders that affect hypothalamic function and impair synthesis or transport of hypophysiotropic hormones. Besides granuloma, these disorders include trauma, infection, hydrocephalus, and congenital malformation.

MEDICAL MANAGEMENT
Effective medical management of anterior pituitary disorders requires various radiologic and blood tests to confirm the diagnosis and to help direct treatment.

Radiologic tests detect tumors
Since hyperpituitarism usually results from hormone-secreting tumors, radiologic tests—X-rays, computerized tomography (CT), sellar tomography, and carotid arteriography—are

necessary to determine possible gross structural changes of the bone, sella turcica, or pituitary fossa. Radiologic tests are also useful in diagnosing hypopituitarism due to nonfunctioning pituitary tumors.

X-rays. In hyperpituitarism, skull X-rays may show the effects of a tumor on the pituitary—sella turcica enlargement and erosion, demineralization, displacement of bony boundaries, suprasellar calcification, elevation or destruction of anterior or posterior clinoids, depression of the sella floor, or ballooning of the fossa. X-rays may also show enlargement of the pituitary fossa, which occurs in many, but not all, intrasellar and suprasellar tumors. If skull X-rays reveal sellar enlargement, a CT scan is necessary to distinguish a tumor from empty-sella syndrome. (See *Empty-sella syndrome,* page 53.)

In acromegaly, skull X-rays show sellar enlargement, bone thickening, enlargement of the paranasal sinuses, and mandibular angle widening with prognathism (jaw projection). X-rays of the hands show increased soft tissue mass and phalangeal tufting.

In GH deficiency, particularly in patients with postpartum necrosis or pituitary dwarfism without a tumor, skull X-rays show a small pituitary fossa. Hand and other X-rays can determine bone age. In pituitary dwarfism, X-rays also usually show epiphyseal maturation retarded to the same extent as height.

CT scan. This is the preferred noninvasive test for determining sellar and parasellar tumor extension. When CT scan isn't available, sellar tomography and carotid arteriography are used.

Sellar tomography. In hyperpituitarism, this test helps clarify questionable skull X-ray findings. If a tumor is present, sellar tomography shows local areas of sellar erosion or thinning that may not appear on skull X-rays.

Carotid arteriography. This test helps differentiate carotid artery aneurysm from pituitary tumor, since both disorders may cause sellar enlargement and erosion.

Radioimmunoassays and provocative tests evaluate hormone levels

Radioimmunoassays measure plasma hormone levels directly; provocative tests measure hormone levels after administration of substances that stimulate or suppress hormonal secretion. However, unlike radiologic tests, these tests can't determine tumor size.

GH tests. In adults, elevated plasma GH levels confirm acromegaly when supported by unchanged, inadequately suppressed, or rising GH levels on suppression tests, such as glucose loading.

In children, plasma GH levels that fail to respond to more than one type of stimulation test confirm pituitary dwarfism. In adults, depressed GH levels usually indicate hypopituitarism from a tumor. However, this diagnosis requires confirmation by a provocative test such as an insulin tolerance, levodopa, or glucagon stimulation test.

PRL tests. Elevated levels of PRL on several occasions indicate an abnormality. However, the presence or absence of a tumor is determined radiologically. PRL deficiency is not clinically significant, so testing for deficiency is rare.

ACTH tests. Because reliable direct measurement of plasma ACTH is expensive, plasma cortisol, one of the regulators of ACTH, and urinary 17-hydroxycorticosteroids (17-OHCS), an index of cortisol secretion, help evaluate ACTH secretion. In an ACTH-secreting tumor, plasma ACTH, urinary 17-OHCS, and both urinary free cortisol and plasma cortisol levels are elevated; also, normal diurnal variation in ACTH secretion is absent.

To support these findings, a dexamethasone suppression test is performed to detect altered feedback control of the hypothalamic-pituitary-adrenal axis. In the normal individual, administration of dexamethasone depresses ACTH and, consequently, cortisol levels. Absence of cortisol suppression may indicate Cushing's syndrome or Cushing's disease.

Decreased morning plasma cortisol levels indicate ACTH deficiency when supported by increased cortisol levels after administration of cosyntropin, a synthetic analogue of ACTH. However, in patients with chronic ACTH deficiency due to adrenal atrophy, cortisol levels may fail to rise initially but may rise after prolonged stimulation.

A depressed response to administration of metyrapone also indicates ACTH deficiency. In the normal individual, metyrapone inhibits 11-beta hydroxylase (the last enzymatic step in cortisol synthesis), thus reducing plasma cortisol levels and stimulating ACTH secretion. Also, in the normal individual, 11-deoxycortisol (the precursor of cortisol) rises after metyrapone administration; in the patient with ACTH deficiency, 11-deoxycortisol doesn't rise.

TSH tests. TSH tests may help differentiate between primary hypothyroidism and pituitary or hypothalamic insufficiency. In primary hypothyroidism, TSH levels rise. In pituitary or hypothalamic insufficiency, TSH levels are normal or low.

After exogenous administration of TRH, TSH levels usually increase. In primary hypothyroidism, this increase is exaggerated. In secondary hypothyroidism and in hyperthyroidism, TSH levels fail to rise in response to TRH.

FSH-LH tests. Elevated FSH-LH levels, an exaggerated response to administration of luteinizing hormone-releasing hormone (LH-RH) and inadequate suppression of FSH-LH in response to testosterone administration, indicate excessive FSH-LH secretion. Depressed FSH-LH levels may accompany deficient FSH-LH secretion; however, it's difficult to differentiate depressed FSH-LH levels from normal levels. An inadequate rise of FSH-LH in response to LH-RH administration indicates hypothalamic-pituitary dysfunction.

Treatment: Surgery, radiation, or drugs

Treatment of anterior pituitary disorders aims to restore or limit loss of pituitary function. If a space-occupying tumor is present, treatment also aims to prevent such complications as visual deficit from compression of the optic chiasm. In severe pituitary apoplexy, emergency surgery may be needed to prevent irreversible blindness.

Surgery. Using a transsphenoidal or a transfrontal approach, surgical excision is the standard treatment for pituitary tumors. (See *Transsphenoidal adenomectomy,* page 56.) Depending on preoperative evaluation, the extent of surgery can range from adenomectomy, leaving the pituitary intact, to almost complete removal of the anterior lobe. Preferably, a small amount of secretory tissue is left.

Surgery offers important advantages, including immediate results, low mortality, and the ability to treat radioresistant tumors. Its disadvantages include occasional postoperative complications—frontal lobe damage, pituitary hemorrhage, infection, and CSF rhinorrhea—particularly with the transsphenoidal approach. Also, surgery may necessitate lifelong hormonal replacement and may cause visual damage.

Radiation therapy. Occasionally, radiation is needed postoperatively to treat residual tissue that was left to preserve healthy secretory tissue. Because it avoids surgical complications, radiation may even be preferred to surgery. However, the disadvantages of radiation

Empty-sella syndrome

Normal pituitary

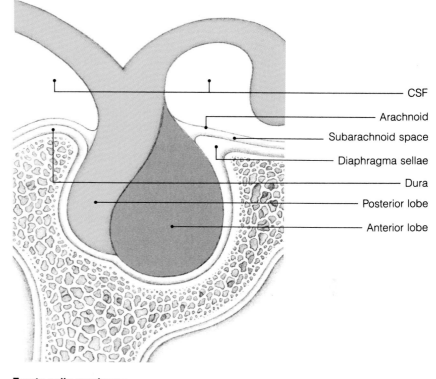

CSF
Arachnoid
Subarachnoid space
Diaphragma sellae
Dura
Posterior lobe
Anterior lobe

Empty-sella syndrome

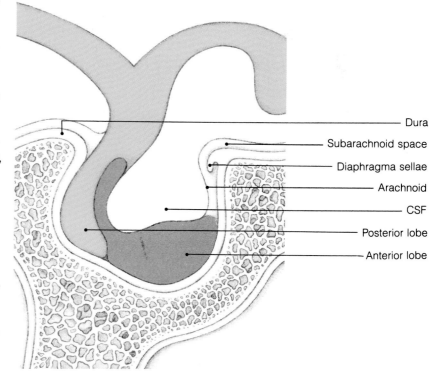

Dura
Subarachnoid space
Diaphragma sellae
Arachnoid
CSF
Posterior lobe
Anterior lobe

In empty-sella syndrome, the subarachnoid space extends into the intrasellar region, enlarging the sella turcica. Subarachnoid extension can result from necrosis, from resorption of a previous tumor, or, as shown at bottom, from an incompetent diaphragma sellae that permits cerebrospinal fluid to enter and fill the sella. Eventually, the pressure exerted by this fluid flattens the anterior pituitary and makes the sella appear empty.

include the radioresistance of some tumors, prolonged duration of therapy, danger of pituitary apoplexy, damage to surrounding neural tissue, and possible hypopituitarism resulting from radiation damage to normal pituitary tissue.

Two forms of external radiation—conventional (super voltage) and heavy particle (proton beam) therapy—are currently used. Conventional therapy usually delivers radiation in divided doses over several weeks. Heavy particle therapy delivers a slightly greater single dose and is often preferred for ACTH-secreting adenomas, unless complications, such as severe involvement of the optic chiasm, require surgery. Both forms of radiation may be used concurrently with corticosteroid therapy.

Drug therapy. Hyperpituitarism requires drugs that suppress hormone secretion; hypopituitarism requires replacement with natural hormones (such as GH for correcting growth retardation) or synthetic hormones (such as corticosteroids for ACTH deficiency).

For GH disorders. When excessive secretion of GH is present, bromocriptine may normalize GH levels. However, its long-term effects are unknown, and excessive GH secretion recurs after drug therapy ends.

In children with severe growth retardation

from GH deficiency, GH replacement is required. Human pituitaries at autopsy provide the standard, but scarce, source of GH. Some centers now use synthetic GH, created by recombinant DNA technology using bacteria bearing the gene for GH. Other promising sources of GH may evolve from development of synthetic placental lactogen and the isolation of a GH-releasing factor.

For PRL disorders. In hyperprolactinemia, bromocriptine decreases PRL levels, suppresses galactorrhea, and normalizes the menstrual cycle. In hypoprolactinemia, PRL replacement is unnecessary because this disorder is not clinically significant.

For ACTH disorders. Therapy is directed at the adrenals, the target organ, rather than the pituitary tumor. Before surgical removal of an ACTH-secreting adenoma, metyrapone and dexamethasone are given together to normalize cortisol secretion. Occasionally, cyproheptadine hydrochloride, a serotonin antagonist, is given instead, but its effects aren't predictable. When given concurrently with radiation therapy, cyproheptadine usually improves therapeutic response time.

Complete ACTH deficiency requires lifelong hormone replacement with cortisone or hydrocortisone (cortisol). With increased stress, such as fever or trauma, the maintenance

Arteriogram shows pituitary tumor

Normal

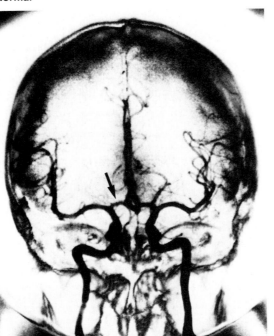

Abnormal

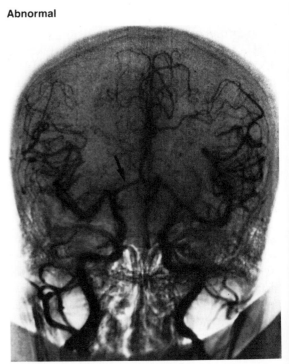

Compare the normal arteriogram (at left) to the abnormal arteriogram (at right). The latter shows superior and

lateral displacement of both anterior cerebral arteries from extensive suprasellar extension by a pituitary tumor.

EMERGENCY MANAGEMENT

Pituitary apoplexy

Pituitary apoplexy is caused by the sudden infarction or enlargement of a pituitary tumor or hemorrhage into a tumor. It occurs in up to 10% of pituitary tumors, but its exact cause is unknown.

Pituitary apoplexy requires early diagnosis and immediate treatment. Its first sign is sudden, excruciating headache. Other common signs and symptoms include blurred vision, diplopia, altered level of consciousness, nausea and vomiting, extraocular palsies, and hyperpyrexia. Less common signs and symptoms include nuchal rigidity, loss of vision, facial paresthesia, seizures, and hemiparesis. With the onset of deepening coma and severe neurologic deficits, the risk of mortality increases.

Diagnosis of pituitary apoplexy requires lumbar puncture and radiologic tests. Typically, lumbar puncture initially reveals elevated cerebrospinal fluid pressure and the presence of red blood cells. The skull X-ray shows an enlarged sella turcica; a CT scan shows suprasellar extension.

After diagnosis, cortisol administration helps reduce intracranial swelling and corrects coexisting hypocortisolism from lack of ACTH. Then, if visual acuity continues to deteriorate, emergency surgery is needed to prevent irreversible blindness.

---

dose of these drugs may need to be doubled. As stress subsides, the dose can be gradually reduced. In partial ACTH deficiency, administration of cortisone or hydrocortisone only during stress may prove effective.

For TSH disorders. For TSH-secreting tumors, antithyroid agents—propylthiouracil or methimazole—prevent further increase in thyroid hormone levels. In TSH deficiency, L-thyroxine replaces thyroid hormone after serial measurements of serum thyroxine levels and the patient's clinical picture determine the appropriate dose.

For FSH-LH disorders. In women, therapy for FSH-LH deficiency is aimed at correcting ovarian hormone secretion. Estrogen may be given. To avoid the risk of thromboembolism and hyperlipidemia, it's given in small doses. In men, FSH-LH deficiency requires periodic intramuscular administration of androgen to enhance muscle strength, libido, and beard growth. In both sexes, menotropins and human chorionic gonadotropin (HCG) may restore fertility. However, these fertility-restoring hormones may cause multiple births in women, may be successful in only 50% of men, and are costly.

Drug therapy in FSH-LH disorders usually offers significant benefits but may cause problems for the patient. For example, a patient with longstanding hypogonadism who has become accustomed to the consequences of hormone imbalance may find considerable difficulty in coping with drug-induced changes in libido, appearance, and social behavior. Typically, the benefits of normal hormone balance outweigh the potential disadvantages of drug therapy.

NURSING MANAGEMENT

Because the anterior pituitary influences so many complex functions, managing anterior pituitary disorders requires special expertise. Such expertise begins with knowing the right questions to develop a relevant patient history and must include the ability to recognize the subtle signs of anterior pituitary dysfunction.

Take patient history

Because many anterior pituitary disorders produce subtle symptoms that progress so gradually, getting a relevant and revealing patient history can challenge your assessment skills as sharply as the physical exam. So you'll have to plan your interview carefully to pick up subtle physical and psychological changes. Also, to obtain as much information as possible, you'll need to interview the patient's family as well.

The following questions about signs and symptoms should help you recognize clues to these elusive disorders.

• Does the patient experience any paresthesia (abnormal sensations), such as burning or prickling? Does he have joint pain? Has he needed to change his hat, shoe, glove, or ring size recently? Has the fit of his dentures changed recently? These conditions or changes may suggest excessive secretion of GH.

• Has the patient's muscle strength decreased recently? Decreased muscle strength occurs with GH excess and deficiency, FSH-LH deficiency, and ACTH excess and deficiency.

• Do the patient's wounds heal slowly? Impaired wound healing occurs with GH excess and ACTH excess.

Transsphenoidal adenomectomy

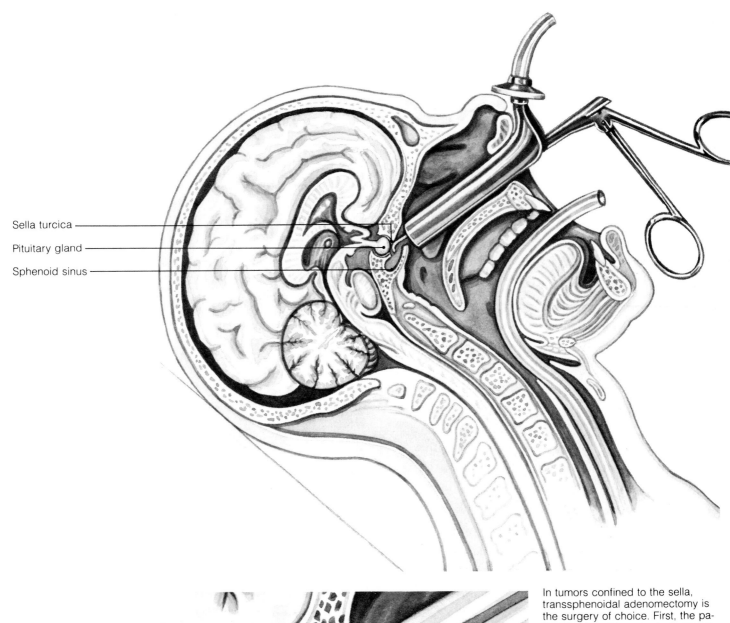

Sella turcica
Pituitary gland
Sphenoid sinus

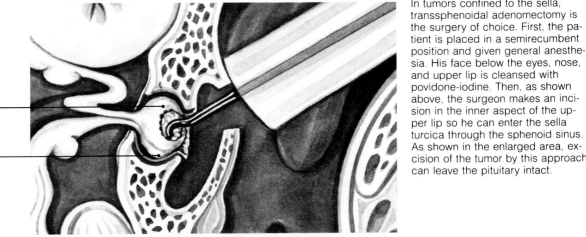

Anterior pituitary
Posterior pituitary

In tumors confined to the sella, transsphenoidal adenomectomy is the surgery of choice. First, the patient is placed in a semirecumbent position and given general anesthesia. His face below the eyes, nose, and upper lip is cleansed with povidone-iodine. Then, as shown above, the surgeon makes an incision in the inner aspect of the upper lip so he can enter the sella turcica through the sphenoid sinus. As shown in the enlarged area, excision of the tumor by this approach can leave the pituitary intact.

• Does the patient frequently experience fatigue? Constant fatigue may occur with GH deficiency and ACTH deficiency or excess.
• Has the patient noticed unusual intolerance to cold? This may be a sign of TSH deficiency.
• Has he noticed unusual intolerance to heat? Does he sweat profusely? Does he experience palpitations or dyspnea? These signs and symptoms occur with TSH excess.
• If the patient is a child, ask his parents to review his growth patterns so you can compare them to normal.

Next, ask about nutritional status.
• Have the patient's eating or drinking habits changed recently? Such changes occur with GH excess.
• Has the patient's urination or bowel pattern changed recently? Such changes occur with GH excess; constipation occurs with TSH deficiency.
• Has the patient suddenly gained weight? Rapid weight gain occurs with GH excess, ACTH excess, and panhypopituitarism.
• Has he experienced nausea and vomiting? This can result from ACTH deficiency.

Now, proceed with questions to evaluate psychological status and sexual development and function.
• Has the patient noticed recent personality changes (lethargy, depression), impotence, or decreased libido? Such changes suggest GH and PRL excess and FSH-LH deficiency; decreased libido may suggest ACTH deficiency.
• Has he experienced milk discharge from his breasts? This results from PRL excess.
• Has the female patient experienced menstrual abnormalities or infertility? These disorders may reflect excessive secretion of GH, PRL, ACTH, FSH, or LH.

To detect possible pituitary damage, ask the patient:
• Has he ever undergone head or neck radiation or cranial surgery? Has he recently sustained a head injury?
• Review the female patient's obstetric history. Has she ever experienced postpartum hemorrhage? Did she fail to lactate postpartum? Did she have persistent postpartum amenorrhea?

To determine possible tumor and pituitary apoplexy, ask these questions:
• Does the patient experience recurring headaches? If so, determine their location, severity, quality, duration, precipitating factors, and effective treatment.
• Does he suffer from visual disturbances, such as double vision, photophobia, or loss of peripheral vision? In one or both eyes? Have

these changes occurred suddenly or gradually?

Finally, take a thorough drug history. Be sure to ask about use of phenothiazines, which stimulate PRL secretion, and vincristine, which can cause hypopituitarism.

Physical exam: Helpful in advanced stages
Unfortunately, physical examination is unlikely to reveal significant physical changes until anterior pituitary dysfunction has become severe and advanced. Typically, you can't detect any prodromal changes. So check for overt dysfunction as follows:

First, inspect the skin for abnormal pigmentation, striae, thickening, and excessive oiliness or wrinkling, particularly premature wrinkling. These changes may indicate GH or ACTH excess. Also, look for hirsutism and acne, signs of ACTH excess.

Check for abnormal growth patterns and distribution of fatty tissue or hair, indicating GH excess or deficiency. In adults, check for signs of acromegaly—coarsening and enlargement of facial features, prognathism from overgrowth of facial bones, and overgrowth of bones in the extremities. (See *Signs of acromegaly,* page 60.) In children, look for features of pituitary dwarfism—immature facial features, inappropriate body proportions for age, and excess facial and truncal fat. (See *Pituitary dwarfism: Before and after treatment,* page 58.)

Check for visual field defects, which can indicate a pituitary tumor. First, instruct the patient to cover his right eye with his right hand. Then, stand back about 2' and cover your left eye with your left hand. Tell the patient to stare at your right eye while you move two waving fingers into his visual field from each quadrant. Ask him to report when he first sees your fingers. If your visual fields are normal, the patient should see your fingers at the same time you do.

Next, palpate the thyroid for enlargement, a sign of TSH excess. To examine the thyroid, stand in front of the patient and observe the lower half of his neck, first in the normal position and then with his neck slightly extended.

Auscultate the heart for tachycardia, indicating TSH excess, or bradycardia, indicating TSH deficiency. Also, check for hypertension, which may occur in a mild form in GH excess.

Assess the patient for absence of secondary sex characteristics, a sign of FSH-LH deficiency. In men, evaluate pubic and axillary

Psychosocial dwarfism

A reversible form of GH deficiency, psychosocial dwarfism results from extreme neglect, abuse, or social isolation. Typically, along with showing delayed growth, the child with this condition appears apathetic and withdrawn and may occasionally exhibit temper tantrums. He overeats and drinks excessively and may experience incontinence and insomnia, which can cause night wandering, sometimes in search of food.

If such a child is placed in a happy, supportive environment, normal growth and behavior begin within a few weeks. However, if the child returns to his original environment, relapse is possible, so his progress needs monitoring every 4 to 8 weeks.

Pituitary dwarfism: Before and after treatment

Before treatment, this 6-year-old girl with dwarfism secondary to craniopharyngioma showed infantile chubbiness and immature facial features in addition to short stature—37" (94 cm). After approximately 15 months of treatment, 2.5 mg of human growth hormone twice weekly, her height increased to 48.25" (122.5 cm). Note that she also lost her infantile fat and her facial features matured.

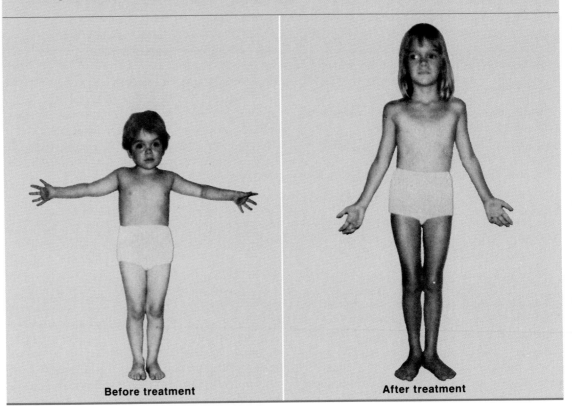

Before treatment

After treatment

hair growth, deepening of the voice, and genital development. In women, evaluate breast development and growth of pubic and axillary hair.

Inspect the breasts for discharge, a sign of PRL excess, by compressing the patient's nipple between your thumb and index finger. If this produces a discharge, milk the breast along the radii to locate its source. Document the color, consistency, amount, and site of discharge.

Palpate the abdomen for visceromegaly, a prominent feature of acromegaly. Also, palpate the liver and spleen to detect early stages of visceromegaly, during which the intestines may not be palpable.

Nursing diagnosis

Because the physical signs of anterior pituitary disorders are often quite subtle, you must consider your assessment findings in light of laboratory data. Then, to monitor any changes in the disorder and effectiveness of therapy, keep your assessment data current. The resulting nursing diagnoses will help you plan appropriate treatment goals and interventions. In patients with anterior pituitary disorders, your integrated assessment will

typically lead to the following diagnoses, goals, and interventions:

Disturbances in self-concept, behavior, sexuality, or body image related to hormonal imbalance. Such hormonal imbalance may stem from hypersecretion, hyposecretion, or initial exogenous replacement. Your goals are *to identify related disturbances in self-concept, behavior, sexuality, or body image and to help the patient cope with them*. Explain the psychological effects of hormonal imbalance. For example, you may explain that FSH-LH deficiency or GH excess causes depression and mood swings and that ACTH deficiency causes lethargy and reduces stress tolerance.

Explain the effects of hormonal imbalance on sexuality. Help the patient understand that decreased libido or impotence has a physiologic cause, and that hormone replacement can improve sexual response.

Expect the patient with long-term hypogonadism to have considerable difficulty adjusting to changes in libido and behavior after hormone replacement. To ease this adjustment, explain the anticipated changes and encourage the patient to discuss any sexual difficulties with his doctor.

Review the causes of any physical changes

that could affect body image. Then explain these causes to the patient and, if appropriate, use illustrations to show the expected effects of treatment. Be open to questions and encourage the patient to express his concerns. Also discuss external factors, such as stress, that can aggravate hormonal imbalance. Promote socialization with other patients and, if necessary, refer the patient and his family to a social worker, therapist, or support group.

After effective teaching, the patient should be able to identify changes in self-concept, behavior, sexuality, or body image that stem from hormonal imbalance; to describe the expected physical changes from treatment; and to identify external factors that aggravate hormonal imbalance. The patient should also ask appropriate questions, freely express his concerns, interact effectively with others, and attend scheduled therapy sessions.

Potential for injury from visual deficit. Such deficit results from compression of the optic

Clinical findings in hyperpituitarism and hypopituitarism

Causative hormone	Hyperpituitarism	Hypopituitarism
Growth hormone	• *Gigantism* (in children): increased skeletal growth before puberty (closure of epiphyseal plates), leading to acromegaly. • *Acromegaly* (in adults): soft tissue hypertrophy of the extremities and face; thickening, lengthening and proliferation of bone, causing enlarged hands and feet and prognathism; coarsened facial features; arthropathy, ranging from mild arthralgia to crippling arthritis; thickened, leathery, oily skin; cyst formation; generalized hirsutism; increased skin pigmentation; increased sweating; heat intolerance; deepening of the voice; peripheral neuropathy (paresthesia and sensory losses); proximal muscle weakness; enlarged viscera; weight gain, but not obesity; glucose intolerance, diabetes; hypertension, cardiomegaly, and increased cardiovascular disease. Also, galactorrhea, amenorrhea, infertility, decreased vaginal secretion, and decreased libido in women; impotence and decreased libido in men.	• *Pituitary dwarfism* (in children): normal appearance at birth, delayed growth, increased truncal fat, delayed development or absence of secondary sex characteristics, immature body proportions and facial features, high-pitched voice, hypoglycemia, wrinkled skin giving appearance of aging. • Usually, no significant clinical symptoms in adults; possible delayed wound healing, anemia, and decreased muscle strength.
Prolactin	• Galactorrhea in adults of both sexes. • In women: amenorrhea, infertility, decreased vaginal secretions, and decreased libido from estrogen deficiency. • In men: impotence and loss of libido.	• Absence of postpartum lactation.
Adrenocorticotropic hormone	• *Excessive adrenocortical function* (Cushing's syndrome): truncal obesity, moon face, buffalo hump; diabetes; amenorrhea; hirsutism; acne; osteoporosis; muscle wasting; purple striae; capillary fragility; impaired wound healing; increased skin pigmentation over pressure points, genitalia, and sites of new scars; euphoria, reduced sleep requirements, and psychoses.	• *Diminished adrenocortical function*: weakness, postural hypotension, dehydration, nausea, vomiting, hyperthermia, hypoglycemia, possible depigmentation. In women: decreased libido and loss of axillary and pubic hair.
Thyroid-stimulating hormone	• *Thyrotoxicosis*: heat intolerance, excessive sweating; tachycardia, congestive heart failure, palpitations; nervousness, tremors; fatigue, weakness; warm, moist skin; fine, brittle hair or alopecia; increased appetite; exophthalmos, weight loss.	• Severe growth retardation in children. • *Secondary pituitary hypothyroidism* in adults—cold intolerance, constipation, dry skin, pallor, mental slowing, bradycardia, hoarseness, myxedema, lethargy. In women—decreased or increased menstrual bleeding.
Follicle-stimulating hormone and luteinizing hormone	• FSH-LH excess is rare and when it does occur, symptoms are vague.	• *Hypogonadism* in adults: in women—amenorrhea, breast atrophy, dry skin, decreased vaginal secretions and libido from estrogen deficiency; in men—small testes, decreased libido, impotence, decreased pubic hair growth, muscle weakness. In children: partial or complete impairment of secondary sexual development and, if GH secretion isn't impaired, eunuchoid appearance.
All of the above hormones	• Excess of all hormones has never been documented.	• *Panhypopituitarism*: causes all the signs and symptoms listed above under hypopituitarism.

Signs of acromegaly

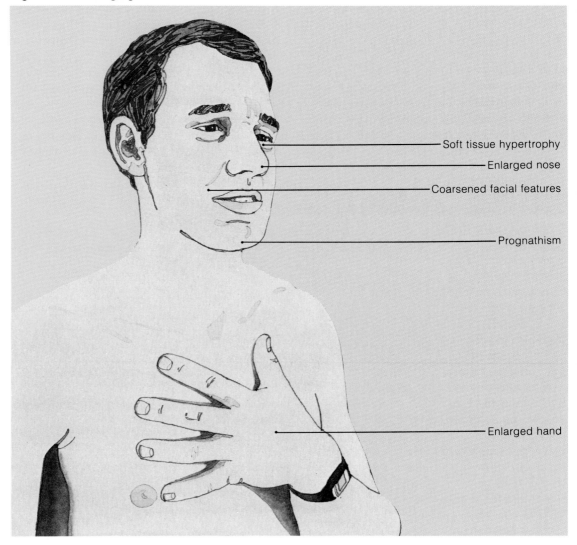

Soft tissue hypertrophy

Enlarged nose

Coarsened facial features

Prognathism

Enlarged hand

chiasm and usually begins with narrowing of visual fields (tunnel vision). Your goals are *to prevent injury, if possible, and to help the patient adjust to and accept visual deficit.*

Teach the patient about his visual deficit and its causes. Familiarize him with his environment. Show him the location of furniture and the bathroom, and introduce him to his roommate. Keep the patient's personal items, such as dentures, in a set place. Encourage the patient to express his concerns. Listen and provide emotional support. If the patient has a permanent visual deficit, refer him to a support group for the visually impaired.

After effective teaching, the patient should be able to identify his visual deficit and describe its cause and to understand the need for safety precautions. If the patient's deficit is permanent, he should be aware of support groups and be able to discuss his feelings and possible life-style changes.

Menstrual abnormalities related to hormonal imbalance. Your goals are *to teach the patient about the effects of hormonal imbalance and its treatment on her menstrual cycle and to help her verbalize her anxieties and fears.*

To achieve these goals, instruct the patient to keep a detailed record of her menstrual cycle. Review the cause of her specific menstrual abnormality; its implications, such as infertility; and its responsiveness to treatment.

Allow the patient to express any feelings of inadequacy, guilt, fear, or worry. Provide emotional support. After effective teaching, the patient should be able to relate her menstrual abnormality to hormonal imbalance and be able to cope with its implications.

Knowledge deficit related to treatment. Your goal is *to teach the patient about treatment.* First, assess the patient's readiness to learn and his current knowledge level. If the patient is scheduled for a transsphenoidal adenomectomy or other surgery, explain the procedure, including any pre- and postoperative care. Emphasize ways to prevent postoperative complications, such as CSF leakage. For instance, tell the patient to avoid coughing and sneezing. To avoid pulmonary complications, encourage deep breathing. Tell the patient, to avoid infection, he should practice good oral hygiene using a soft toothbrush. To reinforce teaching, introduce him to another patient who had similar surgery, if possible.

If the patient is scheduled for radiation therapy, explain irradiation and its goal. Arrange for him to visit the radiation therapy unit. Explain that he'll be alone during therapy. Emphasize that radiation therapy won't expose him to harmful levels of radioactivity. Stress the importance of complying with concurrent corticosteroid therapy according to the prescribed schedule. Explain that this schedule reflects his individual sleep and activity level. Explain the expected outcome and possible side effects of drug therapy. If the patient needs lifelong corticosteroid replacement, tell him to wear a Medic Alert bracelet.

After effective teaching, the patient should understand the prescribed treatment, its side effects and potential complications, and its expected benefits. Make sure the patient who's receiving radiation therapy knows the importance of complying with concurrent corticosteroid therapy.

Pain related to intrasellar pressure on the sella turcica. Your goal is *to promote patient comfort.* Give analgesics as ordered. Provide dim lighting and quiet. To prevent central nervous system depression from analgesics, watch for signs of neurologic deficit, such as unusual somnolence, apathy, and decreased level of consciousness. Report such changes to the doctor.

When the patient is comfortable, begin appropriate teaching. For example, you may use an illustration of the brain to show him and his family the location of the tumor. Help them realize that pain results directly from the pressure of the tumor. Consider your intervention effective if the patient is as comfortable as possible, you've reported any neurologic deficit, and the patient and his family can identify the cause of pain.

Potential discomfort from meningitis related to surgical invasion of the sella turcica. Your goals are *to promote patient comfort and to maintain adequate nutrition and bodily functions.*

During the acute period, monitor neurologic status (pupil checks, level of consciousness) and fluid status (intake and output, urine specific gravity) every 2 hours. Give analgesics as ordered. To ease the discomfort of fever and severe headaches, give sponge baths and apply an ice cap to the patient's head. Maintain bed rest and elevate the guard rails to prevent falls during possible seizures. Give range-of-motion exercises and skin care as needed and maintain adequate nutrition by providing high-calorie, high-protein meals and adequate fluids.

As the patient improves, decrease the frequency of neurologic checks. Also, increase the patient's activity as tolerated, always making sure to plan for rest periods. Consider your intervention effective if the patient is stable and as comfortable as possible.

Hormonal imbalance related to failure of compliance with therapy. Your goals are *to detect failure to follow prescribed treatment, to identify its cause, and, if possible, to correct it.*

To achieve these goals, find out exactly how and when the patient is taking prescribed drugs. If he isn't following the prescribed schedule, try to find out why. If the schedule is difficult to follow, help him set up a more convenient, realistic one that he can discuss with his doctor. Consider your intervention successful if you've identified and corrected the reason for failure of compliance.

Evaluate your teaching

To help the patient cope with the wide-ranging and often devastating physical and psychological effects of anterior pituitary disorders, you'll need to provide comprehensive patient teaching and timely emotional support. You can be sure your teaching has been successful when the patient:
• can identify and cope with changes in his self-concept, behavior, sexuality, or body image that stem from hormonal imbalance or hormone replacement
• understands his treatment, whether it be surgery, radiation therapy, or drug therapy
• follows his treatment regimen faithfully and achieves optimal pituitary function.

Keep working with the patient until you achieve all these goals. Because anterior pituitary disorders affect the patient's family as well, be sure to include his family in your teaching plan. The patient with an anterior pituitary disorder can't eliminate all of its often devastating effects. But effective treatment and nursing care can help him understand, cope with, and reduce them.

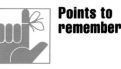

Points to remember

• The anterior pituitary secretes growth hormone (GH), prolactin (PRL), adrenocorticotropic hormone (ACTH), follicle-stimulating hormone (FSH), luteinizing hormone (LH), and thyroid-stimulating hormone (TSH). Because these hormones regulate growth, sexual development, and metabolic activity, anterior pituitary disorders cause wide-ranging physical and psychological effects.
• Because signs and symptoms of anterior pituitary disorders can be insidious in onset and difficult to identify, you must polish your interviewing and physical assessment skills. For example, be ready to spot signs of GH excess—inappropriate body proportions, soft tissue hypertrophy, and coarsened facial features.
• Transsphenoidal adenomectomy, the preferred surgery, allows for complete removal of a pituitary tumor while leaving the pituitary intact.
• Thorough teaching and emotional support help the patient cope with the wide-ranging and often devastating physical and psychological effects of anterior pituitary disorders.

5 IDENTIFYING POSTERIOR LOBE DYSFUNCTION

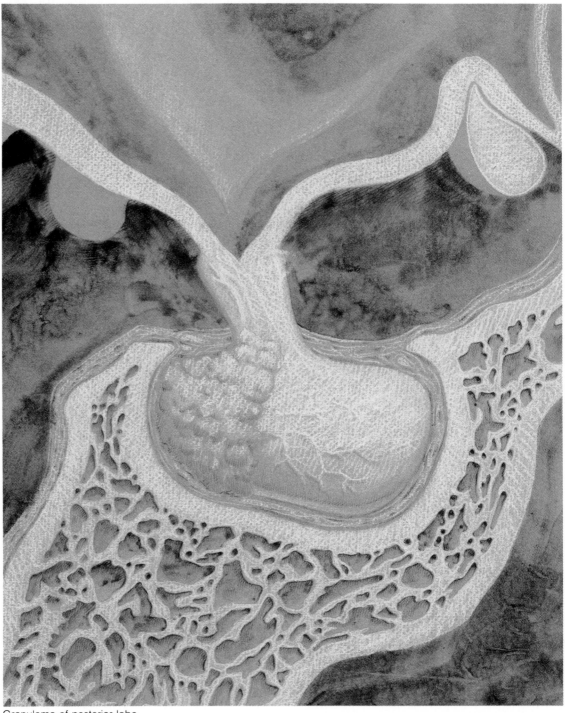

Granuloma of posterior lobe

Disorders of the posterior lobe of the pituitary—diabetes insipidus and syndrome of inappropriate antidiuretic hormone (SIADH)—are often as difficult to identify as they are uncommon. Because they typically produce clinical effects that mimic those of other disorders, mastering precise assessment skills is essential. A thorough patient history and complete physical exam can often provide valuable clinical data that make differential diagnosis possible. After diagnosis, continuing assessment helps you plan appropriate care to maintain electrolyte balance and prevent complications. Of course, accurate assessment rests on a thorough understanding of these disorders, including their pathophysiology, diagnosis, and treatment.

What causes posterior pituitary disorders?

Simply stated, these disorders result from a defect in the production or secretion of antidiuretic hormone (ADH). This hormone is produced in the hypothalamus along with oxytocin. Both hormones travel along nerve fibers in the pituitary stalk to the posterior pituitary, where they're stored until neural stimuli signal the need for their secretion. Oxytocin is important in pregnancy and lactation (see *Effects of oxytocin,* page 64); it has not been implicated in disease. ADH maintains normal serum osmolality and fluid balance.

ADH insufficiency. Decreased production or secretion of ADH—the result of a defect in the hypothalamus, pituitary stalk, or posterior pituitary—causes diabetes insipidus. This disorder typically strikes young male adults, but increasing prevalence of hypophysectomies and radiation treatments has spread it to a wider population. Central diabetes insipidus has two forms: primary and secondary. In *primary diabetes insipidus,* the defect may be familial, congenital, or idiopathic (in about 50%). In about 4% of patients with idiopathic diabetes insipidus, the disease begins in early childhood and may be familial.

Secondary diabetes insipidus may develop as a complication of basal skull fracture or of neurosurgery, such as hypophysectomy. Its symptoms may be transient, and the severity of ADH insufficiency depends on the location and extent of the trauma. However, in more than 30% of patients with secondary diabetes insipidus, this disorder results from primary or metastatic tumors. Rarely, it may result from aneurysm of the circle of Willis; cerebrovascular hemorrhage; granulomatous diseases, such as sarcoidosis, tuberculosis, or meningovascular syphilis; and histiocytosis X. Secondary diabetes insipidus occasionally subsides with successful treatment of the underlying disease.

Nephrogenic diabetes insipidus, a hereditary disorder, results from renal tubule resistance to ADH. A similar form of diabetes insipidus may also develop during treatment with lithium or demeclocycline. Also, renal resistance to ADH is partially responsible for the polyuria of hypercalcemia and hypokalemia.

ADH excess. SIADH results from excessive release of ADH, causing water retention. First described in 1951, this syndrome is now being recognized more often in acute-care settings.

SIADH occurs secondary to disorders that affect the osmoreceptor of the hypothalamus. Its most common cause is oat cell carcinoma of the lung, but it may also result from pancreatic and duodenal carcinoma, Hodgkin's disease, and thymoma. Malignant cells from patients with SIADH have been shown to synthesize, store, and release a substance that is physiologically and immunologically indistinguishable from ADH.

Because nonmalignant pulmonary tissue can also synthesize ADH, SIADH can occur in viral and bacterial pneumonia, tuberculosis, and lung abscess. Possibly, the changes in intrathoracic pressure secondary to diffuse pulmonary disease promote ADH secretion by stimulating baroreceptors in the lung that are sensitive to fluid shifts and osmotic pressure changes.

In addition, SIADH can result from certain central nervous system disorders, such as head trauma, brain abscess and tumor, meningitis, encephalitis, Guillain-Barré syndrome, subarachnoid hemorrhage, and acute intermittent porphyria. SIADH has recently been reported in patients with acute psychosis.

Drugs can also cause SIADH. For example, chlorpropamide, vincristine sulfate, and cyclophosphamide are known to stimulate secretion of ADH; so can nicotine, morphine, barbiturates, phenothiazines, vasopressin, oxytocin, carbamazepine, and general anesthetics. Thiazides and other diuretics can produce hyponatremia, with all the clinical signs of SIADH.

Finally, hypothyroidism, adrenal insufficiency, positive-pressure ventilation, and even physical or emotional stress and pain can cause SIADH.

Effects of oxytocin

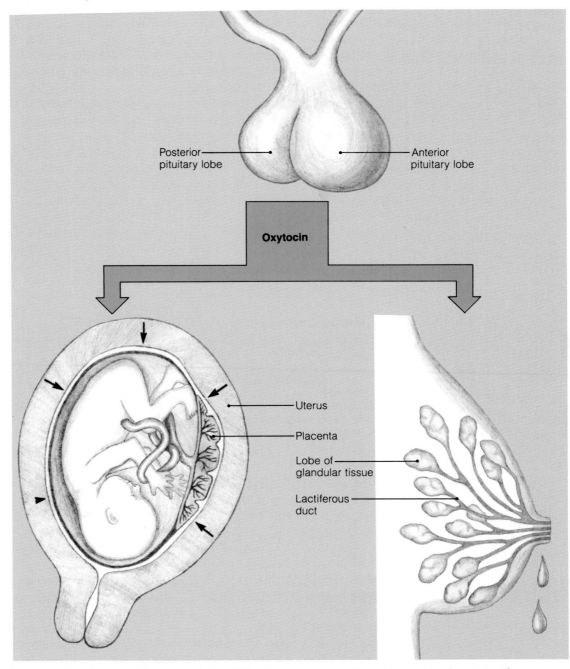

Posterior pituitary lobe

Anterior pituitary lobe

Oxytocin

Uterus

Placenta

Lobe of glandular tissue

Lactiferous duct

Oxytocin, which is secreted by the posterior pituitary lobe, promotes milk ejection and uterine contraction.

PATHOPHYSIOLOGY

ADH acts on the distal tubules and collecting ducts of the kidneys, increasing their permeability to water. (See *ADH release and regulation,* page 66.) This promotes reabsorption of water and reduces urine output. Although researchers don't yet know the precise mechanism of ADH activity, they do know that ADH binds to specific receptor sites in the collecting ducts and stimulates production of cyclic adenosine monophosphate. This, in turn, activates the enzyme protein kinase and even-

tually causes the collecting duct's epithelium to become more permeable to water. The resulting reabsorption of water reduces urine volume and leads to concentrated urine.

Stimuli for ADH secretion

Depletion of blood volume and plasma hyperosmolality are the most important stimuli for ADH release. These changes in blood volume stimulate special pressure-sensitive receptors in the atria and aortic arch. When plasma volume drops suddenly, as in hemorrhage, increased secretion of ADH helps restore volume. (See *Cellular effects of ADH,* page 67.) Similarly, congestive heart failure, nephrotic syndrome, and cirrhosis, in which effective arterial blood volume is decreased, are also marked by increased levels of ADH. Conversely, increased circulating volume inhibits release of ADH, with resulting diuresis.

Plasma osmolality also affects ADH secretion. When osmoreceptors in the hypothalamus detect increased plasma osmolality, the thirst mechanism promotes increased fluid intake, and the posterior pituitary secretes ADH, which promotes fluid retention. Both ADH and the thirst mechanism respond to hyperosmolality by trying to increase extracellular fluid. When increased fluid intake and fluid retention have diluted the extracellular fluid to normal osmolality, ADH secretion falls to a baseline level, and thirst disappears. When plasma osmolality is low, the osmoreceptors do not trigger secretions of ADH; consequently, diuresis allows plasma osmolality to rise to normal levels.

ADH insufficiency

In central and nephrogenic diabetes insipidus, ADH deficiency or lack of response reduces the renal tubule's permeability to water, causing diuresis. This water loss, in turn, elevates plasma osmolality, which stimulates the thirst mechanism, a compensatory physiologic mechanism to reduce plasma osmolality to normal levels.

In central diabetes insipidus, ADH deficiency may be complete, partial, or a transient complication of pituitary or hypothalamic surgery. A surgical lesion at or near the posterior pituitary may cause only partial deficiency of ADH, since it leaves intact fibers in the pituitary stalk that end at the median eminence. However, if the lesion occurs higher on the pituitary stalk, retrograde degeneration of all fibers in the stalk may follow, causing complete absence of ADH secretion.

If more than 85% of the secretory capacity of the posterior pituitary is lost, severe polyuria may follow. Fortunately, such permanent severe polyuria is rare because irreversible injury to the neurons is rarely so extensive.

If diabetes insipidus results from injury caused by hypothalamic or pituitary surgery, initial polyuria lasts 1 to 6 days because of ADH deficiency resulting from transient paralysis of posterior pituitary function. Then, if injured neurons have degenerated, initial polyuria may be followed by 4 to 5 days of normal urine output, probably resulting from release of stored ADH from within the injured neurons.

Excessive ADH secretion

In SIADH, excessive ADH secretion increases renal tubular permeability. Consequently, water that's normally excreted is reabsorbed into the circulation; water retention and, eventually, water intoxication may result. As retained water expands extracellular fluid volume, plasma osmolality declines, the glomerular filtration rate rises, and sodium levels decline to hyponatremia. (See *What happens in SIADH,* page 68.) At first, hyponatremia reflects dilution of body fluids by retained water, but subsequently hyponatremia may reflect increased renal excretion of sodium. Such excretion may reflect secondary hypoaldosteronism that results from the expanded extracellular space, the effect of the increased filtered sodium load related to an increased glomerular filtration rate, and suppressed proximal tubular reabsorption of sodium in response to expansion of extracellular fluid volume.

Body weight increases in proportion to retained water, but usually without extreme hypervolemia. Such water retention usually produces nonspecific signs and symptoms that often relate to the gastrointestinal tract (abdominal cramps, anorexia, nausea, vomiting) and to the central nervous system (disorientation, lethargy, confusion, headache, and possible hemiparesis, coma, or seizures).

MEDICAL MANAGEMENT

Diagnosis of posterior pituitary disorders requires a careful patient history, especially related to fluid and electrolyte status; thorough physical examination; and laboratory studies to exclude other disorders.

Diabetes insipidus: Difficult diagnosis

Confirming diabetes insipidus first requires ruling out other causes of polyuria and polydipsia, such as diabetes mellitus, solute diuresis (involving sodium chloride, sodium bicarbonate, mannitol, or glycerol), or postobstructive diuresis. Then diagnostic tests, such as urinalysis, osmolality and dehydration tests, and radiography, can be used to distinguish central diabetes insipidus (partial or complete) from nephrogenic diabetes insipidus or primary (psychogenic) polydipsia. Posttraumatic or surgically induced diabetes insipidus tends to be transient, lasting from

ADH release and regulation

Neural impulses signal the supraoptic nuclei of the hypothalamus to secrete antidiuretic hormone (ADH). This hormone moves along nerve fibers of the pituitary stalk to the posterior pituitary lobe, where it's stored until needed to maintain fluid balance. In the kidneys, ADH binds to receptors in the tubular epithelial cells, promoting water retention.

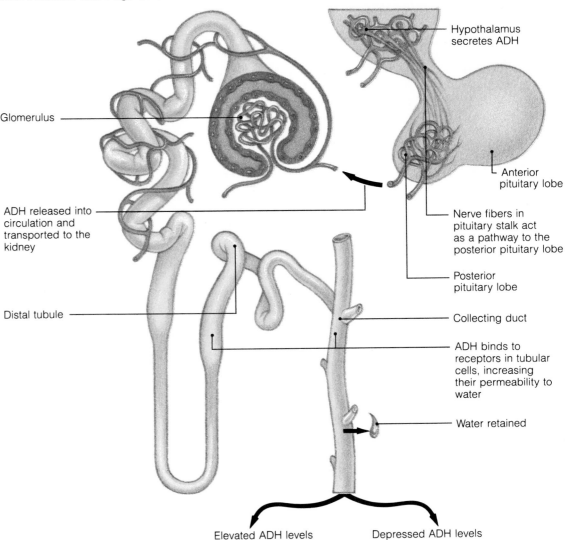

Glomerulus

ADH released into circulation and transported to the kidney

Distal tubule

Hypothalamus secretes ADH

Anterior pituitary lobe

Nerve fibers in pituitary stalk act as a pathway to the posterior pituitary lobe

Posterior pituitary lobe

Collecting duct

ADH binds to receptors in tubular cells, increasing their permeability to water

Water retained

Elevated ADH levels decrease urine output

Depressed ADH levels increase urine output

a few hours to several months; it seldom persists longer than 6 months after the onset of polyuria. Other types of central diabetes insipidus are usually permanent, changing little in severity or therapeutic requirements with time. Drug-induced nephrogenic diabetes insipidus disappears shortly after withdrawing the causative drug. Drugs that cause nephrogenic diabetes insipidus include lithium, demeclocycline, tolazamide, colchicine, and vinblastine sulfate.

Complete diabetes insipidus produces polyuria of at least 10 to 12 liters/day and a urinary osmolality below 100 mOsm/kg water. If concurrent illness, such as viral gastroenteritis, prevents adequate fluid intake, life-threatening hypernatremia may develop rapidly. Also, a hypothalamic lesion may involve the patient's thirst center, causing hypodipsia and hypernatremia. However, the thirst mechanism is usually left intact, so that polydipsia and adequate fluid intake together maintain a normal plasma sodium concentration (osmolality). A patient with partial diabetes insipidus has less-pronounced polydipsia and polyuria.

Urinalysis. In diabetes insipidus, urinalysis reveals almost colorless urine with low osmolality (50 to 200 mOsm/kg) and low specific gravity (less than 1.005). Plasma osmolality may be normal if the thirst mechanism remains intact, but it may rise slightly if fluid intake doesn't compensate for urine loss. Urine output varies but may exceed 5 to 10 liters/day. Even less severe polyuria may cause dehydration if fluid intake is inadequate.

Tests for osmolality. A rapid, easy-to-perform test for diabetes insipidus correlates several simultaneously determined levels of plasma and urine osmolality. It's performed postoperatively by reducing the infusion rate of I.V. fluids to determine if urine osmolality rises proportionately to serum osmolality. If results are equivocal, plotting plasma and urine osmolalities on a graph for several hours after fluid deprivation provides more definitive information. In diabetes insipidus, urine osmolality increases only slightly and plateaus at an inappropriately low level, while plasma osmolality increases, sometimes to hyperosmolar levels.

Dehydration test. This test detects diabetes insipidus and helps identify its form. (See *Detecting diabetes insipidus,* page 70.) Normally, the body responds to dehydration or fluid deprivation by releasing ADH and conserving water, thereby elevating urine osmolality. As a result, subcutaneous injection of ADH after dehydration doesn't significantly raise urine osmolality in a healthy patient because endogenous ADH is already present in sufficient amounts, concentrating urine. However, in central diabetes insipidus, subcutaneous injection of ADH after dehydration raises urine osmolality an average of 28% in partial diabetes insipidus and at least 100% in the complete form.

Hypertonic saline infusion test. After confirmation of ADH deficiency, this test may be used to verify osmoreceptor dysfunction.

Nonosmotic stimulus tests, using nicotine or glycopenic agents, are also used to test ADH secretion, but these tests have no advantages over the dehydration and saline infusion tests.

Radiographic tests. An intravenous pyelogram may reveal severe bladder distention, hydroureter, hydronephrosis, and renal insufficiency—possible findings in nephrogenic diabetes insipidus. Skull X-rays may reveal a lesion in the pituitary fossa, and a CT scan may reveal hypothalamic or pituitary disease in central diabetes insipidus.

SIADH: Electrolytes and osmolalities

Because congestive heart failure, dehydration, hypovolemia, cirrhosis, nephrosis, and renal insufficiency produce similar clinical syndromes, confirming SIADH requires exclusion of hyponatremia associated with hyperglycemia, hypertriglyceridemia, or hyperproteinemia. It also requires evaluation of fluid volume and of cardiac, hepatic, and renal functions. Similarly, hypothyroidism and adrenal insufficiency must also be excluded. Because both affect fluid balance and ADH secretion, tests detect hypothyroidism or ad-

Cellular effects of ADH

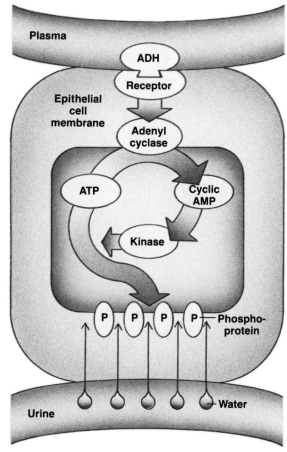

Initially, antidiuretic hormone (ADH) binds to specific receptor sites in the membrane of the collecting duct's epithelial cells. The receptor-ADH complex activates adenyl cyclase and promotes conversion of adenosine triphosphate (ATP) to cyclic adenosine monophosphate (AMP). Cyclic AMP then activates protein kinase to form phosphoprotein. Phosphoprotein, in turn, increases membrane permeability, allowing water to move along the osmotic gradient. The resultant reabsorption of water from the tubules increases urine concentration and decreases urine excretion.

renal insufficiency. These disorders must be corrected before SIADH can be confirmed.

Electrolyte levels. Extracellular fluid volume affects electrolyte levels in all body fluids. Typically, urine sodium levels rise above 20 mEq/liter, and serum sodium levels fall below 130 mEq/liter. Serum potassium and calcium levels may be low as a result of the dilutional effect of the expanded extracellular volume, or they may be normal.

Osmolality determinations. In SIADH, fluid retention causes inappropriately elevated urine osmolality (usually greater than 150 mOsm/kg) and reduced plasma osmolality (less than 280 mOsm/kg). To detect these characteristic differences, the most frequently performed test for SIADH involves serial determinations of urine and serum osmolalities after delivery of an exogenous water load to evaluate renal capacity. In SIADH, the kidneys excrete less than 40% of the water in 5 hours without diluting urine to hypotonic levels. Also, ADH levels remain inappropriately elevated, confirming SIADH unless concurrent severe stress, pain, hypovolemia, or hypotension have stimulated ADH release. (Such stimuli may

What happens in SIADH

Excessive antidiuretic hormone (ADH) secretion increases the permeability of the renal tubules, promoting water retention. As the extracellular fluid volume expands, plasma osmolality falls. The glomerular filtration rate (GFR) rises, and aldosterone secretion decreases, eventually causing hyponatremia.

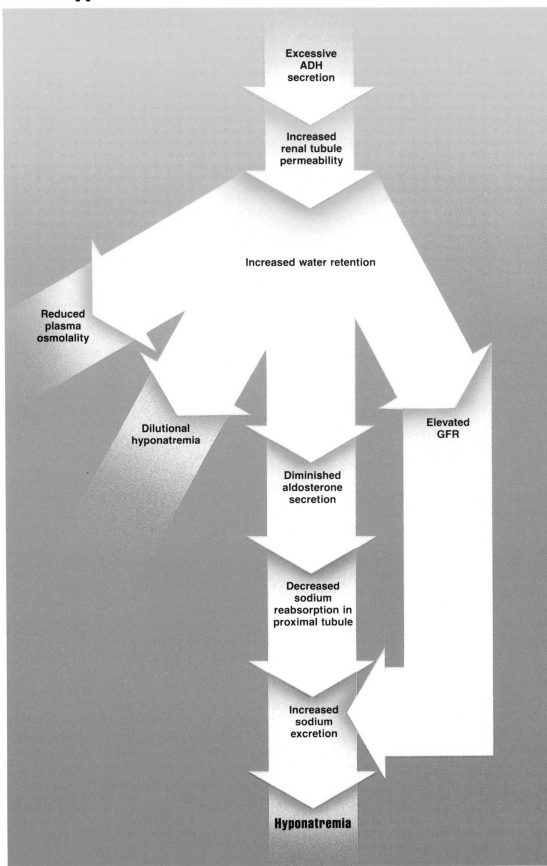

Excessive ADH secretion

Increased renal tubule permeability

Increased water retention

Reduced plasma osmolality

Dilutional hyponatremia

Elevated GFR

Diminished aldosterone secretion

Decreased sodium reabsorption in proximal tubule

Increased sodium excretion

Hyponatremia

evoke physiologic release of ADH, even with hypotonicity.)

Treatment to control symptoms

ADH replacement may control symptoms in diabetes insipidus. Long-acting vasopressin tannate oil suspension was once the treatment of choice for central diabetes insipidus, but it's seldom prescribed today because it requires painful I.M. injections, and accurate dosage is difficult to achieve. The short-acting aqueous solution may be administered by I.V. drip or subcutaneously to relieve symptoms after neurosurgery.

Desmopressin acetate (DDAVP), a nasal inhalant form that's active for 12 to 24 hours, is used more commonly today. Lypressin, another intranasal preparation, is less costly than DDAVP and may be used as an adjunct to other therapy because its antidiuretic effect lasts only 4 to 6 hours.

Chlorpropamide and clofibrate, primarily useful for other disorders, are also effective in treating partial central diabetes insipidus. Both drugs have an antidiuretic effect and consequently reduce polyuria and polydipsia. They may stimulate ADH release and enhance its effects on the renal tubular cells. However, both drugs are ineffective in treating nephrogenic diabetes insipidus.

Paradoxically, thiazide diuretics reduce polyuria in central and nephrogenic diabetes insipidus. Thiazides act by a different mechanism than chlorpropamide and clofibrate. They decrease plasma volume and deplete sodium, causing an increase in renal water and sodium reabsorption.

Adjunctive therapy for diabetes insipidus may include sodium restriction, which requires frequent monitoring of serum osmolality to detect dehydration.

In the rare instance of an advanced hyperosmolar state with symptoms of encephalopathy, emergency treatment includes rapid administration of fluids and hourly monitoring of urine and plasma osmolalities and serum sodium levels. If this treatment is ineffective after 2 to 3 hours, administration of aqueous ADH is necessary.

Treatment to correct SIADH

Surgical resection, radiation, or chemotherapy may alleviate water retention in SIADH caused by malignancy. When the cause is unknown, treatment consists of restricting water intake, giving diuretics to promote water excretion, and giving other drugs that block the action of ADH, which usually corrects hyponatremia. Typically, water intake should not exceed urinary output until serum sodium levels are normal and symptoms subside. Then fluid intake should equal urinary output. Administration of demeclocycline hydrochloride or lithium inhibits the renal effects of ADH.

NURSING MANAGEMENT

Because signs and symptoms of posterior pituitary disorders frequently mimic those of other disorders, a careful patient history and physical exam are invaluable for developing accurate nursing diagnoses, setting care goals, and planning interventions. When developing these nursing diagnoses, be sure to include psychosocial and cultural aspects of the patient's life.

The history

Begin by gathering specific information about the patient's chief complaint. How long has he had this complaint? Was its onset related to any specific event?

Did symptoms come on gradually or suddenly? Although posterior pituitary disorders may develop suddenly after a traumatic event, onset is more gradual if they result from a secondary disorder.

How much fluid does the patient drink each day? Six to eight glasses of water is considered normal. In diabetes insipidus, the patient may drink 45 to 50 glasses of water daily!

Ask the patient about changes in voiding habits. How often does he urinate during the day and night? What were his normal voiding patterns before his present complaint began?

Does nocturia disturb the patient's sleep so much that he's fatigued and irritable during the day? This may interfere with job performance.

Has he noticed any change in the amount of urine voided? Has urine color changed? Patients with diabetes insipidus usually have dilute, clear urine.

Have the patient's bowel habits changed? Dehydration eventually leads to constipation.

Has the patient gained weight recently? This can indicate fluid retention even without overt edema. Has he noticed that his clothing feels restrictive? Do his arms or legs swell or his eyes feel puffy? The presence of edema may rule out posterior pituitary disorders.

Has the patient experienced anorexia, nausea, or vomiting? In SIADH, gastrointestinal disturbances may result from fluid retention. Since fluid retention may also cause cerebral

Detecting diabetes insipidus

The dehydration test measures urine osmolality after a period of dehydration and after subcutaneous injection of vasopressin. Plasma osmolality is determined just before the injection. Comparison of the two urine osmolalities allows diagnosis of diabetes insipidus and helps to identify its form.

Plasma osmolality (mOsm/kg) after dehydration	Urine osmolality (mOsm/kg) after dehydration	Change in urine osmolality after vasopressin injection	Clinical significance
288 to 291	700 to 1,400	None	Normal
310 to 320	100 to 200	100% or greater	Complete central diabetes insipidus
295 to 305	250 to 500	9% to 67%	Partial central diabetes insipidus
310 to 320	100 to 200	None	Nephrogenic diabetes insipidus

edema, the patient may report headaches, dizziness, lethargy, or, possibly, personality changes. His family may report that he's had seizures.

Check recent or current health problems. Once you've thoroughly investigated the patient's chief complaint, explore his past and current health history. A current health problem can interfere with the diagnosis, obscure symptoms, or affect the patient's recovery. For instance, an immobilizing injury can interfere with the patient's voiding or drinking habits, leading to dehydration. This factor should have priority when you plan nursing care.

Check for trauma or unrelated diseases. Because posterior pituitary disorders may result from trauma or unrelated systemic disease, ask if the patient has undergone a recent neurosurgical procedure or suffered a head injury. Does he have any type of cerebrovascular disease?

Does he have a history of recent infection, tuberculosis, or other pulmonary disease? Does he have cancer? Malignant cells tend to stimulate or mimic ADH secretion.

Rule out other causes of polyuria or fluid retention. Does the patient have a history of cardiac, renal, or thyroid disorders; adrenal insufficiency; or diabetes mellitus?

Does he have a history of low serum potassium levels resulting from inadequate dietary intake or drug therapy? This can lead to polyuria—a renal response to low potassium levels.

Look for evidence of stress. Is the patient attempting to cope with a highly stressful job or emotional problem? Primary polydipsia (resulting in polyuria) can result from mental disorders. Is he taking drugs for depression, anxiety, or stress? Has he been treated for emotional or psychiatric disorders?

Thoroughly check current medication. Why is he taking it? How long has he been taking it? What is the dosage? Remember that certain drugs cause polyuria. Is the patient taking lithium, demeclocycline, Dilantin, or adrenergic or anticholinergic agents? Does he use alcohol excessively? Alcohol can also cause polyuria.

Check the patient's life-style. A person's life-style and value system affect his response to illness. What is the patient's daily routine? What is his occupation, his position in the family structure? Is he the sole or chief provider for the family? How will prolonged illness or hospitalization affect other family members? What is the patient's philosophy of health? A person who believes that he shares responsibility for his health may recover earlier or adjust better to illness. What coping mechanisms have the patient and his family used to deal with stress in the past? What is the impact of the illness on current life-style?

Physical examination

During the physical examination, give special attention to the patient's neurologic and hydration status. Begin by checking vital signs, both supine and standing, for orthostatic changes. If volume depletion has occurred, blood pressure may be low, and heart and respiratory rates may be elevated. Record weight as a baseline.

Examine the skin and mucous membranes for dryness, and check for muscle wasting.

Palpate the skin for moisture and turgor. Check for edema to rule out other causes of SIADH-like symptoms.

Check for neurologic signs of fluid imbalance. These include headache, lethargy, confusion, stupor, nervousness, or irritability.

Nursing diagnoses: Keys to good care

After completing the history and physical examination, correlate this information with diagnostic test findings. Then formulate nursing diagnoses, set care goals, and plan interventions. Ideally, you should share these diagnoses with the patient so that you may both work toward reasonable and achievable goals.

Potential for dehydration related to polyuria. Your goals are to promote skin integrity and moist mucous membranes, to ensure adequate fluid intake, to achieve normal serum electrolyte levels, to maintain normal vital signs and normal weight, and to provide thorough patient teaching.

To achieve these goals, check the skin for poor turgor, dryness, and flaking. Also check the mucous membranes for dryness and cracking. Check for poor muscle tone, weakness, and flaccidity. Observe and record the patient's fluid intake and output, daily weight, urine specific gravity, and vital signs. Note any orthostatic hypotension. Monitor serum studies for abnormal electrolyte values. Provide a constant supply of fluids, preferably ice water. Ensure that I.V. fluids are given as ordered if the patient can't drink. Check patency of I.V. lines and time the infusions.

Teach the patient about the effects of dehydration, its signs and symptoms, and preventive measures, such as evaluating fluid status by recording intake and output.

Consider your interventions successful if signs and symptoms of dehydration are absent, the patient has good skin turgor and moist mucous membranes, vital signs have stabilized, fluid intake equals fluid output, the serum electrolyte levels do not reflect dehydration, and the patient can understand and describe the effects of dehydration and knows how to prevent it.

Potential for constipation related to dehydration. Your goal is to ensure normal bowel function. Check for regularity and stool characteristics (amount, size, consistency). Ensure adequate fluid intake, and encourage the patient to eat high-fiber foods. Promote a regular exercise program, and give stool softeners or laxatives, as ordered. Consider your interventions successful if the patient's bowel movements are regular, without constipation.

Potential for anxiety related to diagnostic tests, chronicity, complications, and treatment. Your goal is to reduce the patient's anxiety. To achieve this goal, explain all diagnostic tests beforehand, and remain with the patient during tests, providing instruction, reassurance, and emotional support. Teach the patient and his family about the disease and its complications and how to avoid them. Explain the treatment regimen, its rationale, and expected responses to the drugs and fluid restriction. Instruct the patient about necessary hormone injections or about using the nasal spray properly, and teach him and his family to recognize the signs and symptoms of ADH deficiency or excess.

Consider your interventions successful if the patient can describe the mechanisms and possible complications of his disorder; can state the rationale for and the benefits expected from treatment; adheres to the drug regimen and to prescribed fluid restriction in SIADH; demonstrates skill in using nasal spray; and shows improved weight control, fluid status, and mental status.

Potential for discomfort related to therapeutic fluid restriction in SIADH. Your goal is to promote patient comfort while controlling fluid intake. To achieve this goal, teach the patient to measure fluid output carefully to determine the appropriate daily fluid intake, to evenly distribute prescribed fluid intake over 24 hours, and to vary his fluid selection. To moisten the mucous membranes, encourage oral rinsing without swallowing, and suggest sugarless hard candy to suck on, unless contraindicated.

Consider your interventions successful if signs of water retention or water intoxication are absent and if the patient accepts and follows prescribed fluid restriction.

Keep your care plan current

Caring for a patient with a posterior pituitary disorder requires special efforts to support, teach, and motivate, and these are part of a good care plan. Depending on the severity and underlying cause of your patient's disorder, some aspects of his care plan may require greater emphasis than others. The care plan itself may need revision as your patient's condition changes. Only continuing assessment of the patient's condition can provide a reliable data base to evaluate your care plan and ensure its success.

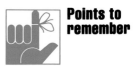

Points to remember

• Posterior pituitary disorders can result from a deficiency or excess of antidiuretic hormone (ADH).
• ADH affects the body's water balance since it helps regulate urine output.
• ADH deficiency causes diabetes insipidus, which can lead to water depletion. An excess of ADH causes syndrome of inappropriate antidiuretic hormone (SIADH), which promotes water retention.
• Treatment consists of exogenous administration of ADH or of water restriction to compensate for excessive ADH secretion.

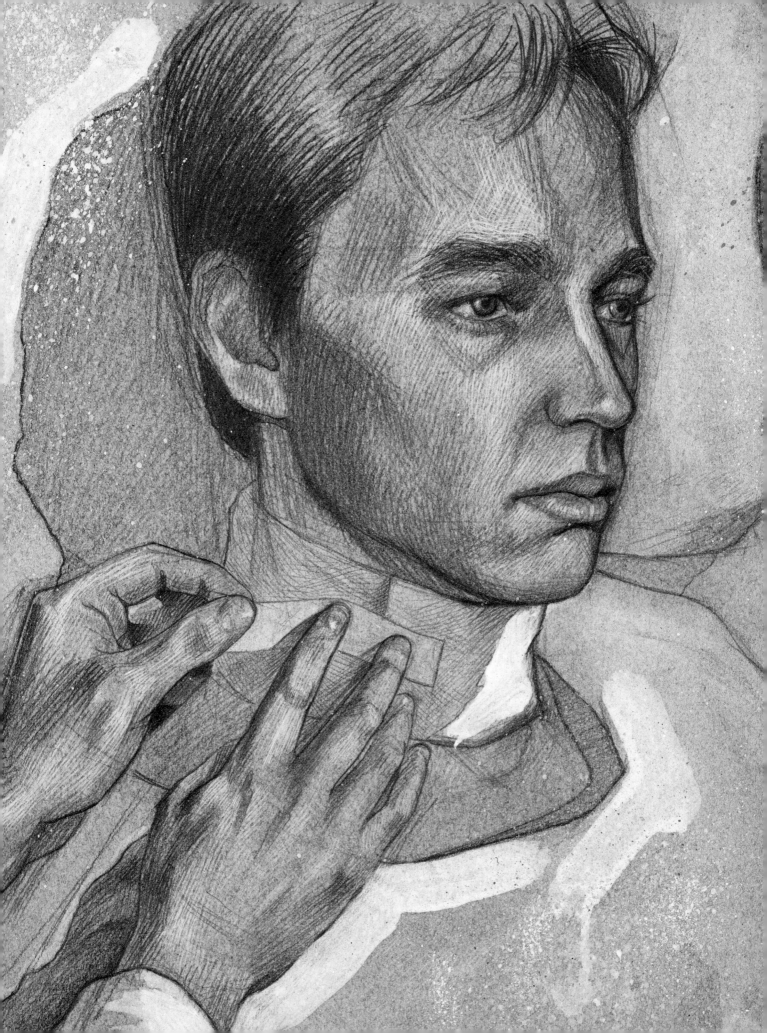

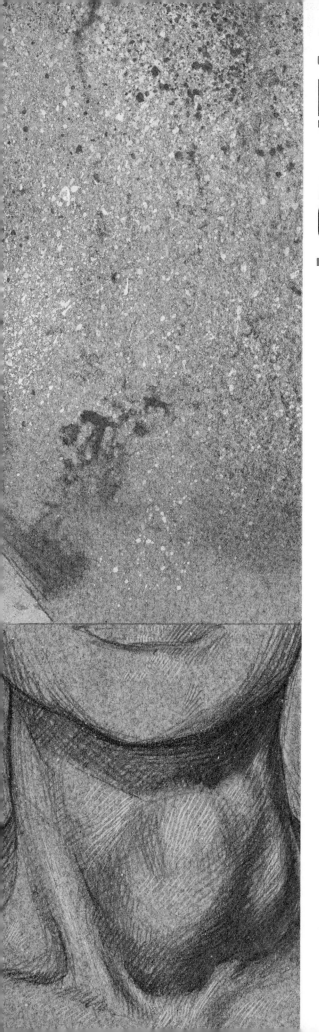

DISORDERS OF THE THYROID AND PARATHYROID GLANDS

6 CONTROLLING ABNORMAL THYROID SECRETION

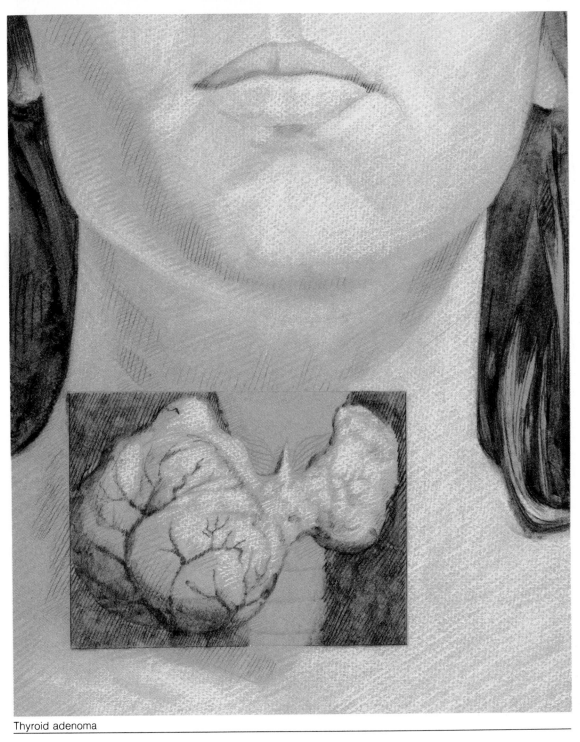

Thyroid adenoma

Thyroid disorders strike up to 20% of the population and profoundly affect virtually every body system. Because of their widespread and sometimes nonspecific effects, thyroid disorders may initially be mistaken for disorders of other body systems. Thyrotoxicosis, for example, can cause significant cardiovascular abnormalities, such as tachycardia and widened pulse pressure. That's why detection of thyroid disorders requires sound knowledge of thyroid pathophysiology and complete assessment of all body systems. Most important, timely detection and treatment of these disorders can help forestall potentially life-threatening complications, such as thyroid storm and myxedema coma.

Thyroid disorders: Excess or deficiency?

Thyrotoxicosis and *hypothyroidism* result from thyroid hormone imbalance. Thyrotoxicosis, an umbrella term for disorders caused by excessive thyroid hormone, includes Graves' disease (diffuse toxic goiter), toxic multinodular goiter, thyroiditis, excessive intake of thyroid hormone, and various rare disorders. (See *Classifying thyrotoxicoses.*) Hyperthyroidism, a term used inexactly as a synonym for thyrotoxicosis, refers only to those disorders in which the thyroid gland produces or secretes excessive hormone.

Hypothyroidism results from insufficient thyroid hormone and may be primary or secondary. Primary hypothyroidism results from reduced functional thyroid tissue mass or impaired hormonal synthesis or release. Secondary hypothyroidism, which accounts for about 5% of cases of hypothyroidism, results from inadequate stimulation of the gland because of pituitary disease or from peripheral tissue resistance to thyroid hormone.

Both thyrotoxicosis and hypothyroidism affect four times as many women as men and tend to affect several members of a family. Usually, they're detected between the ages of 30 and 60.

PATHOPHYSIOLOGY

Thyroid disorders result primarily from functional or structural changes of the thyroid gland, or both. Functional changes result in excessive or deficient levels of thyroid hormone, which stimulate or depress cellular metabolism. Structural changes in the thyroid gland result from inflammatory, hyperplastic, or neoplastic disease. The most common structural change is goiter—an enlarged thyroid gland, which may be diffuse or associated with nodule formation. (See *Goiter: Types and causes,* page 76.)

Thyrotoxicosis: Expect Graves' disease

Graves' disease, also known as Parry's or Basedow's disease, accounts for more than 85% of cases of thyrotoxicosis. It may result from an immunogenetic defect, leading to production of abnormal thyroid-stimulating antibodies. These antibodies, called thyroid-stimulating immunoglobulins (TSIs), appear in the serum of roughly 80% of patients with active Graves' disease. This antibody stimulation causes pervasive structural and functional changes in the thyroid: goiter, increased hormonogenesis and vascularity, and lymphoid tissue infiltration of the gland.

Effects of thyrotoxicosis

Thyrotoxicosis accelerates the metabolic rate, causing changes in almost every body system.

Central nervous system (CNS) effects. Hallmarks of thyrotoxicosis include nervousness, emotional lability, hyperkinesis, and tremors. Similarities between these symptoms and the effects of adrenergic stimulation suggest that thyroid hormone exerts effects similar but additive to those of catecholamines.

Cardiovascular and respiratory effects. Enhanced adrenergic stimulation increases cardiac contractility and cardiac rate, thereby increasing cardiac output. It also causes dysrhythmias, particularly atrial fibrillation, premature ventricular contractions, and paroxysmal atrial tachycardia. In the elderly and those with heart disease, it can cause congestive heart failure.

Weakness of respiratory muscles results in breathlessness and mild hypoventilation.

Cutaneous effects. The skin, hair, and nails show obvious effects of excessive thyroid stimulation. Capillary dilatation—causing warm, flushed, moist skin—results from increased cardiac output and adrenergic stimulation. Other effects of thyrotoxicosis include heat intolerance (due to hypermetabolism); separation of the fingernail from the nail bed (onycholysis); hyperpigmentation; palmar erythema; fine, soft, easily broken hair; and increased hair loss. In Graves' disease, up to 10% of patients develop infiltrative dermopathy (pretibial myxedema), which causes violet indurations over the pretibial areas.

Ocular effects. Irreversible infiltrative ophthalmopathy occurs in about 50% of patients with Graves' disease but doesn't affect

Classifying thyrotoxicoses

Graves' disease (diffuse toxic goiter). Most common type of thyrotoxicosis. Believed to be an autoimmune disorder caused by an abnormal thyroid stimulator.

Hashitoxicosis. Transient manifestation of stored hormone leakage in acute phase of chronic lymphocytic thyroiditis (Hashimoto's thyroiditis).

Silent thyroiditis. Self-limiting and transient, with no inflammatory symptoms.

Subacute nonsuppurative thyroiditis (de Quervain's thyroiditis). Transient, apparently viral-induced granulomatous inflammation.

Toxic multinodular goiter and uninodular goiter (toxic adenoma). Autonomous function of slowly growing nodules, which synthesize thyroid hormone.

Pituitary-hypothalamic dysfunction. Autonomous function of the pituitary gland, a pituitary tumor that produces thyroid-stimulating hormone (TSH), or hypothalamic dysfunction, resulting in excess secretion of thyrotropin-releasing hormone.

Choriocarcinoma. Excessive secretion of human chorionic gonadotropin, which weakly mimics the function of TSH.

Follicular carcinoma. Metastatic lesions composed of follicular elements produce thyroid hormone in addition to hormone produced by the thyroid itself.

Struma ovarii. A rare benign tumor of the ovary that contains predominantly thyroid tissue.

Iodine-induced hyperthyroidism (jodbasedow phenomenon). The result of excessive intake of inorganic iodine in susceptible individuals.

Thyrotoxicosis factitia. The result of self-administration of excessive thyroid hormone.

Goiter: Types and causes

Goiter, an enlargement of the thyroid gland, may be classified by consistency and function. Its consistency may be diffuse (uniformly enlarged) or nodular (small, protuberant masses of tissue in its substance). Its function may be nontoxic (euthyroid or hypothyroid) or toxic (hyperthyroid). Nontoxic goiter, however, can become toxic; for example, nontoxic diffuse goiter related to iodine deficiency can become toxic when iodine is added to the diet (jodbasedow phenomenon) or may develop into multinodular goiter, which can become toxic.

Function	Consistency		
	Diffuse	Multinodular	Uninodular
Nontoxic	Iodine deficiency; thyroiditis; biosynthetic or enzymatic defects; excessive ingestion of goitrogenic foods (cabbage, peanuts, kale) or drugs (propylthiouracil, phenylbutazone, lithium); and peripheral tissue resistance to thyroid hormone	Long-standing nontoxic diffuse goiter, resulting from autonomous function of slowly growing nodules	Neoplasms, cysts, thyroiditis, hemorrhage
Toxic	Abnormal thyroid stimulators produced by the immune system (Graves' disease)	Autonomous or semiautonomous function of slowly growing nodules, occurring most often in long-standing nontoxic multinodular goiter	Autonomous function of a nodule that produces thyroid hormone or, rarely, thyroid carcinoma

patients with other types of thyrotoxicosis. Its signs include weakness of the extraocular muscles, resulting in poor convergence; occasionally, paralysis of upward gaze; increased retroorbital fat, resulting in exophthalmos; lid edema, increased tearing, and photosensitivity; and possible loss of vision from corneal ulceration or optic nerve involvement.

Spasm and retraction of the upper eyelids, lid lag and tremor, and infrequent blinking may be considered noninfiltrative ophthalmic changes. These eye changes disappear with successful treatment of thyrotoxicosis.

GI effects. Thyrotoxicosis increases the rate of glucose absorption from the intestine and the rate of glucose uptake into fat and muscle cells. Hypermetabolism may cause weight loss, despite a vigorous appetite. Also, increased GI motility accelerates gastric emptying and bowel peristalsis, with possible diarrhea, nausea, and vomiting. Other common effects include gastric achlorhydria and mild fat malabsorption. Severe Graves' disease may cause hepatic dysfunction.

Genitourinary effects. Enhanced rate of renal blood flow and glomerular filtration may cause frequent urination, which may be aggravated by nervousness and restlessness. Other effects include decreased or absent menstrual flow and female infertility.

Musculoskeletal effects. Severe myopathy, particularly of proximal muscles, may affect mobility virtually to the point of paralysis (called Basedow's paraplegia when thyrotoxicosis causes paralyzing muscle weakness). Periodic paralysis, which is associated with hypokalemia, may be intermittent, developing over several hours and lasting up to a day.

Thyroid storm: A life-threatening complication
Thyroid storm, the fulminating onset of all signs and symptoms of thyrotoxicosis, results from untreated or inadequately treated thyrotoxicosis. Its precipitating factors include trauma, surgery, infection, embolism, diabetic acidosis, and discontinuation of antithyroid drugs. Despite vigorous treatment, thyroid storm causes death in about 20% of affected patients.

Hypothyroidism and autoimmunity
Primary hypothyroidism commonly results from chronic lymphocytic thyroiditis (Hashimoto's thyroiditis), an autoimmune disorder. Unlike Graves' disease, in which circulating antibodies stimulate thyroid secretion, Hashimoto's thyroiditis produces antibodies that cause fibrosis of the thyroid gland, which interferes with thyroid hormone production. Primary hypothyroidism can result from treatment of thyrotoxicosis with radioactive iodine (^{131}I), from surgery, or from a metastasizing tumor.

Feedback mechanisms control hormonal secretion

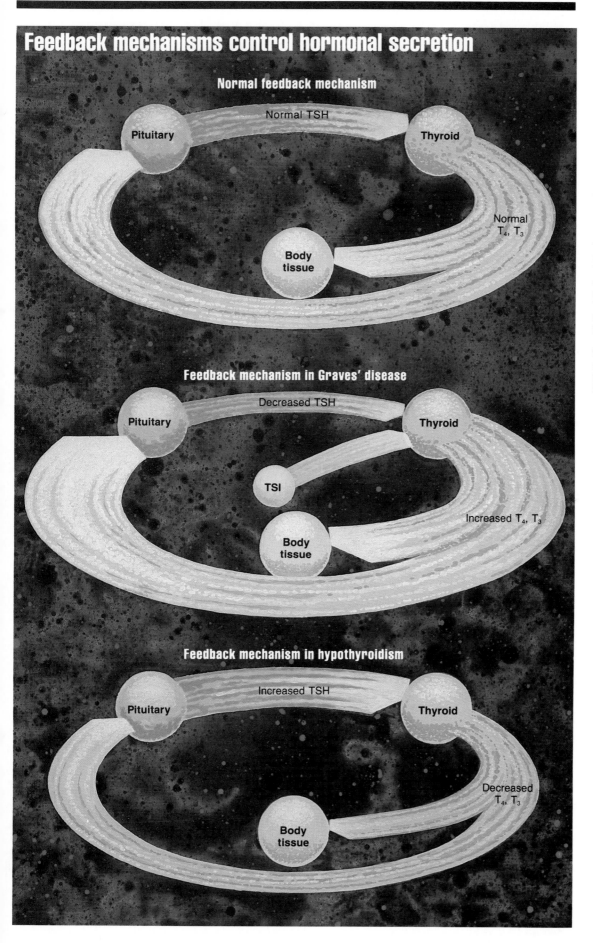

Normal feedback mechanism

Pituitary — Normal TSH — Thyroid

Body tissue

Normal T4, T3

Feedback mechanism in Graves' disease

Pituitary — Decreased TSH — Thyroid

TSI

Body tissue

Increased T4, T3

Feedback mechanism in hypothyroidism

Pituitary — Increased TSH — Thyroid

Body tissue

Decreased T4, T3

Normally, a negative feedback system regulates hormonal balance. Thyroid-stimulating hormone (TSH), secreted by the pituitary in response to low levels of thyroxine (T4) and triiodothyronine (T3), stimulates production and secretion of T4 and T3. As T4 and T3 levels rise, the pituitary stops secreting TSH.

In Graves' disease, thyroid-stimulating immunoglobulin (TSI) acts like TSH, causing excessive T4 and T3 secretion. In response to elevated T4 and T3 levels, TSH secretion decreases, but TSI secretion continues.

In hypothyroidism due to reduced thyroid tissue mass, insufficient production of T4 and T3 causes increased TSH secretion.

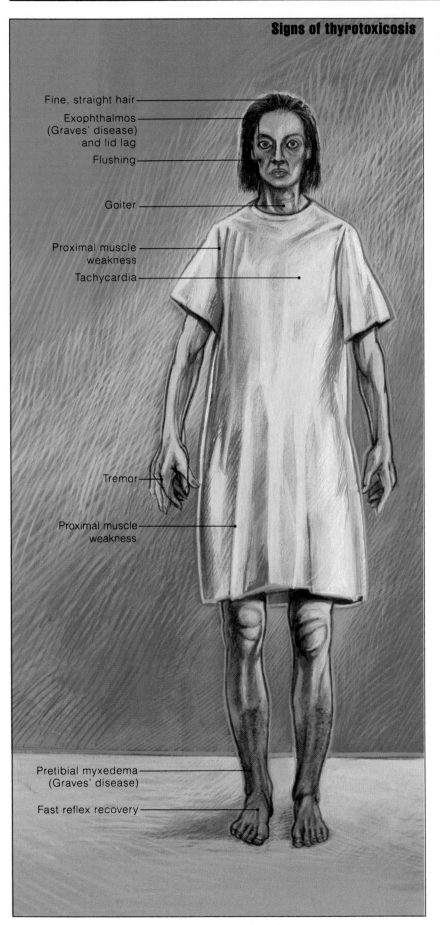

Signs of thyrotoxicosis

Fine, straight hair

Exophthalmos (Graves' disease) and lid lag

Flushing

Goiter

Proximal muscle weakness

Tachycardia

Tremor

Proximal muscle weakness

Pretibial myxedema (Graves' disease)

Fast reflex recovery

Primary hypothyroidism can also result from impaired synthesis and release of thyroid hormone. Such impairment may result from iodine deficiency, which leads to compensatory hypersecretion of thyroid-stimulating hormone (TSH) and to goiter. However, if this compensatory mechanism is inadequate, hypothyroidism results. Iodine deficiency has been virtually eliminated in developed countries through the availability of iodized salt and seafoods, but it's still the major cause of hypothyroidism in many underdeveloped countries.

Impaired synthesis of thyroid hormone can also result from use of thyroid hormone antagonists in treating thyrotoxicosis, but such impairment subsides when antithyroid treatment is stopped. It can also stem from excessive ingestion of goitrogens (in vegetables, such as cabbage, turnips, and kale). Goitrogens chemically resemble thyroid hormone antagonists and block iodine organification; however, they don't usually cause hypothyroidism when iodine intake is adequate.

Finally, primary hypothyroidism can result from excessive iodine intake, impairing secretion of thyroid hormone, and from prolonged lithium therapy (in up to 30% of patients).

Secondary hypothyroidism, in which the thyroid is normal, results from lack of TSH stimulation. Its most common causes are pituitary insufficiency, postpartum pituitary necrosis, and pituitary tumor.

Effects of hypothyroidism
Hypothyroidism depresses the metabolic rate, causing related signs and symptoms in many body systems.

CNS effects. Decreased adrenergic activity and myxedematous infiltration of the tongue and larynx result in slowed speech and hoarseness. Decreased cerebral blood flow slows mental function, causing loss of interest in routine activities, poor short-term memory, and, in severe cases, myxedema madness or paranoid schizophrenia. In the elderly, these mental changes can be severe enough to be confused with senile dementia.

Cardiovascular effects. Decreased cardiac contractility and output may lead to bradycardia and congestive heart failure (CHF). Hypertension may develop, and serum cholesterol triglyceride levels may rise.

Cutaneous effects. The skin, hair, and nails are particularly vulnerable to the effects of a lowered metabolic rate. Cold intolerance and slightly lower body temperature also result from a lowered metabolic rate. Decreased cardiac output and myxedematous infiltration of tissues cause cool, dry, and scaly skin, particularly over the elbows and knees; nonpitting edema of the hands and feet, with facial puffiness, especially in the eyelids; and coarse, broken hair and thick, brittle nails. Impaired degradation and synthesis of protein cause poor wound healing. Since thyroid hormones promote synthesis of vitamin A from carotene, increasing levels of carotene in thyroid hormone deficiency may cause distinct yellowing of the skin. Decreasing vitamin A levels cause night blindness.

GI effects. A slow metabolic rate prolongs GI transit time, causing anorexia and constipation. Hypothyroidism is commonly associated with other autoimmune disorders, such as pernicious anemia.

Reproductive effects. Decreased secretion of luteinizing hormone may result in heavy and irregular menses. Other effects include decreased libido in both sexes, infertility in females, and impotence in males.

Musculoskeletal effects. Muscles show edema and mucinous deposits, slowed contraction and relaxation, and stiffness. Backache is a common symptom.

Myxedema coma: Frequently fatal
This life-threatening complication of hypothyroidism develops in patients with chronic, untreated hypothyroidism; typically, it follows exposure to cold, trauma, infection, or use of CNS depressants. It causes severe hypothermia, respiratory depression, prolonged relaxation phase of the tendon reflexes, seizures, and hyponatremia.

MEDICAL MANAGEMENT
The wide-ranging effects of thyroid dysfunction mimic those of other disorders and can make accurate diagnosis difficult. Consequently, diagnosis requires careful interpretation of physical findings in light of laboratory test results.

Laboratory tests valuable
Many tests are available for evaluating thyroid function. Serum tests measure concentration and binding of thyroid hormones and evaluate thyroid function and regulatory mechanisms. Radiologic, sonographic, and biopsy studies are used to detect and evaluate nodules and distinguish types of thyroiditis.
   Measurement of concentration and binding. *The protein-bound iodine (PBI) test* indirectly

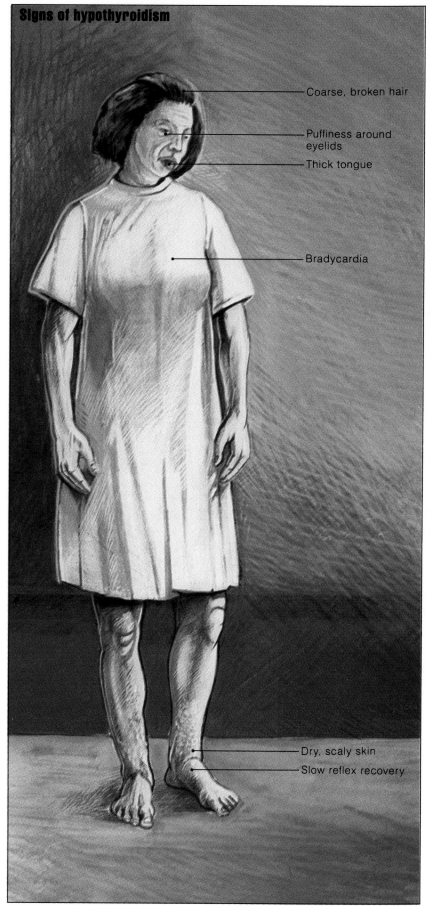

Signs of hypothyroidism

- Coarse, broken hair
- Puffiness around eyelids
- Thick tongue
- Bradycardia
- Dry, scaly skin
- Slow reflex recovery

Thyrotoxicosis in pregnancy

Pregnancy complicates diagnosis of thyrotoxicosis because its characteristic physiologic changes resemble the pathologic changes of thyrotoxicosis. These changes include increased metabolic rate, cardiac output, and appetite; emotional lability; easy fatigability; and, at times, an enlarged thyroid. As a result, diagnosis of thyrotoxicosis relies on a history of complaints before and exaggerated symptoms during pregnancy, or on the development of ophthalmopathy.

Pregnancy also complicates drug therapy for thyrotoxicosis, because thyroid hormone antagonists readily cross the placenta. Typically, the lowest effective dose is given since high doses may cause fetal hypothyroidism.

estimates thyroxine (T_4) levels by measuring the iodine content of serum proteins. Because many nonthyroidal factors can alter PBI levels (for example, liver and kidney disease, testosterone, displacement of T_4 from its binding site by phenytoin and salicylates), this test has now been replaced by direct measurement of T_4 using radioimmunoassay (RIA). However, it's still useful in detecting abnormal iodoprotein released by the thyroid.

Radioimmunoassay is the most precise and the most frequently used technique for measuring serum T_4 and T_3 (triiodothyronine) levels. T_4 RIA shows depressed levels in hypothyroidism and elevated levels in thyrotoxicosis. T_3 levels usually parallel T_4 levels in thyrotoxicosis. Reverse T_3, generated from the conversion of T_4 to T_3, can be measured by RIA. It helps to differentiate the sick euthyroid patient from the truly hypothyroid. Reverse T_3 is elevated in thyrotoxicosis and depressed in hypothyroidism.

Measurement of free T_4 and free T_3 evaluates the minute portions of T_4 and T_3 not bound to thyroxine-binding globulin and other serum proteins. As the active components of total serum T_4 and T_3, these unbound hormones enter target cells and are directly responsible for the thyroid's effect on cell metabolism. Consequently, free T_4 and free T_3 levels provide the best indication of thyroid function. However, these hormone levels are infrequently tested because the laboratory methods they require are expensive, cumbersome, and time-consuming.

The *T_3 resin uptake test* measures free T_4 levels indirectly by showing the number of unoccupied serum protein-binding sites for T_4. In hypothyroidism, excess binding sites result in diminished T_3 uptake; in thyrotoxicosis, the opposite occurs.

Many nonthyroid disorders cause decreased conversion of T_4 to T_3 in the peripheral tissues; therefore, T_3 may fall below normal (low T_3 syndrome), even though the patient is euthyroid.

Evaluation of thyroid function. *The ^{131}I uptake test* measures the amount of orally ingested ^{131}I that accumulates in the thyroid after 2, 6, and 24 hours. This test is not useful in detecting hypothyroidism. Increased dietary iodine has raised circulating iodine levels in the average American with consequent suppression of ^{131}I uptake in most patients. A low uptake cannot reliably distinguish hypothyroidism. However, the test can help to determine the cause of thyrotoxi-

cosis, especially when combined with a thyroid scan.

Evaluation of thyroid regulatory mechanisms. *Serum TSH* and *thyrotropin-releasing hormone stimulation tests* distinguish primary from secondary hypothyroidism. In primary hypothyroidism, serum TSH also helps monitor thyroid replacement therapy.

The *thyroid suppression test* is used in suspected Graves' disease when diagnosis is unclear and in euthyroid Graves' disease (ophthalmopathy without thyrotoxicosis). Suppression of TSH by exogenous T_3 results in suppression of ^{131}I uptake by the normal thyroid gland. Failure to suppress ^{131}I uptake indicates an autonomously functioning thyroid.

Evaluation of nodules and thyroiditis. The *thyroid scan* visualizes the size and shape of the thyroid gland after administration of a radioisotope, usually ^{131}I. It can reveal "hot" spots—functioning nodules that readily take up the radioisotope—and "cold" spots—nodules that fail to take it up. Roughly 20% of cold spots are malignant. This test can also detect small nodules that are not palpable.

Thyroid ultrasonography, a safe, noninvasive test, evaluates thyroid structure and can differentiate between a cyst and a solid lesion. It's especially useful for evaluating nodules during pregnancy since it doesn't expose the fetus to radiation.

Thyroid aspiration and needle biopsy help differentiate between benign and malignant thyroid disease and aid diagnosis of Hashimoto's thyroiditis, subacute granulomatous thyroiditis, and hyperthyroidism.

Immunologic tests can also demonstrate Hashimoto's thyroiditis and Graves' disease and help to detect silent thyroiditis. These tests may include RIA for human antithyroglobulin antibodies, tanned erythrocyte hemagglutinin test for thyroglobulin antibodies, complement fixation test for microsomal antigen, microsomal fluorescent antibody test, and colloid fluorescent antibody test.

Drug therapy in thyrotoxicosis

Thyroid hormone antagonists prevent thyroid hormone formation by preventing oxidation of trapped iodine, iodination of tyrosine, and coupling of iodotyrosines. Propylthiouracil (PTU) has replaced thiouracil in the treatment of thyroid disorders. Roughly 75% as potent as thiouracil, PTU carries less risk of agranulocytosis. PTU also prevents peripheral conversion of T_4 to T_3. Methimazole, another commonly used thyroid hormone antagonist, is 10 times more potent than thiouracil. Its use is similar to PTU.

PTU is used as a primary treatment, before surgery for 2 to 3 months, or before treatment with ^{131}I to control symptoms of thyrotoxicosis and to render the patient euthyroid. Such treatment lessens the risk of thyroid storm during or after these procedures.

PTU is also used in long-term treatment (12 to 24 months) of thyrotoxicosis; symptoms usually begin to subside in 10 to 20 days, with euthyroidism in 6 to 10 weeks. Unfortunately, thyrotoxicosis recurs in 50% to 60% of patients after drug therapy ends. To prevent overtreatment and hypothyroidism, some doctors concomitantly administer levothyroxine; others closely monitor thyroid hormone levels during treatment.

Administration of inorganic iodine, which inhibits release of thyroid hormone, reduces vascularity of the gland in thyroid storm and before surgery. However, iodine is contraindicated before ^{131}I therapy because it interferes with uptake of the isotope.

Administration of propranolol controls tachycardia, dysrhythmias, and tremor in thyrotoxicosis until more specific treatment can take effect.

Drug therapy in hypothyroidism

Thyroid hormone replacement therapy includes levothyroxine sodium, liothyronine sodium, liotrix, thyroglobulin, and thyroid USP. Levothyroxine (synthetic T_4) has uniform potency and can be injected I.V. during myxedema coma. This drug has replaced liothyronine (synthetic T_3) for replacement therapy because of the body's ability to convert T_4 to T_3, as needed. Liothyronine is useful, however, in athyroid patients with a history of thyroid cancer who require radioiodine scans. The shorter half-life of T_3 allows discontinuation of therapy for 2 to 3 weeks, compared with 4 to 6 weeks for T_4. (See *Therapeutic effectiveness of thyroid hormones,* page 82.)

For thyrotoxicosis: [131]I and surgery

[131]I is the preferred treatment for thyrotoxicosis because it avoids the complications of surgery. For 3 months before treatment with ^{131}I, patients receive PTU to deplete stored thyroid hormones and to prevent their sudden release into the circulation after ^{131}I radiation. In mild to moderate thyrotoxicosis, patients receive ^{131}I without pretreatment with PTU. Patients are a radiation hazard for about 1 week, depending on the strength of the dose.

Treatment with ^{131}I frequently causes hypothyroidism.

Thyroidectomy

Thyroid surgery is indicated in primary thyroid cancer, in severe Graves' disease, and for relief of symptoms in Riedel's thyroiditis, where extensive fibrosis of the thyroid and surrounding tissues occurs. Total thyroidectomy is the surgery of choice for thyroid cancer. It eliminates the possibility of recurrent thyrotoxicosis but requires lifetime thyroid replacement therapy.

Today, subtotal thyroidectomy is a standard treatment for Graves' disease. It restores euthyroidism. Its disadvantages include an up to 30% risk of permanent hypothyroidism, required lifetime thyroid replacement therapy, a 20% risk of recurring thyrotoxicosis, and a greater risk of complications if surgery is required to correct recurring thyrotoxicosis.

Possible complications of thyroidectomy include hemorrhage, airway obstruction from hematoma or injury to the recurrent laryngeal nerves, and hypoparathyroidism (transient or permanent). Hemorrhage and hematoma may require surgical treatment; if removal of a hematoma fails to relieve airway obstruction, intubation is required. Transient hypoparathyroidism occurs in about 3% to 5% of thyroidectomy patients in the first 7 postoperative days, usually because of inadvertent resection of the parathyroids or impaired circulation during surgery. In any case, the resulting hypoparathyroidism causes tetany, which can be relieved by I.V. injection of calcium gluconate. Recurring episodes of tetany may indicate permanent hypoparathyroidism.

Thyroid emergencies

Thyroid storm and myxedema coma are life-threatening emergencies that require immediate, vigorous treatment. Thyroid storm requires administration of a thyroid hormone antagonist (such as PTU), propranolol, iodine, and corticosteroids. If hypoadrenalism is suspected, hydrocortisone may be given. (See *Thyroid storm,* pages 86-87, for full details on treatment.)

In myxedema coma, effective treatment supports vital functions and restores euthyroidism. It includes I.V. or nasogastric administration of T_4, corticosteroids, glucose, and antibiotics. Hyponatremia usually responds to thyroid replacement therapy and fluid restriction. Respiratory acidosis responds to oxygen, tracheotomy, and assisted ventilation, if

Neonatal hypothyroidism: Early detection crucial

Hypothyroidism affects roughly 1 in 5,000 neonates, occurring in three times as many girls as boys. This disorder can result from thyroid dysgenesis or hypoplasia, congenital goiter, severe maternal iodine deprivation, or use of thyroid inhibitors during pregnancy. If untreated, it can lead to permanent mental deficiency. Because clinical signs are few, in the past, most cases of hypothyroidism in the newborn went undetected until cretinism became apparent. Today, radioimmunoassays for thyroxine and thyroid-stimulating hormone effectively screen neonates for hypothyroidism, allowing prompt replacement of missing thyroid hormone.

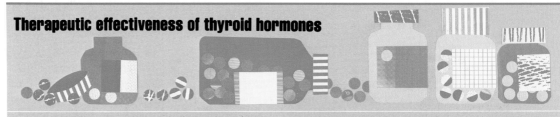

Therapeutic effectiveness of thyroid hormones

In hypothyroidism, drug therapy includes thyroxine (T₄), triiodothyronine (T₃), or combinations of these hormones. Although most T₄ is converted to T₃, the prolonged action and long half-life of T₄ make it the treatment of choice. T₃, a short-acting drug, requires more frequent administration, and combinations of T₃ and T₄ have varying durations of action, depending on their relative concentrations.

Drug	Equivalent dose	Contents	Relative duration	
levothyroxine	100 mcg	T_4	Long	
liothyronine	25 mcg	T_3	Short (multiple daily doses)	
liotrix	62.5 to 75 mcg	T_4 and T_3 in 4:1 ratio	Intermediate	(Those with higher T_4 concentrations are longer acting; those with lower T_4 concentrations are shorter acting.)
thyroglobulin	65 mg	T_4 and T_3 in 2.5:1 ratio	Intermediate	
thyroid USP	65 mg	T_4 and T_3 in variable ratios	Intermediate	

needed. Hypothermia requires blankets to prevent loss of body heat, but rapid warming causes vasodilatation and may lead to shock.

NURSING MANAGEMENT
In thyroid disorders, the goal of nursing management is prevention or correction of thyroid crisis and complications.

A thorough patient history
Begin the patient history by recording the patient's chief complaint—or by noting its absence. Consider that a patient with myxedema may be so apathetic that a family member or friend must urge him to seek help. This patient may have neither the energy nor the mental clarity to volunteer any information. So ask him simple, direct questions and give him time to formulate his answers. Speak loudly, if necessary, because such a patient can develop deafness from fluid accumulation.

Once you've recorded the chief complaint and decided that the patient doesn't require immediate treatment, proceed with specific questions that will help you define the patient's metabolic state. Ask the patient how many hours he sleeps. The hypothyroid patient usually sleeps more than average, the thyrotoxic patient less. Also ask about fatigue, irritability, and difficulty in concentrating (common in both thyrotoxicosis and hypothyroidism); forgetfulness (in hypothyroidism); and nervousness and mood swings (in thyrotoxicosis). If a family member is present, ask if he's noticed personality changes in the patient.

Inquire about palpitations, chest pain, and exercise tolerance. Weakness and atrial fibrillation may be present in thyrotoxicosis in the elderly (masked thyrotoxicosis).

Ask about temperature tolerance. Typically, you may ask the patient: Do other family members complain that you keep the room too hot or too cold? Do you prefer hot or cold weather, and why? Does the weather strongly affect how you feel? Thyrotoxic patients complain about heat and prefer cool temperatures; hypothyroid patients complain about feeling cold and prefer warmer temperatures.

Ask if the patient's collar size has increased. This change may indicate goiter growth. Also ask about dry skin, changes in hair texture, eye irritations, complaints of double vision, and muscle and joint aches. Dry, rough skin, coarse and broken hair, and muscle and joint aches suggest hypothyroidism. Moist, smooth skin, fine and silky hair, eye irritation, and double vision suggest thyrotoxicosis.

Ask the patient to classify his appetite as small, average, or large; then ask if he's noted any weight gain or loss. Thyrotoxic patients may complain of weight loss despite a large appetite. Ask the patient about the frequency and consistency of bowel movements. Constipation commonly accompanies hypothyroidism; soft stools accompany thyrotoxicosis.

Ask female patients about the frequency, duration, and quality of their menses—often scant in thyrotoxicosis and heavy in hypothyroidism. Also ask if they've noticed a change in menstrual flow. Be sure to ask about pregnancy, which could influence diagnosis and treatment. Has the patient delivered in the past year? Silent thyroiditis classically occurs during the first postpartum year.

Ask if thyroid disorders have occurred in other family members. Graves' disease and Hashimoto's thyroiditis, for example, frequently affect more than one family member. Ask if there is a family history of other autoimmune disorders, such as systemic lupus erythematosus, myasthenia gravis, Addison's disease, or pernicious anemia. Autoimmune disorders may run in families but may cause different disorders in each member.

Ask the patient about irradiation of the head or neck, which has been linked to thyroid cancer. When interviewing elderly patients, remember that in the early 1900s the thymus of children was irradiated for such conditions as tonsillitis.

Ask the patient about previous ^{131}I treatment, thyroid surgery, and use of lithium (in treating manic depressive illness; acts as a thyroid hormone antagonist) or iodine-containing drugs (for example, in expectorants). Such treatment can influence diagnostic test results and prescribed treatment.

Find out about the patient's other medical, psychiatric, and drug histories. In myxedema, slowed drug metabolism can cause a routine dose of a sedative, narcotic, or anesthetic to be fatal.

To help you plan patient care, your interview should help you determine how the patient copes with the changes caused by thyroid disorders and how these changes affect his relationships with family and friends. To help you understand and deal with his expectations, you should assess his current knowledge of his disease. With all of this information in mind, you're ready to proceed to the physical examination.

First impressions count
As you're preparing to perform a complete physical exam, carefully consider the impressions you formed during the interview. You may have noticed the bright-eyed stare characteristic of thyrotoxicosis, marked hearing loss, or nervousness. Keep these impressions firmly in mind—they may help confirm findings from the physical exam.

Check vital signs. In thyrotoxicosis, you'll find resting pulse rate greater than 100 beats/minute or an irregular pulse and widened pulse pressure. In myxedema, you'll find slow pulse and respiratory rates, a narrow pulse pressure, and a possible subnormal body temperature.

Observe the patient's skin. In thyrotoxicosis, you'll find skin that's salmon-colored, fine, moist, smooth, and warm. You may also detect onycholysis, dirt under the nail of the fourth finger, and palmar erythema. In myxedema, you'll find skin that's pale or slightly yellow, rough, dry, scaly, and cool.

Pass your hand over the patient's head and rub a few strands of his hair between your fingers to determine its texture: fine and silky in thyrotoxicosis, coarse and thin in hypothyroidism.

Observe the patient's face. In myxedema, you'll note a masklike expression, puffy eyelids, hair loss in the eyebrows, thick lips, and a broad tongue. In thyrotoxicosis, you'll note a fine tremor of the tongue.

Ask the patient to perform extraocular range-of-motion exercises. Standing about 2′ from the patient, look for upper lid lag in inferior gaze, lower lid lag in the superior gaze, and strabismus or paralysis, particularly in the superior lateral gaze. Test for poor convergence as the patient follows your finger when you move it toward the bridge of his nose. Ask the patient to tell you when he sees double, and note that distance from the bridge of the nose. The thyrotoxic patient sees double much sooner than the euthyroid patient, demonstrating poor convergence.

Observe, auscultate, and palpate the thyroid (see Chapter 2). Then auscultate the heart for atrial fibrillation (in thyrotoxicosis) and for S_3 (in thyrotoxicosis and myxedema). Auscultate the lungs for rales, occurring in CHF.

To help you gauge the patient's muscular strength, ask him to grip your hand. Then, to check for the fine tremor of thyrotoxicosis, place a piece of paper on the dorsal surface of the patient's hand. Continue to test the strength of your patient's extremities: Ask him to fold his arms on his chest and get up from a chair several times. Or ask him to extend his leg while sitting. He should be able to do this for 60 seconds. These tests and repeated squatting or stair climbing can help detect the proximal muscle weakness associated with thyrotoxicosis.

Observe the pretibial and tibial areas for erythematous, brawny, violet-colored, or pigskinlike nonpitting edema—the pretibial myxedema of Graves' disease.

Test deep tendon reflexes (brachial, brachioradialis, triceps, patellar, and Achilles) with a percussion hammer. In thyrotoxicosis, reflexes are usually quick. In myxedema, reflexes show an exaggeratedly slow relaxation phase. Expect to see delayed Achilles tendon reflex time in hypothyroidism, but remember that diabetes mellitus, peripheral vascular disease, and pernicious anemia also delay this reflex. Also keep in mind that certain drugs, such as morphine, propranolol, quinidine, and procainamide, can also prolong relaxation time.

Formulate nursing diagnoses

Integrating subjective data from the interview and objective data from the physical examination, you can formulate appropriate nursing diagnoses to help you set goals and plan effective interventions. Unless the patient is gravely ill, involve him in your care plan and be flexible in adjusting it to meet his needs. The following sample nursing diagnoses and interventions are commonly appropriate in thyroid disorders.

Self-care limitation related to insufficient knowledge of thyroid disorders. To promote self-care, teach the patient about his thyroid disorder and its effects, using short teaching sessions with written handouts. Define the disorder and discuss its expected course. Describe its signs and symptoms, and point out which ones are reversible and which are not. Explain the purpose of and describe the procedure for diagnostic tests and treatments. Also explain the dosage schedule and side effects of prescribed drugs. Because of the potential for agranulocytosis with PTU, instruct the patient to immediately report any severe sore throat, high fever, or other sign of infection and to stop this drug. Also tell the patient what to expect before and after thyroidectomy and during treatment with [131]I. (See nursing diagnoses: *Self-care limitation related to knowledge deficit about postoperative care* and *Concern for self and others over potential radiation exposure after treatment with* [131]*I.*) Emphasize the importance of treatment and medical follow-up. Reassure the patient that the risk of thyroid cancer is not increased in treated or untreated patients. Finally, suggest that the patient write down any questions for the doctor.

Evaluate your teaching. At the time of discharge, does the patient understand his disease and how to care for himself? Have you given him written information about prescribed drugs, signs and symptoms of thyroid disorders, and potential crises?

Anxiety related to altered body image, chronic disease, and possible changes in lifestyle. Help relieve the patient's anxiety and provide emotional support. Allow him to express his concerns over his loss of health and independence because of the need for lifetime treatment. Also, encourage the patient to express his feelings about his appearance. Remember, some people base their self-worth on their appearance; others, on their strength or earning capacity. Reassure the patient about his self-worth, and help him to see his strengths. Also help the patient and his family anticipate the life-style changes as treatment takes effect. Provide information about low-cost community follow-up services, if needed.

Before discharge, has the patient begun to accept his disorder? If so, he interacts more frequently with others and shows a more positive attitude about himself. He's also begun to anticipate necessary changes in life-style.

Alteration in neurologic function related to thyroid hormone excess or insufficiency. Help the patient with thyrotoxicosis understand that such symptoms as irritability, nervousness, and hyperactivity are, to a degree, beyond his control. Acknowledge the hyperactive patient's need to be busy. If possible, provide a quiet environment, without a roommate, and limit visitors to those who don't excite the patient. Educate the patient about the body's need for rest. Schedule short rest periods (if the patient is not on bed rest) until nervousness and hyperactivity subside and his normal endurance level returns. While he rests, provide mental diversions, such as reading, quiet conversation, TV, or crafts.

Approach the patient with hypothyroidism unhurriedly, and give him time to answer your questions. Help him make choices by limiting their number. Remember to attend to his needs; patients with hypothyroidism make few demands. Limit sleep to 8 hours a day, and don't hesitate to wake him for visitors. Help the patient develop appropriate interest in routine activities.

In evaluating your care of the thyrotoxic patient, check for an improved attention span, less hyperactivity, and less sensitivity to external stimuli. Does he now report a normal correlation between mental and physical fatigue? (He's no longer tired from the neck down.) If an outpatient, can he do a normal day's work without fatigue? In evaluating your care of the hypothyroid patient, notice if he answers questions more quickly, without repeating them or asking you to repeat them.

Does the patient show improved interest in routine activities, such as dressing himself and initiating conversation? Of course, you may not observe all these changes in patients hospitalized for short periods.

Visual disturbances related to thyrotoxicosis. The patient risks vision loss from an exposed cornea that results from exophthalmos with lid retraction. To prevent visual disturbances, don't stand for long periods where the patient must use the superior lateral gaze to see you. This can precipitate strabismus. Instruct the patient to do range-of-motion eye exercises twice a day. Give eye drops (methylcellulose), as ordered, to keep corneas moist. Advise the patient to wear sunglasses. Explain that surgery can relieve eyelid retraction and pressure on the eye. Your care has been successful if the patient reports normal vision with reduced eye irritation.

Temperature intolerance secondary to altered metabolism. Keep the patient comfortable until normal tolerance returns. For the thyrotoxic patient, provide a cool (65° to 68° F., or 18° to 20° C.) environment until he becomes euthyroid. Place the patient with a roommate who likes a cool room, if a private room isn't available. Provide cool clothing and light bed linens. Provide antiperspirant and cornstarch powder, as needed. Avoid using a rubber draw sheet. For the hypothyroid patient, provide a comfortably warm environment (75° F., or 24° C.) until he becomes euthyroid. Provide extra blankets, as needed. While metabolic depression impairs the patient's capacity for self-care, help him with daily hygiene, as necessary. Apply skin lotion to dry, rough skin.

Your care is successful if the patient wears appropriate clothing and indicates he's comfortable.

Alteration in cardiac status secondary to excessive or deficient thyroid hormone. To avert complications, monitor the patient's cardiac function. Monitor vital signs every 4 hours, particularly heart rate and rhythm and temperature. Assess for CHF: auscultate the heart and lungs, weigh the patient daily, and measure intake and output.

When managing the patient with thyrotoxicosis, take precautions to avoid stimulating the sympathomimetic system. Limit caffeine. Administer drugs as ordered, but ensure that the patient with CHF or asthma doesn't receive propranolol. Warn the patient to report symptoms or signs of CHF. Remember that dyspnea related to decreased pulmonary compliance and decreased vital capacity secondary to weakness of respiratory muscles result from thyrotoxicosis. Instruct the patient to report increased or new dyspnea. In hypothyroidism, because the patient is at risk for a cerebrovascular accident and for angina (particularly during initiation of thyroid hormone replacement therapy), instruct him to report chest pains or persistent headaches.

You've given effective care to the thyrotoxic patient if he demonstrates an absence of palpitations, decreased dyspnea, improved exercise tolerance, a sleeping pulse rate of 70 to 80 beats/minute, narrowing of an initially wide pulse pressure, and, in CHF, an absence of pedal edema, S_3, and pulmonary rales. You've given effective care to the hypothyroid patient if he demonstrates increased exercise tolerance, a resting pulse rate of between 70 and 80 beats/minute, wider pulse pressure, decreased signs of CHF, and absence of angina and headaches.

Alteration in GI and nutritional status due to altered metabolism. Provide nutrition appropriate for the patient's metabolic state—high-calorie, nutritious meals for the thyrotoxic patient. Administer vitamins, as ordered. Teach the patient to avoid caffeine, which enhances breakdown of fatty tissue. Instruct him about the relation between thyrotoxicosis and increased GI motility, and tell him which foods may produce diarrhea. Consult the dietitian, and monitor the patient's weight and food intake and the frequency, consistency, and amount of stools. Observe for signs and symptoms of vitamin deficiency.

For the hypothyroid patient, provide low-calorie meals. Encourage roughage, unless contraindicated, and fluid intake. Instruct the patient to avoid salty foods because of the potential for CHF related to myxedema. Monitor frequency and consistency of stools; administer stool softeners, as ordered. Encourage moderate exercise to prevent constipation. Monitor the patient's food intake and weight. Administer vitamins, as ordered: vitamin B_{12}, to treat pernicious anemia, and vitamin A, to prevent night blindness resulting from deficiency of this vitamin. Provide good lighting in the patient's room.

You've helped the patient if his weight stabilizes, his food intake is normal, his bowel function is normal (one or fewer bowel movements a day in thyrotoxicosis, or one every 2 or 3 days in hypothyroidism), and, in hypothyroidism, night vision returns and pernicious anemia is absent.

EMERGENCY MANAGEMENT

Thyroid storm

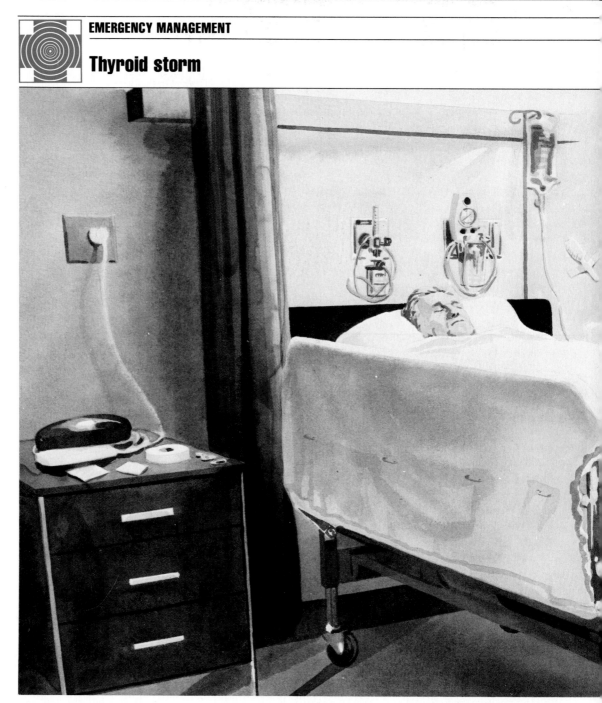

Fever—as high as 106° F. (41.1° C.)—is the classic feature of thyroid storm, a life-threatening exacerbation of thyrotoxicosis. Tachycardia, often accompanied by atrial fibrillation or atrial flutter, may occur along with vomiting, shock, and, at times, coma.

Thyroid storm may develop spontaneously, but in about 60% of patients it results from surgical trauma, severe emotional stress, infection, or metabolic alterations. Untreated, thyroid storm causes death from fever, exhaustion, heart or liver failure, or other complications. Even with prompt treatment, mortality is about 20%.

Early recognition is important: Consider any temperature greater than 100° F. (37.8° C.) in a thyrotoxic patient thyroid storm until proven otherwise.

In thyroid storm, you'll have to act quickly but carefully to support vital functions. Here's what you should do:
• Reduce fever with hypothermia blankets, ice packs, and fans. Monitor the patient's temperature with a rectal probe, and administer acetaminophen, as ordered. Salicylates are contraindicated because they displace thyroid hormones from their binding protein. Notify the doctor if shivering occurs since this raises metabolic demands.
• Administer propylthiouracil (PTU) before iodine, if possible, to prevent further synthesis and release of thyroid hormones. If the patient remains unresponsive, assist with plas-

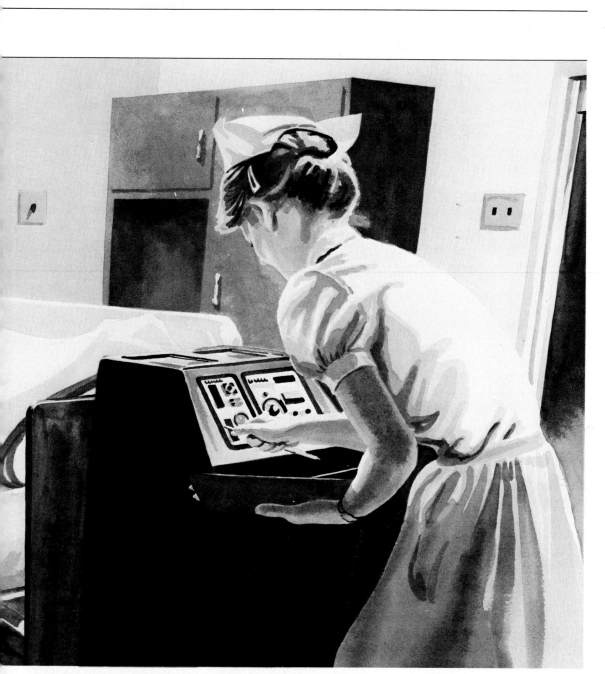

mapheresis, if necessary, to remove excess circulating thyroid hormone. Monitor cardiac function.
• Administer propranolol, reserpine, or guanethidine to block sympathetic effects, as ordered. Monitor the patient closely, and keep atropine available.
• Provide a calm, cool, protected environment. Reassure the patient, explain all procedures to him, and orient him, if necessary. Pad side rails, institute seizure precautions, and

employ vest or cloth wrist restraints, if needed.
• Administer I.V. fluids, as ordered, and monitor intake and output to detect dehydration or fluid overload. Encourage small, frequent feedings to prevent nausea and vomiting. Administer vitamin B_{12} and folic acid, as ordered. Continue to assess the patient for subtle changes in his condition. Check laboratory results frequently for electrolyte imbalances: hyperglycemia from insulin resistance,

hypokalemia from GI losses, hyponatremia from water toxicity, and hypercalcemia from accelerated bone metabolism.

After the crisis
Give the patient information about thyroid storm—its causes, signs and symptoms, and medical follow-up. Emphasize adherence to the prescribed drug regimen, since abrupt withdrawal of PTU or overuse of thyroid replacement hormones can precipitate thyroid storm.

Potential for infertility resulting from hormone imbalance. Provide emotional support and encourage the patient to express his feelings. Inform the patient that fertility can decrease in thyrotoxicosis and hypothyroidism but returns with euthyroidism. Encourage the female patient to discuss family planning with her doctor since certain forms of thyroid therapy are contraindicated in pregnancy.

After effective teaching, the patient can relate infertility to thyroid disease and understands the risks of certain forms of treatment during pregnancy.

Potential for development of thyroid storm and myxedema coma. Prevent thyroid storm; if thyroid storm is unavoidable, give proper care. Precipitating factors include infection, surgical trauma, metabolic alterations, and severe stress. Administer thyroid hormone antagonists, as ordered, and educate the patient about the importance of continuing his medical regimen. (See *Thyroid storm,* pages 86 and 87.)

To prevent myxedema coma, know its predisposing factors: exposure to cold, infection, and administration of CNS depressants. Question the patient about the use and dosage of sedatives, analgesics, and anesthetics, if appropriate, since normal doses of these drugs can be fatal in myxedema coma. Protect the patient from infection (because of his inability to meet its metabolic demands). Since proper self-care helps prevent myxedema coma, emphasize the importance of continuing thyroid medication, getting regular medical follow-up, and avoiding exposure to cold.

Consider myxedema coma in all patients with unexplained coma, even those with no known history of hypothyroidism. Myxedema coma can develop within hours in an untreated patient. In some patients, psychotic symptoms signal onset of coma. Early recognition is important. Despite prompt treatment, myxedema coma is fatal in about 50% of patients.

If myxedema coma occurs, maintain adequate ventilation. Check arterial blood gases for indications of hypoxia and respiratory acidosis and for the need for ventilatory assistance. Clear any airway obstruction. Provide emergency ventilatory support with an Ambu bag.

Provide blankets to prevent further heat loss. Frequently monitor temperature with a rectal thermometer. A temperature as low as 75° F. (24° C.) is possible, but in infection it may be normal.

Recognize the signs of hypoglycemia (in about 25% of patients with myxedema coma), and prepare to administer $D_{50}W$ I.V. immediately. In hyponatremia (in about 50% of patients with myxedema coma), administer hypertonic saline solution I.V.; restrict fluids, as ordered; and monitor intake and output. Also monitor cardiac function for signs of CHF and possible dysrhythmias.

Administer thyroid hormone replacement drugs and vasopressor amines (for hypotension), as ordered. Check blood pressure frequently. Expect improved mental status with thyroid hormone replacement and improved tissue oxygenation.

Check neurologic status, as ordered, and maintain seizure precautions. Prevent bed-rest complications (such as pressure sores and thrombi). Turn the patient every 2 hours. Apply compression-gradient stockings, as ordered. To prevent adrenal crisis, hydrocortisone may be ordered. Check for worsening hypotension. Observe strict sterile technique for invasive procedures.

After the crisis, give the patient written information about myxedema coma. Include information about precipitants, signs and symptoms, and the importance of getting medical follow-up and taking medication as prescribed.

You've cared effectively for the patient with myxedema coma if his temperature returns to normal after the crisis, if complications are prevented, and if he understands the cause of the crisis and the importance of continuing medical treatment and follow-up.

Potential for drug overdose, secondary to decreased metabolism in hypothyroidism. To prevent overdose, check all medication orders carefully for appropriate reduction of dosage to prevent toxicity in the hypothyroid patient. Observe for signs of toxicity; routine doses of sedatives, analgesics, and anesthetics can cause death in patients with hypothyroidism. Check that the patient is protected from drug overdose or oversedation.

Concern for self and others over potential radiation exposure after treatment with [131]**I.** Provide emotional support, and reassure the patient that treatment with ^{131}I doesn't carry an increased risk of leukemia or thyroid cancer. Also tell the patient that children of parents treated with [131]I (but not treated during pregnancy) show no increased incidence of birth defects. After treatment, instruct the patient to avoid close contact with pregnant women, infants, and children for 1 week. Since the patient's urine and saliva are radioactive, instruct him to carefully flush urine and to use disposable plates and cutlery for the first 48 hours after treatment. When the patient is treated with less than 30 millicuries of ^{131}I, contact with a spouse poses no hazard for the spouse, except for contact with body secretions for the first 48 hours. If treatment is greater than this dose, the patient is hospitalized. The hospital's radiation safety officer can then advise the patient, family, and nursing staff about precautions.

Evaluate your teaching effectiveness. Do the patient and family show less anxiety about treatment with ^{131}I? Does the patient follow prescribed precautions? If he's an outpatient, did he resume normal physical contact with family members after precautions were lifted?

Potential for hypothyroidism after treatment with ^{131}I. Tell the patient that many patients treated with ^{131}I later develop hypothyroidism (about 40% to 70% of patients develop hypothyroidism within 10 years after treatment). Teach him its signs and symptoms and the importance of long-term medical follow-up. Check that the patient understands the signs and symptoms of hypothyroidism and accepts the need for follow-up.

Self-care limitation related to knowledge deficit about postoperative care. Before surgery, prepare the patient to care for himself after thyroidectomy. Teach coughing and deep-breathing exercises and the proper position to prevent abnormal neck extension; show him how to support the neck with his hands to reduce stress on the incision. Also tell the patient what to expect regarding oxygen administration, swallowing, suctioning, voice checks, and the need to rest his voice. Provide emotional support.

To evaluate your interventions, notice if the patient asks appropriate questions about postoperative self-care, can show mastery of necessary techniques, and actively participates in postoperative care.

Potential for developing postoperative complications. Prevent thyroid storm in the postoperative period with correct presurgical treatment. Administer PTU and iodine, as ordered, to achieve euthyroidism. If iodine treatment continues for 7 to 10 days, observe for signs of iodine escape (recurring signs and symptoms of thyrotoxicosis). Also observe for signs of iodine toxicity (excessive salivation, swelling of the buccal mucosa, coryza, or skin eruptions).

Be alert for hemorrhage: monitor blood pressure, observe the suture site and amount of drainage on the dressing, and check under the patient's neck and shoulders for drainage. Note complaints of sensations of pressure and fullness in the neck. Check respiratory rate frequently. Observe for dyspnea, crowing respirations, and supraclavicular retractions. Report these to the doctor immediately. Administer humidified oxygen, as ordered.

To reduce postoperative swelling, place the patient in semi-Fowler's position. Position the neck to prevent hyperextension or flexion. Position sand bags at both sides of the head to prevent movement. Administer narcotics, as ordered, and use other pain-relieving techniques, as appropriate. Teach the patient to support his neck with his hands during movement. Apply an ice bag to prevent swelling and promote comfort. To help prevent pneumonia, encourage coughing and deep breathing every 2 hours after surgery for 48 hours. If coughing is ineffective, suction the trachea, as needed; also suction oral secretions, as needed. Notify the doctor if you detect a weak, breathy voice or any difficulty swallowing, speaking, or coughing. This can indicate laryngeal nerve injury, which may lead to respiratory distress.

Because inadvertent removal of the parathyroid glands during surgery can cause hypocalcemia, observe for hyperreflexia, tetany, Chvostek's sign (spasm of facial muscles when tapped), Trousseau's sign (carpopedal spasm induced by occluding circulation in a limb with a blood pressure cuff), and laryngeal stridor. Early signs include numbness and tingling of extremities and perioral tissue, malaise, or anxiety. For emergency treatment of tetany, keep calcium gluconate available for 72 hours after surgery. Report any signs of hypocalcemia immediately.

Replace fluids, prevent thrombi, and ensure good nutrition. After suture removal, instruct the patient to perform active range-of-motion exercises of the neck several times daily, as ordered, to prevent keloid scar formation.

To evaluate postoperative care, consider if complications were prevented or quickly resolved.

A measure of effectiveness

Effective nursing management of thyroid disorders must emphasize educating the patient to comply with a lifetime medical regimen, preventing thyroid crises, careful monitoring during crises, and helping the patient adjust to a changing self-image and life-style.

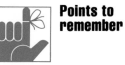

Points to remember

- Thyroid disorders develop from the effects of excess or insufficient thyroid hormone on peripheral tissues or from pathologic changes in the thyroid gland itself, or both.
- Thyroid disorders affect up to 20% of the population and occur more commonly in women than in men.
- Graves' disease, an immunogenetic disorder caused by an abnormal thyroid stimulator, is the most common cause of thyrotoxicosis.
- Reduced thyroid tissue mass or interference with thyroid hormone synthesis or release causes hypothyroidism.
- Because thyroid disorders are cyclic and chronic, treatment typically must continue for life.
- Nursing management of thyroid disorders requires a thorough interview, careful physical exam, prevention or correction of thyroid crises and complications, and patient education about prescribed treatment and potential life-style changes.

7 DETECTING PARATHYROID DISORDERS

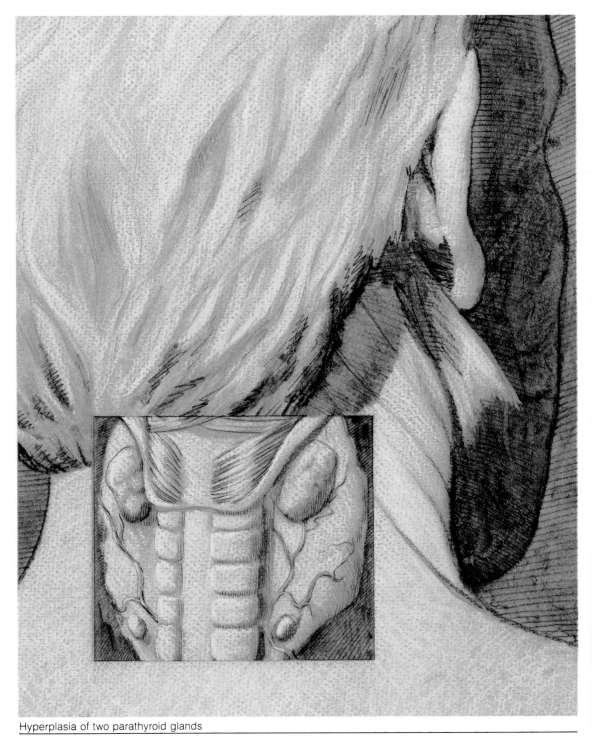

Hyperplasia of two parathyroid glands

More often than you'd expect, you'll see parathyroid disorders in acute-care and postoperative patients, because these disorders can result from diseases and certain surgeries. Unless you know what to look for, you can easily miss the sometimes subtle signs and insidious onset of parathyroid disorders. Yet, because the parathyroid glands control the body's calcium and phosphorus levels, early treatment is crucial to prevent irreversible or long-term damage to kidneys and bones and to avoid such crises as tetany. To provide effective care, you'll need to understand the pathophysiology, signs, and medical management of parathyroid disorders.

Parathyroid hormone: Too much or too little

Hyperparathyroidism—excessive secretion of parathyroid hormone (PTH)—upsets calcium, phosphate, and bone metabolism. Hyperparathyroidism may be primary, secondary, tertiary, or ectopic. Primary hyperparathyroidism occurs in about 1 of every 1,000 people. This disorder typically results from a benign adenoma in one of the four parathyroid glands (in 85% of patients), but may also result from multiple gland hyperplasia (in 15%). A familial form of primary hyperparathyroidism may result from diffuse multiple gland hyperplasia. Commonly, primary hyperparathyroidism strikes people ages 30 to 60 and affects women about twice as often as it does men.

Secondary hyperparathyroidism may accompany chronic renal failure or vitamin D deficiency; the parathyroids adapt to prolonged hypocalcemia by secreting excess PTH. Tertiary hyperparathyroidism may occur following chronic parathyroid stimulation in renal failure; autonomous neoplastic parathyroid hypersecretion results in hypercalcemia.

Ectopic hyperparathyroidism occurs most commonly with lung or kidney carcinomas: Nonparathyroid neoplastic tissue produces PTH.

Hypoparathyroidism—deficient secretion of PTH—also upsets mineral metabolism. It may be surgically induced or idiopathic. Surgically induced hypoparathyroidism may be purposeful or inadvertent in anterior neck surgery; temporary hypoparathyroidism may result from impaired blood supply to the parathyroid glands during surgery or from chronic suppression of nonpathologic tissue after pathologic tissue is removed.

Idiopathic hypoparathyroidism generally occurs in children; it may be familial or associated with an autoimmune factor. It may also occur with thymic aplasia (DiGeorge's syndrome). Acquired hypoparathyroidism may result from hypomagnesemia and treatment with radioactive iodine for Graves' disease. A rare, hereditary form of hypoparathyroidism, pseudohypoparathyroidism produces developmental and skeletal defects. It occurs twice as commonly in women as in men.

PATHOPHYSIOLOGY

Usually, adenoma of one gland or chief cell hyperplasia of all parathyroid glands causes primary hyperparathyroidism, resulting in excessive PTH secretion and elevated calcium levels. Excessive PTH secretion remains controlled by a feedback mechanism, achieving a hypercalcemic equilibrium. Evidently, excess PTH results from alteration in the level at which calcium exerts feedback control or from growth of a parathyroid mass with its own feedback mechanisms. In adenomas, both factors are apparently involved. In hyperplasia, the factor appears to be excessive functioning tissue with normal feedback control. If calcium levels rise above this equilibrium point, PTH secretion is suppressed. (See *Normal feedback mechanism between calcium and parathyroid secretion,* page 93.)

Excessive PTH levels adversely affect the bones, kidneys, and intestines. In the bones, excessive PTH stimulates osteoclastic activity in the presence of vitamin D, enhances osteoblastic activity, and may raise serum alkaline phosphatase levels. All this results in subperiosteal bone resorption, lessened bone density, cyst formation, and generalized bone weakness. In severe bone disease, fibrous tissue replaces the marrow, causing anemia.

In the kidneys, high calcium levels overwhelm the renal tubular calcium reabsorptive mechanisms, and hypercalciuria results. That and the large amounts of phosphate excreted in the urine can lead to formation of calculi. Recurrent renal calculi can cause obstruction, urinary tract infection, and progressive renal failure. Because excessive loss of calcium impairs renal water conservation by interfering with the action of antidiuretic hormone, polyuria may occur.

High serum chloride levels commonly cause mild-to-moderate metabolic acidosis with urinary bicarbonate loss. Acidosis aggravates existing hypercalcemia because it impairs albumin's ability to bind with ionic calcium, raising ionic calcium levels. Also, hyperchloremia creates an acid environment where bone readily demineralizes.

In the intestines, increased production of vitamin D by the kidneys enhances intestinal calcium absorption, further raising serum calcium levels. Hypercalcemia may cause anorexia, nausea, vomiting, and constipation. It also causes high gastrin and pepsin secretion, leading to an increased incidence of peptic ulcers. Incidence of pancreatitis also increases in hyperparathyroidism.

Secondary hyperparathyroidism: Bone demineralization

Excessive compensatory production of PTH that stems from a hypocalcemia-producing abnormality outside the parathyroid gland causes secondary hyperparathyroidism. Abnormalities, such as chronic renal failure, vitamin D deficiency, and osteomalacia, can cause resistance to the metabolic action of PTH. In renal failure, marked hyperphosphatemia occurs because of the kidneys' inability to filter phosphate. When the glomerular filtration rate drops below 10%, no phosphate is filtered despite high PTH levels. Consequently, elevated phosphorus levels depress ionized calcium levels, promoting PTH secretion.

High PTH levels cause excess osteoclastic stimulation. Renal osteodystrophy, due to calcium and phosphorus resorption from the bone matrix, causes bone demineralization. The chronic acidosis of renal failure augments the process. The damaged kidneys inadequately activate vitamin D, which normally promotes calcium absorption from the intestine. Also, impaired calcium absorption results from ineffective vitamin D activity and excess phosphorus, which binds with calcium in the intestine.

Metastatic calcification and calcitonin secretion: Compensatory mechanisms

To lower extracellular calcium levels when serum calcium–phosphorus product exceeds 60 to 70 mg/dl, metastatic calcification causes deposition of calcium phosphate crystals in the soft tissues. This compensatory process causes discomfort and dysfunction that may include muscle weakness, ocular band keratopathy and itching, hypertension and eventual heart failure, lethargy, drowsiness, paresthesias, psychosis, fever, and headache.

Calcitonin, which is secreted by the thyroid parafollicular cells, also lowers serum calcium levels by decreasing osteoclastic activity, pre-

venting new osteoclast formation, and increasing osteoblastic activity. In fact, calcitonin and PTH work synergistically to maintain normal serum calcium levels.

Hypoparathyroidism: Its causes

Surgery, with purposeful or inadvertent removal of functioning parathyroid tissue, is the most common cause of hypoparathyroidism. Surgery in adjacent sites may lead to hypoparathyroidism even if it leaves these glands intact. If their blood supply is impaired, they may slowly atrophy because of ischemia; then PTH secretion diminishes, causing symptoms of hyposecretion several days, weeks, or months postoperatively. If the glands have been injured or suppressed by chronic hypercalcemia, they may recover, or a small remnant of remaining parathyroid tissue may hypertrophy to eventually produce adequate levels of PTH. In such patients, postoperative hypoparathyroidism may be transient.

An autoimmune defect is believed to be associated with one type of idiopathic hypoparathyroidism. Parathyroid antibodies have been implicated, since the titer is sixfold greater in patients with this type of idiopathic hypoparathyroidism than in control patients. Also, antibodies in high titers against other endocrine glands and resultant gland failure occur frequently in this type of idiopathic hypoparathyroidism.

Prolonged, severe magnesium depletion, occurring in alcoholism or malabsorption syndromes, inhibits PTH secretion and use.

Any disorder that limits vitamin D availability may cause hypoparathyroidism. Gastric or intestinal surgery, pancreatitis, or malabsorption from small intestine disease or vitamin D-losing nephropathies can cause vitamin D deficiency. Hepatic or renal disease may prevent adequate vitamin D activation. Certain drugs, such as phenobarbital and phenytoin, accelerate metabolic breakdown of vitamin D; therefore, treatment with these drugs may require large concomitant doses of vitamin D to ensure adequate calcium balance.

Hypoparathyroidism: Its effects

Low PTH levels lead to decreased bone resorption, renal phosphate excretion, vitamin D activation and intestinal calcium absorption, and to increased urinary calcium excretion. Hypocalcemia and mild metabolic alkalosis then result from decreased bicarbonate secretion, causing symptoms of neuromuscular excitability and tetany, the hallmark of acute

Normal feedback mechanism between calcium and parathyroid secretion

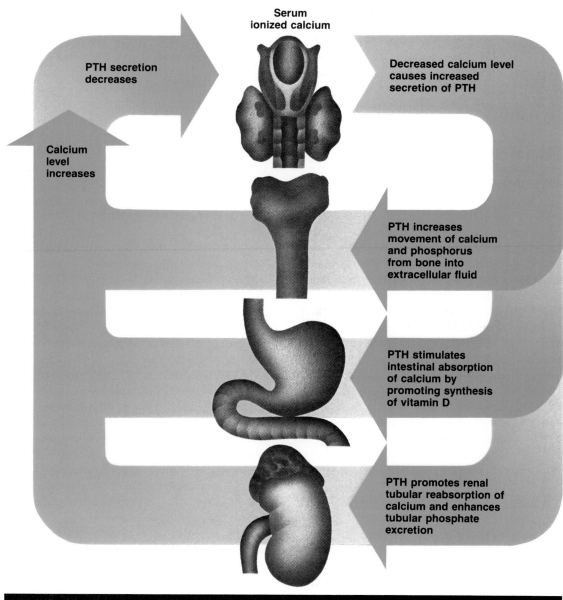

Serum ionized calcium

PTH secretion decreases

Decreased calcium level causes increased secretion of PTH

Calcium level increases

PTH increases movement of calcium and phosphorus from bone into extracellular fluid

PTH stimulates intestinal absorption of calcium by promoting synthesis of vitamin D

PTH promotes renal tubular reabsorption of calcium and enhances tubular phosphate excretion

hypocalcemia. When serum calcium levels fall gradually, other symptoms, such as dry skin, mental changes, or Parkinson-like symptoms appear more frequently.

Pseudohypoparathyroidism: A matter of genetics

Pseudohypoparathyroidism resembles hypoparathyroidism but is due to a genetic defect from a lack of PTH receptor in the appropriate target organ or from a defect that makes the target cell unresponsive to PTH. Skeletal and renal tubular resistance to PTH cause hypocalcemia, despite normal or high PTH levels. In fact, prolonged target organ resistance and

the resulting hypocalcemia can lead to hyperplasia and secondary hyperparathyroidism, usually with hyperphosphatemia because of decreased renal tubular phosphate secretion.

In pseudohypoparathyroidism, congenital growth and skeletal defects usually accompany signs of hypoparathyroidism: mental retardation; stocky build; round face; shortened first, fourth, and fifth metacarpal and metatarsal bones; and ectopic bone formation. Family members may show these developmental defects but without hypocalcemia and hyperphosphatemia. This syndrome, called "pseudopseudohypoparathyroidism," may result from an X chromosome abnormality.

Additional causes of calcium imbalance

Hypercalcemia
• Vitamin D excess
• Milk-alkali syndrome (Burnett's syndrome)
• Malignancy with metastasis
• Malignancy without metastasis
• Sarcoidosis
• Prolonged thiazide therapy
• Immobilization
• Acute renal failure (diuretic phase)
• Hyperthyroidism
• Addison's disease
• Idiopathic hypercalcemia of infancy

Hypocalcemia
• Vitamin D insufficiency
• Small-bowel disease
• Inadequate total parenteral nutrition
• Starvation
• Diarrhea
• Certain malignancies in which bone metastases stimulate a marked increase in osteoblastic activity
• Drugs, such as Dilantin
• Sepsis
• Burns
• Massive blood transfusions
• Markedly increased serum phosphate levels, such as in uremia, after chemotherapy for leukemia, or after phosphate infusion
• Autoimmune disease
• Acute pancreatitis
• Severe liver disease
• Calcium malabsorption
• Hypomagnesemia
• Postoperative abdominal or neck surgery

MEDICAL MANAGEMENT

Differential diagnosis of parathyroid disorders can be difficult. Because these disorders often cause vague symptoms, careful correlation of the history, physical exam, and laboratory data becomes especially important.

Diagnostic tests

Serum calcium and PTH radioimmunoassay are the primary diagnostic tools for detecting parathyroid disorders. Other tests include cyclic AMP and serum phosphorus.

Serum calcium. In asymptomatic patients, serum calcium levels may be high, intermittently high, or normal. In more than 95% of patients with primary hyperparathyroidism, calcium levels consistently exceed 10 mg/dl. In secondary hyperparathyroidism, calcium levels are usually low but occasionally normal (although kidney disease or intestinal malabsorption is present). In hypoparathyroidism, calcium levels are usually less than 8.5 mg/dl.

PTH radioimmunoassay. This test can help diagnose parathyroid disorders more accurately than urine calcium and phosphorus tests. In more than 80% of patients with hyperparathyroidism, the PTH level rises. Depressed PTH levels in the presence of low serum calcium levels and elevated serum phosphorus levels indicate hypoparathyroidism. In pseudohypoparathyroidism, PTH levels are normal or high; serum calcium levels, low or normal; and serum phosphorus levels, high.

Urine cyclic AMP. PTH primarily controls nephrogenous cyclic AMP production and secretion. Nephrogenous cyclic AMP measurements can distinguish between normal and low parathyroid function and can measure rapid changes in parathyroid function. In more than 97% of patients with primary hyperparathyroidism, cyclic AMP levels rise. They fall in hypoparathyroidism. In pseudohypoparathyroidism, cyclic AMP levels may be low, if the defect lies in the PTH receptor level; or elevated, if the defect lies beyond the generation of cyclic AMP in the renal cell. In both cases, urinary phosphate excretion is low.

Serum phosphorus. Because of its inverse relationship to calcium levels, serum phosphorus provides a clue to parathyroid function. In hyperparathyroidism, serum phosphorus usually falls below 3 mg/dl. In hypoparathyroidism, it exceeds 4.5 mg/dl. These changes do not always reliably confirm hypo- or hyperparathyroidism because many factors influence serum phosphorus. However, hypo-

parathyroidism is usually present if hyperphosphatemia and hypocalcemia exist without renal failure. In malignancy with metastasis to bone or without PTH-like activity, serum phosphorus levels are normal or elevated.

Serum magnesium. Serum magnesium directly affects PTH secretion. When magnesium levels fall below 1 mEq/liter, PTH secretion is impaired, even with hypocalcemia. Serum magnesium is always measured in suspected hypoparathyroidism because this disorder can result from primary magnesium deficiency.

Serum chloride. In primary hyperparathyroidism, serum chloride levels usually exceed 102 mEq/liter because of high urinary bicarbonate losses and metabolic acidosis. In hypoparathyroidism, serum chloride levels fall because of low bicarbonate excretion leading to mild alkalosis.

Serum alkaline phosphatase. This test aids differential diagnosis of hyperparathyroidism, because alkaline phosphatase mediates some of the complex reactions of bone formation. However, elevated levels in bone disease are nonspecific, since they may be elevated in other diseases associated with hypercalcemia, such as malignancy or hyperthyroidism.

Radiographic tests. Useful in late hyperparathyroidism when bone changes are present, X-rays of the hands, clavicle ends, and skull can show demineralization, decreased bone density, and, possibly, cyst formation. These tests are inaccurate in early hyperparathyroidism when bone changes are not usually present.

Localization studies. These studies, which localize the parathyroid glands, include cervical esophagography, parathyroid ultrasound, computerized tomography, digital subtraction angiography, and bilateral sampling by percutaneous venous catheter of the neck and thorax veins.

Treating hyperparathyroidism

Surgery is preferred for symptomatic hyperparathyroidism but controversial in the asymptomatic form. If surgery is avoided, treatment includes an annual physical exam and history, biannual serum calcium and creatinine clearance tests, and annual X-rays of the hands (to check for subperiosteal bone resorption) and of the abdomen (for renal calculi).

Surgical removal of the parathyroid glands may be complicated by variations in gland location (20% are located in the mediastinum; others, in the thyroid gland), size, and color.

Test results in parathyroid disorders

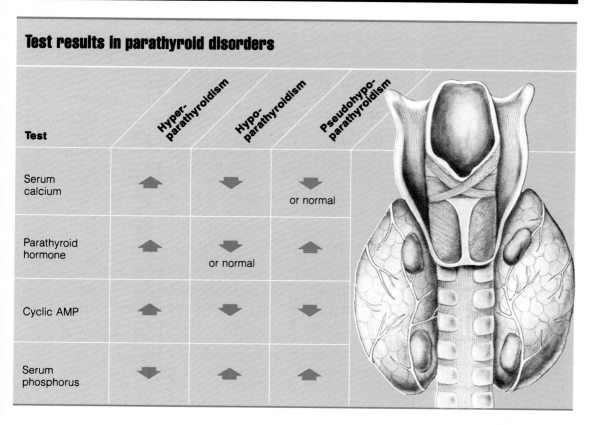

Test	Hyper-parathyroidism	Hypo-parathyroidism	Pseudohypo-parathyroidism
Serum calcium	▲	▼	▼ or normal
Parathyroid hormone	▲	▼ or normal	▲
Cyclic AMP	▲	▼	▼
Serum phosphorus	▼	▲	▲

If only mild symptoms exist and localization studies indicate adenoma, one side of the neck is explored. The adenoma is removed, and the other side of the neck is left untouched. In hyperplasia, all but half of one gland is removed. In parathyroid cancer, the parathyroids are removed entirely because chemotherapy and irradiation are ineffective.

After surgery, calcium levels start to fall within 24 to 48 hours and reach their nadir in 4 to 5 days (but may fall to hypocalcemic levels while the patient is in the recovery room). If not, aberrant parathyroid tissue or ectopic hyperparathyroidism becomes a possibility, requiring extensive diagnostic studies.

Medical treatment of primary hyperparathyroidism, when indicated, involves limiting calcium intake to 400 g/day; encouraging mobility and large quantities of fluid; salt intake of 8 to 10 g/day to replace losses; and phosphorus supplements, except in patients at risk for renal calculi, such as those with persistent urinary tract infection and alkalotic urine.

Hypercalcemia greater than 14 mg/dl, or 12 to 14 mg/dl with symptoms of primary hyperparathyroidism, requires immediate treatment. Saline infusion enhances urinary calcium excretion. Concurrent administration of furosemide aids diuresis and averts fluid overload. Magnesium and potassium supplements prevent depletion of these electrolytes.

Once diuresis has begun, mithramycin, an antihypercalcemic agent, or calcitonin, a rapidly acting hypocalcemic agent with a transient effect, may be given. Inorganic phosphate, which probably lowers serum calcium by complexing it and depositing it in bone, may be used as an adjunct to volume-loading therapy.

Corticosteroids may be given in long-term therapy, especially in malignancies and increased vitamin D states. Indomethacin treats hypercalcemia due to prostaglandins secreted by tumors. Oral sodium cellulose phosphate decreases calcium absorption by increasing fecal calcium excretion. Intravenous phosphates treat severe hypercalcemia unresponsive to other measures. Oral elemental phosphorus, in divided doses, treats chronic hypercalcemia.

Treatment of secondary hyperparathyroidism relies on correcting or controlling the underlying cause of hypocalcemia.

Treating hypoparathyroidism

In acute hypoparathyroidism, treatment aims to control tetany and prevent laryngeal spasm and seizures. Calcium gluconate given by slow I.V. push aims to maintain serum calcium levels over 7 mg/dl. Calcium gluconate can be given I.V. in a dose of 10 to 20 ml of 10% calcium gluconate (contains about 10 mg elemental calcium/ml). If hypocalcemia persists, continuous I.V. calcium infusion follows. Prolonged, symptomatic hypocalcemia despite treatment requires dihydrotachysterol, a synthetic analogue of vitamin D with a similar but faster action. Because it has a shorter duration of action, overdoses can be more quickly corrected than with vitamin D_2.

In chronic hypoparathyroidism, treatment aims to maintain serum calcium levels at 8 to 9 mg/dl to control symptoms and prevent complications and hypercalcemia. Vitamin D replacement is the basis of treatment; however, since vitamin D acts by enhancing intestinal absorption, 1 g/day of dietary calcium is also required. Ineffective treatment of hypoparathyroidism—the result of difficulty in regulating vitamin D levels—can lead to impaired renal glomerular and tubular function, causing nephrolithiasis and nephrocalcinosis.

In mild hypoparathyroidism, treatment includes oral calcium supplements (providing 1,000 to 1,500 mg of elemental calcium) and phosphorus restriction, including phosphate-binding antacids.

If hypoparathyroidism results from hypomagnesemia, treatment includes magnesium replacement. Treatment of pseudohypoparathyroidism also includes calcium supplements and vitamin D.

NURSING MANAGEMENT
In parathyroid disorders, nursing management may include detection of subtle psychological or physical symptoms or immediate treatment of a life-threatening complication. First, take an accurate, carefully focused history and perform a thorough physical exam.

Take a detailed history
What is the patient's chief complaint? Does he even have one? The patient with hyperparathyroidism may be asymptomatic and require laboratory tests to confirm diagnosis. He may have adjusted to the disorder so gradually that he fails to recognize symptoms. If he can pinpoint some, ask about their onset, duration, and severity.

Has the patient's energy level decreased (due to anemia from renal damage or bone marrow destruction)? Easy muscle fatigability, especially proximal and lower extremity weakness, may be the only symptom of hyperparathyroidism. Does he have restless legs at night? Or arthritis (due to intraarticular calcium deposits)? Does he have bone pain, frequent fractures, overly flexible joints (in rare cases, with bone demineralization in advanced hyperparathyroidism)? In hypoparathyroidism, most symptoms are neuromuscular. Has the patient noticed tingling or spasms around the mouth, or in the arms or legs? This signals lowered sensory and motor neuron excitation thresholds, although tetany may not be overt. Cramping, stiffness, or clumsiness may signal covert tetany. The patient may have headaches from cranial spasm. The hypoparathyroid child may suffer convulsions; the hypoparathyroid adult may suffer epileptic-like seizures because of hypocalcemia-induced peripheral and motor neuron excitability.

Early CNS symptoms of hyperparathyroidism include lethargy, drowsiness, myalgia, or paresthesia. Ask about these symptoms. Also ask the patient or his family about emotional lability, memory loss of recent events, depression, somnolence, personality changes, even psychosis.

Rarely, psychiatric disorders also occur in hypoparathyroidism. The patient with hypoparathyroidism may have conjunctivitis, visual problems, or photophobia from calcium deposits in the eye.

Does the patient have polyuria, frequent kidney infections, or kidney stones (in hyperparathyroidism)? Does he have abdominal discomfort, postprandial nausea, epigastric pain, vomiting, constipation? These may signal peptic ulcer disease or pancreatitis.

Ask about intestinal disease or alcohol abuse; both can induce hypomagnesemia and

Effects of chronic hyperparathyroidism
In this X-ray of terminal phalanges, note bone erosion.

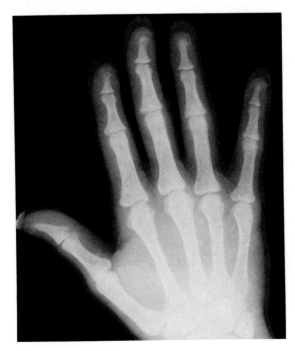

may signal hypoparathyroidism. Also, ask about difficulty in swallowing, abdominal pain, or sharp pain in the upper right quadrant, which may result from smooth muscle spasm because of autonomic ganglia hyperirritability.

Has the patient recently had Graves' disease or undergone neck irradiation or surgery? Does he have a neck tumor?

Ask about use of drugs that alter PTH function: cimetidine, aminoglycoside antibiotics, cytotoxic agents, phosphate salts, theophylline, heparin. Phenobarbital and phenytoin alter vitamin D metabolism.

Check family history. If it's positive for hyper- or hypocalcemia, renal calculi, metabolic bone disease, peptic ulcer, or endocrine tumor, parathyroid dysfunction is likely.

Perform the physical exam

Observe the patient carefully. The patient with chronic hyperparathyroidism may be pale or cachectic and have an enlarged skull; a kyphotic, shortened spine; or irregular deformities of the extremities. The patient with pseudohypoparathyroidism appears short and obese, with a round face and short distal metacarpals.

Look for neuromuscular symptoms. In hypoparathyroidism, the speed at which calcium decreases often determines their severity and rate of development. If serum calcium falls rapidly, neuromuscular symptoms may appear despite higher levels (8 mg/dl). If it falls slowly, symptoms may not appear until 6 mg/dl.

Observe for tetany. Hyperventilation, laryngeal spasm, stridor, loud crowing noises, choking sensation, cyanosis, tachycardia, and sweating may accompany spasms. Test for Chvostek's and Trousseau's signs (in latent hypocalcemia).

In hyperparathyroidism, neuromuscular symptoms may appear as depressed or absent reflexes, lack of coordination, muscle weakness, and hypotonia. Assess the patient's mental status for disorientation, delirium, confusion, paranoia or hallucinations, lethargy, drowsiness, stupor, or coma. In hyperparathyroidism and pseudohypoparathyroidism, mental deficiency or retardation may occur.

Examine the skin. In hypoparathyroidism, look for dry, scaling skin; ridged, brittle nails; coarse, friable hair; alopecia; and cutaneous *Candida* infections (due to poor white cell function). These reflect hypocalcemia.

Check the teeth. Hypoplasia of the tooth enamel with pitting, staining, and caries characterizes hypoparathyroidism.

Examine the eyes. Lenticular cataracts, fully

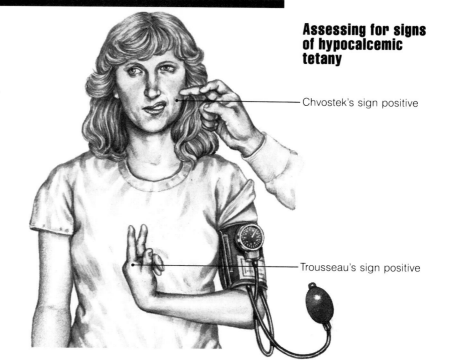

Assessing for signs of hypocalcemic tetany

— Chvostek's sign positive

— Trousseau's sign positive

Positive Trousseau's sign and positive Chvostek's sign are two indications of hypocalcemic tetany. In Trousseau's sign, the patient's hand contracts like this when pressure is applied to the arm. In Chvostek's sign, facial spasm of the lateral muscle results from tapping the side of the patient's face near his lower jaw.

mature and confluent with the entire lens, characterize hypoparathyroidism.

Palpate the parathyroid glands (which may be done if they are very enlarged).

Assess the respiratory and cardiovascular systems. In hypoparathyroidism, the patient may wheeze or be short of breath because of bronchiolar muscle spasm. The EKG shows prolonged QT intervals, particularly in the ST segment. In suspected hyperparathyroidism, check for hypertension and bradycardia.

Form nursing diagnoses

Correlate data from the history and physical exam with laboratory test results to develop nursing diagnoses and an appropriate care plan.

Potential hypercalcemic crisis related to hyperparathyroidism. Your goal: Reduce serum calcium levels. Give fluids, as ordered, using a volumetric infusion pump. Monitor for signs of fluid overload: increased central venous pressure, rales, jugular venous distention, shortness of breath, and pedal edema. Monitor magnesium and potassium levels, and replace urinary losses, as ordered. Monitor for cardiac dysrhythmias (hypercalcemia and hyperkalemia together can cause cardiac irritability).

Give diuretics, except thiazides, as ordered. Maintain intake and output records. Give antihypercalcemic agents, as ordered. With mithramycin, a slow infusion rate minimizes nausea. Monitor for side effects, such as bleeding and a precipitous drop in calcium level. With calcitonin, keep epinephrine close at hand; systemic allergic reactions are possible. Observe for signs of tetany and hypercalcemic relapse. Monitor phosphorus levels. Give phosphate only if the serum phosphorus level is below 3.0 to 3.5 mg/dl.

Once calcium levels have been reduced, limit calcium intake and promote oral hydration. Provide a written diet for the patient. Encourage him to drink 6 to 8 glasses of water a day. Teach the patient with hyperparathyroidism the early signs of calcium toxicity: nausea, vomiting, anorexia, abdominal pain, weakness, thirst, and shortness of breath.

Evaluate your interventions. They were successful if the patient's serum calcium level was reduced; soft tissue calcification was avoided; oral hydration was achieved; and the patient understands his dietary restrictions and knows the signs of calcium toxicity.

Renal abnormalities related to altered fluid and electrolyte balance. Your goal: Prevent or alleviate these renal abnormalities—polyuria, polydipsia, renal calculi, and frequent urinary tract infections. Consult the dietitian for an acid-ash diet to keep urine acidic and avoid formation of renal calculi. Encourage large volumes of fluid (4 liters a day), unless contraindicated by congestive heart failure or renal failure. Turn the immobile patient frequently, and encourage the mobile patient to walk to lessen urinary stasis. Strain all urine for calculi, and record intake and output. Assess for signs of urinary tract infection, such as fever, frequency, urgency, and flank pain, and report them at once.

Evaluate your interventions. They were successful if the patient didn't develop a urinary tract infection, or it was treated at once; maintains adequate fluid; adheres to an acid-ash diet; and passes few or no calculi.

Altered bowel elimination related to impaired smooth muscle function secondary to calcium imbalance. Your goal: Improve intestinal motility. Encourage fluid intake and dietary fruit and fiber. Provide a diet to follow at home. Suggest abdominal exercises and walking to increase intestinal peristalsis. Monitor bowel movements; they should occur at least every other day. Give stool softeners and laxatives judiciously to prevent diarrhea and further electrolyte imbalance.

Evaluate your interventions. They were successful if the patient has regular bowel movements, has a written diet to follow at home, and understands the relationship between exercise and intestinal motility.

Decreased activity and exercise tolerance. This results from the hypercalcemic effects on the neuromuscular system. Your goal: Conserve energy. Tell the patient to allow time to finish tasks. Help him schedule rest periods and shorter periods of activity.

Evaluate your interventions. They were successful if the patient rests between activities and his exercise tolerance has improved.

Impaired mobility related to bone demineralization. Your goal: Prevent complications. Assess for skin breakdown. Turn a bedridden patient every 2 hours. Provide a safe environment during transfers from bed to chair. Warn him that heavy lifting may cause skeletal injury. Demonstrate the proper body mechanics for lifting. Assess for signs of thrombus formation (redness, swelling, tenderness along a leg vein). Encourage the patient to wear antiembolism stockings. Prevent constipation.

Evaluate your interventions. They were successful if the complications did not develop.

Impaired cognitive and perceptual patterns related to hypercalcemic effects on the CNS. Your goal: Decrease the results of such impairment in the patient. Teach him ways to avoid or deal with stress. An individualized exercise program or biofeedback techniques (taught in some hospitals) may reduce stress. Inform the patient that perceptual problems disappear with treatment. Encourage verbalization of fears. Keep the environment quiet until, with the return of normal calcium levels, the perceptual problems disappear.

Evaluate your interventions. They were successful if the patient understands why he experiences stress and can verbalize his fears.

Altered neuromuscular status (tetany) related to hypocalcemia. Your goal: Raise serum calcium levels and prevent cardiopulmonary arrest. Give intravenous calcium: 10 to 20 ml of 10% calcium gluconate in 100 ml of dextrose 5% in water. Be sure the calcium I.V. does not infiltrate; calcium can cause tissue necrosis. If hypocalcemia does not resolve after several calcium doses, start a continuous I.V. calcium infusion. Monitor cardiac function continuously. Keep emergency equipment and a tracheostomy tray and endotracheal tube close by. Auscultate the lungs and elevate the head of the bed.

After serum calcium levels return to normal, maintain them within normal to low-normal limits. Provide a low-phosphorus, high-calcium diet including milk; milk products; green, leafy vegetables; sardines; and salmon.

(Remember, many foods high in calcium are also high in phosphates.) Calcium supplements, given one hour before meals, enhance absorption. If needed, give phosphate binders to raise serum calcium levels indirectly by binding phosphorus in the intestine. Give vitamin D to enhance calcium absorption. Stress frequent monitoring of calcium levels. Remember that hypocalcemia causes insensitivity to digitalis so that, if calcium levels rise rapidly, the patient may become digitoxic. If unstable calcium levels return, tetany could recur. Maintain an ongoing assessment for tetany; be prepared to institute emergency measures.

Evaluate your interventions. They were successful if the serum calcium returned to normal or low-normal levels; cardiac irritability, if any, did not cause dysrhythmia; adequate oxygenation was maintained; resuscitation measures, if needed, were correct; tetany did not return or was treated promptly; the patient understands home treatment measures.

Seizure activity related to profound neuromuscular irritability. Your goal: Prevent patient injury. Pad the bed's side rails. Keep anticonvulsant medications and emergency equipment available.

Evaluate your interventions. They were successful if the patient was free from injury.

Altered integument related to hypocalcemia. Your goal: Prevent complications. Lubricate the patient's skin; turn him frequently. Treat candidiasis with antifungal agents, as ordered. Do not apply heat directly to the skin.

Evaluate your interventions. They were successful if no complications developed.

Mental status changes related to hypocalcemic effects on the CNS. Your goal: Help the patient accept temporary mood swings and apathy. To enhance patient and family acceptance, convey your acceptance of the patient's mental changes. Provide reassurance; a quiet, nonstimulating environment; low lights; comfortable temperature and humidity; and rest alternating with moderate exercise.

Evaluate your interventions. They were successful if the patient conveyed his acceptance of his mental changes to you.

Decreased activity tolerance related to muscle spasm, weakness, and fatigue. Your goal: Increase activity tolerance. Prevent muscle spasm with heat and gentle positioning. Have the patient avoid positions, such as crossing the legs, that aggravate muscle spasm by putting pressure on motor nerves. Alternate periods of mild exercise and rest.

Evaluate your interventions. They were successful if the patient is able to do more than before and he rests between active periods.

Potential for postoperative complications. Your goal: Prevent or promptly correct complications.

Provide adequate oxygenation. Assess for respiratory obstruction because of neck edema resulting from surgery. Monitor for respiratory depth and ease and for dyspnea and cyanosis. Have the patient turn, cough, and use the incentive inspirometer (while you support his head) to prevent atelectasis and pneumonia. Encourage early ambulation. Give pain medications promptly to ease coughing.

Evaluate your interventions. They were successful if adequate oxygenation was maintained and the patient did not develop pneumonia.

Prevent hemorrhage related to surgery. Monitor neck dressings every 2 hours for excessive drainage. Note signs of hypovolemia: restlessness; cyanosis; pallor; cold, clammy skin; decreased urine output; increased pulse and respirations; decreased blood pressure. Monitor hematocrit and hemoglobin levels.

Evaluate your interventions. They were successful if no excessive blood loss occurred.

Prevent hypercalcemic crisis, resulting from PTH secretion during surgical manipulation of the parathyroids. Assess for hypercalcemic crisis (nausea, vomiting, anorexia, abdominal pain, weakness, thirst, dyspnea, and coma). Give nursing care for crisis, if needed.

Evaluate your interventions. They were successful if a hypercalcemic crisis did not occur or was treated properly.

Facilitate communication if laryngeal nerve damage has resulted from surgery. Give the patient paper and pen, and place the call light within his reach. Check the patient's voice quality every hour; damage shows as a low, cracking voice. Report this at once.

Evaluate your interventions. They were successful if no signs and symptoms of laryngeal nerve damage were noted and reported.

In conclusion

Good nursing care of patients with parathyroid dysfunction requires keen assessment skills to detect its early but subtle signs. Such care also requires meticulous attention to laboratory test results and prompt treatment for such complications as tetany. It always requires continuing effort to promote the patient's compliance with treatment and realistic acceptance of his condition.

Points to remember

• Parathyroid disorders result in abnormal secretion of or response to parathyroid hormone (PTH).
• These disorders may show only subtle physical and psychological signs, and they may mimic any number of other conditions. Serum levels of calcium may be the only indication of abnormality.
• Severe hypercalcemia, a medical emergency, needs saline diuresis to speed calcium excretion.
• Calcium gluconate may be needed to treat tetany and prevent seizures in acute hypothyroidism.
• In hypoparathyroidism, the physical exam may more accurately reflect pathology than do the serum calcium levels.

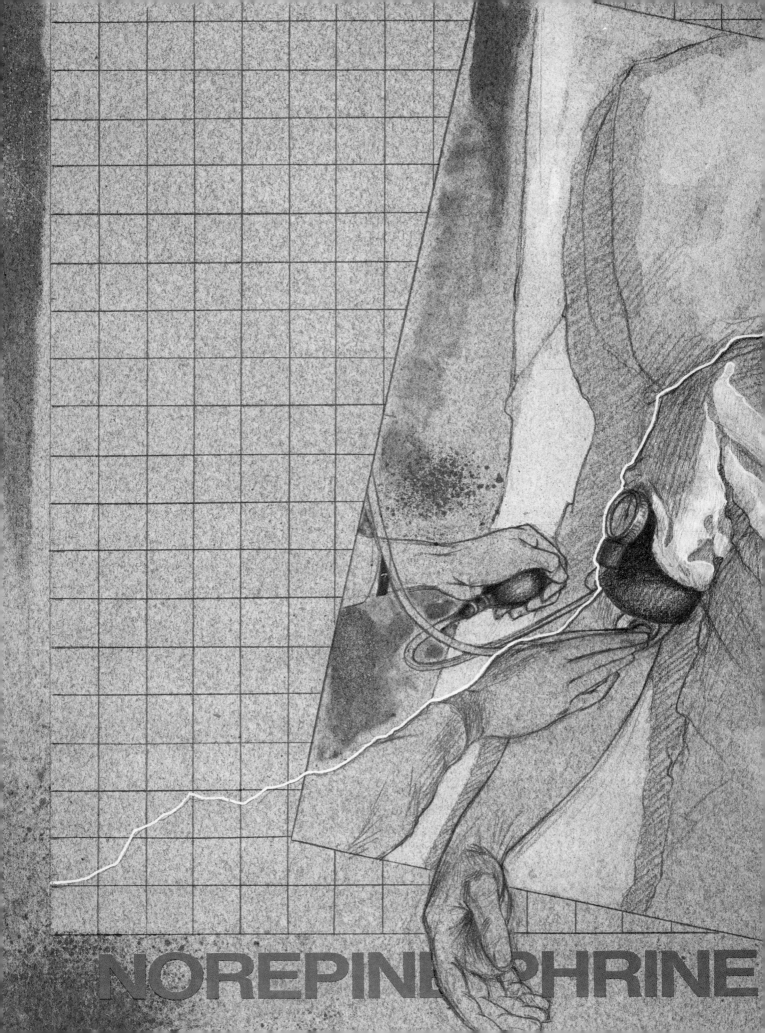

NOREPINEPHRINE

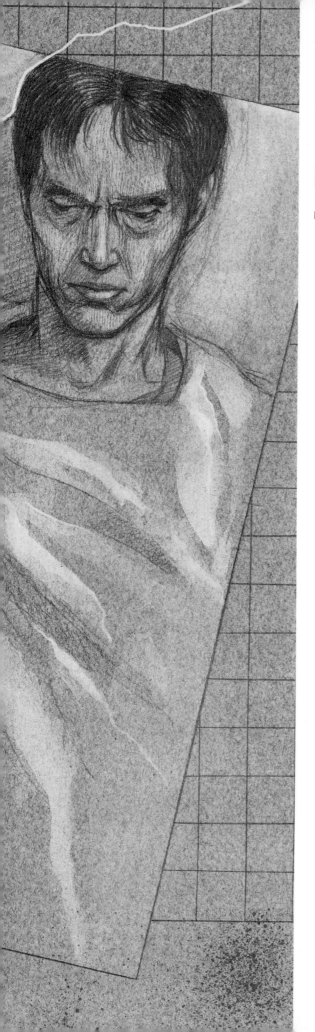

DISORDERS OF THE ADRENAL GLAND

8 FORESTALLING ADRENOCORTICAL EMERGENCIES

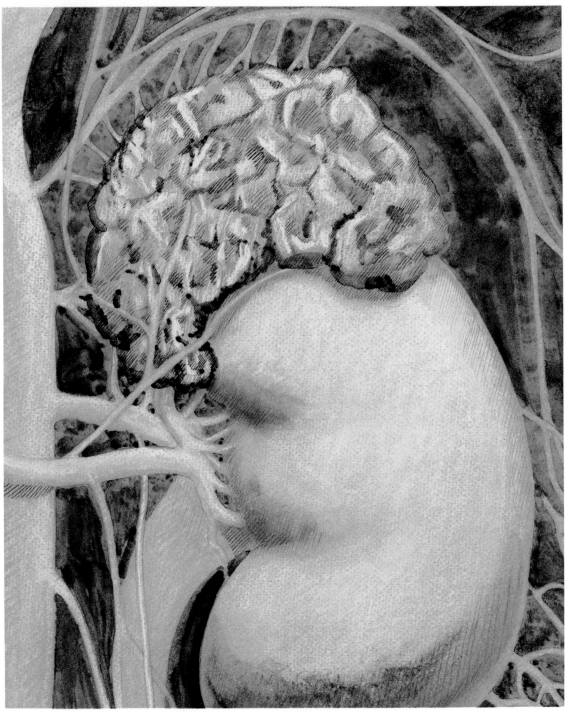

Hyperplasia of the adrenal cortex

The adrenal cortex produces more than 30 different hormones. Most help maintain the body's metabolic processes, and some affect sexual function. Because of this wide hormonal variety, any malfunction of this portion of the adrenal gland carries far-reaching consequences for the patient—social and psychological as well as physical. All these factors can challenge you to the utmost unless you're prepared to meet them with a good understanding of normal and abnormal adrenocortical function and with the necessary skills to achieve thorough assessment and effective intervention.

The adrenal cortex: What it does

The adrenal cortex secretes three types of corticosteroid hormones: glucocorticoids, mineralocorticoids, and sex steroids. *Glucocorticoids* regulate carbohydrate, fat, and protein metabolism and have anti-inflammatory effects; *mineralocorticoids* regulate mineral metabolism (especially electrolytes); and *sex steroids* (androgens and estrogens) have some effect on sexual function, but not nearly as much as the gonads. Of the 30 or more corticosteroids found in the adrenal cortex, only three principal hormones are involved in most cortical dysfunction. These hormones are the glucocorticoid *cortisol,* the mineralocorticoid *aldosterone,* and the *adrenogenital corticoids.* (See *Understanding corticosteroid secretion,* page 104.)

Effects of adrenocortical dysfunction

Adrenocortical *hypersecretion* produces distinct clinical syndromes, which may overlap if two or more hormone groups are involved. The most important hypersecretory disorders are Cushing's syndrome and Cushing's disease, which result from an overabundance of cortisol. Cushing's *disease* results from excessive secretion of adrenocorticotropic hormone (ACTH) by the pituitary. Cushing's *syndrome* results from secretion of ACTH by a nonpituitary neoplasm or from an adrenal tumor that secretes cortisol without ACTH secretion. Iatrogenic Cushing's syndrome may result from therapeutic glucocorticoid administration.

Excessive mineralocorticoid secretion produces primary or secondary hyperaldosteronism. Primary hyperaldosteronism usually results from unilateral adrenal adenoma and, less often, from bilateral adrenal hyperplasia. In secondary hyperaldosteronism, an extra-adrenal stimulus, such as overproduction of renin caused by renal artery stenosis, activates the excessive aldosterone secretion.

Adrenocortical *insufficiency,* also known as Addison's disease, occurs in primary and secondary forms. In primary adrenocortical insufficiency, both glucocorticoid and mineralocorticoid levels tend to be low, reflecting inadequate adrenal secretion of hormones. Its most common cause is idiopathic adrenal atrophy. Rarely, it may result from granulomatous destruction from tuberculosis, disseminated fungal infections, amyloidosis, adrenal infarction, or destruction of the gland by metastatic tumors.

Secondary adrenocortical insufficiency results from inadequate pituitary secretion of ACTH, which, in turn, results from pituitary tumor, infarction, infection, adrenalectomy, or radiation.

Aldosterone deficiency may occur in association with renin deficiency, heparin therapy (due to its inhibiting effect on a layer of the cortex), an inborn error of metabolism, removal of an aldosterone-secreting adenoma, or severe postural hypotension.

PATHOPHYSIOLOGY

Regardless of their causes, adrenal cortex hypersecretion and hyposecretion both produce widespread, significant changes in bodily function.

Cortisol hypersecretion

Excessive cortisol levels cause excess glucose production in the liver and increased destruction of body protein. Tissue proteins are degraded to amino acids, which provide fuel for gluconeogenesis. As larger amounts of mobilized amino acids reach the liver, this organ produces more glucose, which is released into the blood. Increased blood glucose may, in turn, cause hyperglycemia, or *diabetes.* At the same time, cells use less glucose because cortisol also interferes with insulin transport of glucose across the cell membrane.

As protein catabolism increases, protein synthesis decreases, probably because of diminished amino acid transport into extrahepatic tissues. The resultant protein loss can lead to muscular weakness, easy fatigability, and osteoporosis from wasting of the bone matrix (with possible fracture or collapse of vertebrae). In children, it can lead to retarded linear growth.

Renal sodium retention and potassium excretion promote potassium depletion. This combination of protein and potassium loss

Congenital adrenal hyperplasia: Rare causes

Deficiency of 21-hydroxylase
Causes adrenal insufficiency and, in the male fetus, incomplete differentiation of genitalia

Deficiency of 3-beta-hydroxysteroid dehydrogenase
Causes adrenal insufficiency and genital ambiguity in both sexes

Deficiency of 17-alpha-hydroxylase
Causes a curable form of hypertension and sexual infantilism

Deficiency of 18-hydroxysteroid dehydrogenase
Causes impaired aldosterone synthesis, resulting in excessive sodium loss, hypotension, dehydration, and fatigability

causes muscle weakness and atrophy. Potassium deficiency may also lead to cardiac dysrhythmias, such as the appearance of U waves, and renal disorders with impaired renal concentrating capacity. Eventually, hypertension predisposes to left ventricular hypertrophy, congestive heart failure, and stroke.

Protein breakdown also affects connective tissue, and the skin becomes thin and less resistant to trauma. Because of capillary fragility, the skin bruises easily, healing is delayed, and infection is more likely to occur. The face may show redness as facial vessels become visible. Polycythemia may also occur.

Chronic cortisol hypersecretion redistributes body fat, mobilizing it from the arms and legs and depositing it on the face, shoulders, trunk, and abdomen, thus producing the characteristic "moon face," "buffalo hump," and "truncal obesity." Striae develop as large accumulations of fatty tissue unduly stretch the thin skin.

Finally, excess cortisol secretion keeps the body in a chronic stress condition, and otherwise normal, beneficial reactions are so exaggerated as to become harmful. During tissue injury, cortisol stabilizes lysosomal membranes, thereby limiting the damaged cells' release of chemical substances (formed mostly in the lysosomes). Cortisol suppresses leukocyte adherence to the endothelial surface; diminishes leukocyte accumulation at the injury site; and impairs white blood cell migration, antibody formation, and lymphocyte proliferation, lessening the blood cells' ability to limit the spread of infection.

Aldosterone hypersecretion: Renal escape mechanism

Renal tubule epithelial cells respond to increased aldosterone by retaining sodium and excreting potassium, thus raising sodium levels and lowering potassium levels in the extracellular fluid.

Sodium retention increases extracellular volume, elevates blood pressure, and suppresses renin production. Edema seldom becomes overt, because sodium retention ceases after a certain point. Proximal tubular sodium reabsorption decreases; then sodium excretion increases. This is called the "renal escape mechanism." No such compensatory mechanism functions for potassium excretion, which may lead to hypokalemia and nephropathy. Hypokalemic alkalosis—marked by muscular weakness, fatigue, areflexia, tetany, and dysrhythmias—may also occur.

Sodium and potassium exchange transport occurs in other epithelialized organs as well as the kidneys, so that sodium-potassium ratios in perspiration, saliva, and GI secretions tend to be similar.

In addition to potassium, tubular secretion of hydrogen ions may also exchange with sodium, resulting in alkalosis. (See *Effects of hyperaldosteronism,* page 106.)

Congenital enzyme errors

Congenital adrenal hyperplasia results from an inborn error of the enzyme systems needed for cortisol synthesis. This error stimulates pituitary ACTH secretion, causing adrenal hyperplasia and increased steroid production. Within any one family, all the affected members seem to show the same defective enzyme. The most common causes of congenital adrenal hyperplasia are 21- and 11-beta-hydroxylase deficiencies characterized by excessive adrenal androgens under the ACTH drive induced by hypocortisolism. (See *Congenital adrenal hyperplasia: Rare causes.*)

However, many other enzymatic defects are possible, with resulting effects depending on where in the process of hormonal synthesis the defect appears. In virilizing syndrome, hypersecretion of testosterone starts in fetal life and continues after birth. In the female, ambiguous genitalia are evident at birth; in the male, abnormalities aren't evident until later. Rarely hyposecretion of testosterone prevents fusion of the scrotal folds, causing feminization of the male fetus.

Cortisol hyposecretion: Hypoglycemia

Impaired secretion of cortisol slows mobilization of tissue protein, thereby limiting the supply of amino acids available for glucose production. This slows gluconeogenesis, resulting in hypoglycemia; the blood glucose level falls between meals, when carbohydrates are not available.

Both urinary nitrogen excretion and gastric acid production are decreased, causing anorexia, nausea and vomiting, weight loss, weakness, and fatigue. At the same time, the lack of cortisol may sharpen the senses of taste, smell, and hearing.

In primary adrenocortical insufficiency, resulting from adrenal cortex hypofunction, diminished cortisol levels stimulate the pituitary gland to secrete ACTH and melanocyte-stimulating hormone (MSH). The latter causes hyperpigmentation, especially of the mucous

Understanding corticosteroid secretion

When blood corticosteroid levels are low, the hypothalamus secretes corticotropin-releasing factor (CRF), which stimulates the anterior pituitary gland to release adrenocorticotropic hormone (ACTH); this, in turn, stimulates the adrenal cortex to secrete corticosteroids as needed. When the blood contains an adequate or elevated concentration of corticosteroids, a negative feedback mechanism inhibits the hypothalamus from secreting CRF, which would otherwise trigger the sequence of secretion.

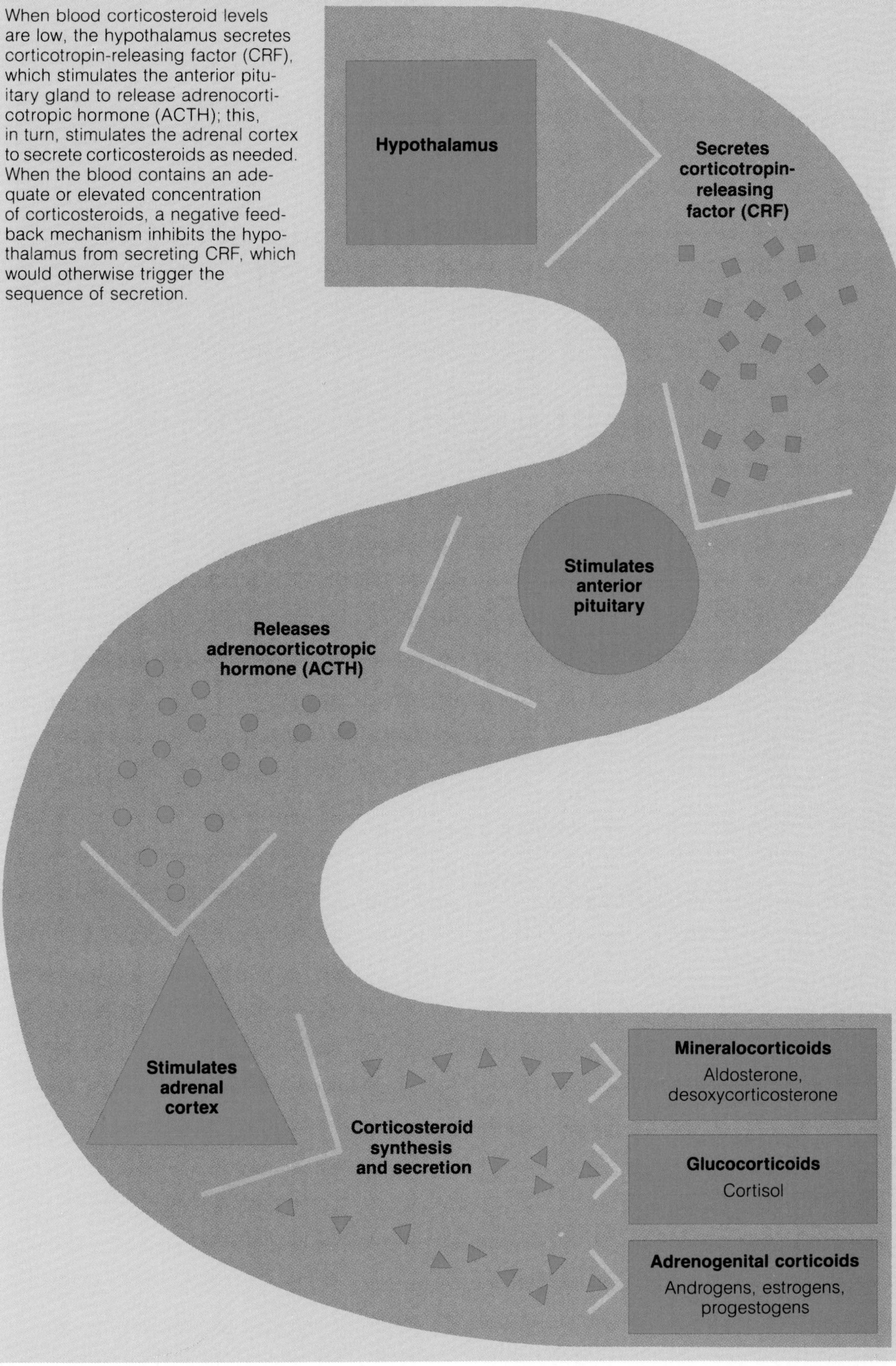

Hypothalamus

Secretes corticotropin-releasing factor (CRF)

Stimulates anterior pituitary

Releases adrenocorticotropic hormone (ACTH)

Stimulates adrenal cortex

Corticosteroid synthesis and secretion

Mineralocorticoids
Aldosterone, desoxycorticosterone

Glucocorticoids
Cortisol

Adrenogenital corticoids
Androgens, estrogens, progestogens

Effects of hyperaldosteronism

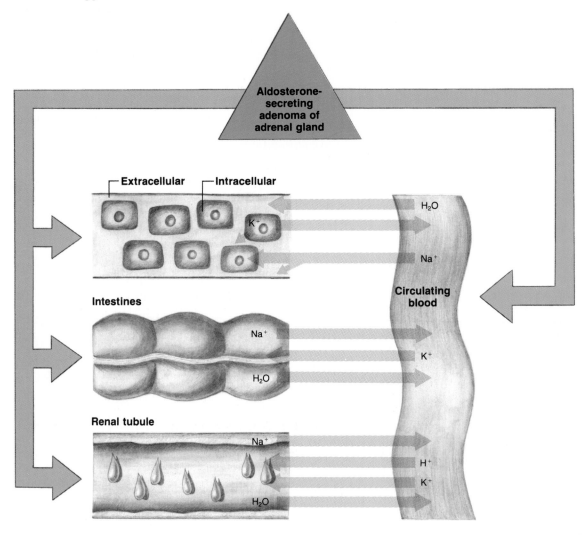

Excessive aldosterone secretion can result from a secreting adenoma (shown here) and many other disorders. Regardless of its cause, excessive secretion results in the movement of water and sodium, potassium, and hydrogen ions as shown. This eventually leads to sodium retention and potassium excretion.

membranes, areolae, and surgical scars. Darker pigmentation appears in skin folds, while blue-black patches appear on the mucous membranes. Other skin areas take on a characteristic tanned appearance. When the disorder results from ACTH deficiency (secondary adrenocortical insufficiency), the skin becomes paler, because MSH may also be diminished.

When adrenal cortex hypofunction decreases both glucocorticoid and mineralocorticoid levels, salt and water depletion may occur. If nausea and vomiting prevent adequate fluid intake, dehydration and hypovolemia may follow, precipitating a crisis in which peripheral vascular collapse leads to hypotension, followed by coma and renal shutdown. Because a patient with adrenocortical insufficiency cannot handle stress, even a simple infection or minor injury can precipitate such a potentially fatal crisis.

Aldosterone hyposecretion: Metabolic acidosis

The adrenal cortex's inability to increase aldosterone secretion in response to diminished sodium levels is the major problem in aldosterone hyposecretion. Sodium is now excreted, potassium is retained, and the potassium clearance decreases greatly. Hyperkalemia can lead to cardiac disturbances; extremely high potassium levels may cause cardiac arrest. Also, potassium retention promotes reabsorption of hydrogen ions, eventually leading to metabolic acidosis.

Aldosterone's absence also affects other organs—sodium and water are lost in the stool, urine, and perspiration. Sodium wasting depletes the extracellular fluid volume, resulting in dehydration and hypotension. Cardiac output falls and heart size may diminish. Hypotension may become so severe and heart action so weak that circulatory collapse and shock occur.

MEDICAL MANAGEMENT

To diagnose adrenal cortex disorders, a thorough history and physical examination are essential. Correct diagnosis also requires a careful assessment of symptoms; X-ray studies; plasma and urine tests; and stimulation, suppression, and pituitary-adrenal responsiveness tests. After diagnosis, treatment can include surgery, radiation, and drug therapy for adrenocortical hyperfunction, as well as hormonal replacement for hypofunction.

Blood tests evaluate adrenal function

Evaluation of adrenal function begins with determination of the plasma cortisol level. Normally, pituitary-adrenal rhythms are governed by a biological clock; in individuals who sleep during the night, ACTH secretions are higher early in the morning. Therefore, cortisol secretion, plasma cortisol concentration, and 17-hydroxycorticosteroid (17-OHCS) excretion normally follow a diurnal rhythm.

In Cushing's syndrome, plasma cortisol levels rise and usually fail to follow their normal diurnal pattern. Remember, however, that plasma cortisol also increases during acute illness, trauma, surgery, or treatment with certain drugs.

In adrenocortical insufficiency, cortisol levels may be low but still within the normal range.

In Cushing's syndrome, a suppressed plasma ACTH level is diagnostic of primary glucocorticoid-producing adrenal gland tumor. With pituitary hypersecretion, plasma ACTH levels are in the normal range but cortisol levels are elevated. With ectopic ACTH syndrome, plasma ACTH concentrations are markedly elevated, just as they are in adrenal insufficiency.

The plasma renin activity (PRA) test may also help identify adrenal dysfunction. Renin catalyzes the conversion of a polypeptide to angiotensin I. Angiotensin I is then converted to angiotensin II, which is responsible for promoting aldosterone synthesis from the adrenal cortex. Therefore, this test can help to determine aldosterone abnormalities. Indexing renin levels against urinary sodium excretion can identify primary aldosteronism. The test

must be done under controlled conditions because dietary sodium and activity influence the results.

In the patient with inappropriate aldosterone secretion, plasma aldosterone levels can be studied along with PRA. In aldosterone-secreting adenoma (Conn's syndrome), plasma aldosterone levels are increased, while in congenital adrenal hyperplasia, levels are usually normal or reduced. In adrenocortical insufficiency, aldosterone secretion is usually low because of adrenal cortex hypofunction.

Precursors of both cortisol and aldosterone (such as 11-deoxycortisol) can be assayed in plasma, although methods to assay cortisol and aldosterone are not widely available. Concentrations of these steroids may be elevated in congenital adrenal biosynthetic defects and adrenal carcinomas.

Electrolyte and glucose levels must be routinely checked in suspected adrenocortical dysfunction. Depressed serum potassium levels can indicate possible hyperfunction, such as occurs in Cushing's syndrome or aldosteronism. Depressed sodium and elevated potassium levels indicate hyposecretion such as occurs in adrenocortical insufficiency. Depressed blood glucose levels suggest adrenal insufficiency, while high levels may indicate Cushing's syndrome.

Urine tests: Clues to steroid production

Twenty-four-hour urine tests reliably measure steroid levels and provide important information about overall steroid production.

For reliable urine test results, renal and hepatic function must be normal. In renal failure, cortisol metabolites are not excreted, and their accumulation inhibits new metabolite formation, so that cortisol production eventually diminishes. Hepatic disease may alter steroid urine test results by favoring abnormal pathways for steroid metabolism.

The 24-hour test for 17-OHCS measures levels of cortisol, cortisone, and 11-deoxycortisol, among other steroids. Elevated urine levels may indicate hyperadrenalism but can appear in many disorders and are also associated with various drugs.

The urine 17-ketosteroids (17-KS) are weak anabolic androgens that are markedly elevated in adrenogenital virilizing syndromes. Thus, both the 17-KS test and suppression tests are required to verify adrenal disorders.

In congenital adrenal hyperplasia in infants and children due to defects in the c-21 hydroxylase enzyme, urine 17-KS excretion in-

Diagnostic test sequence for adrenocortical insufficiency

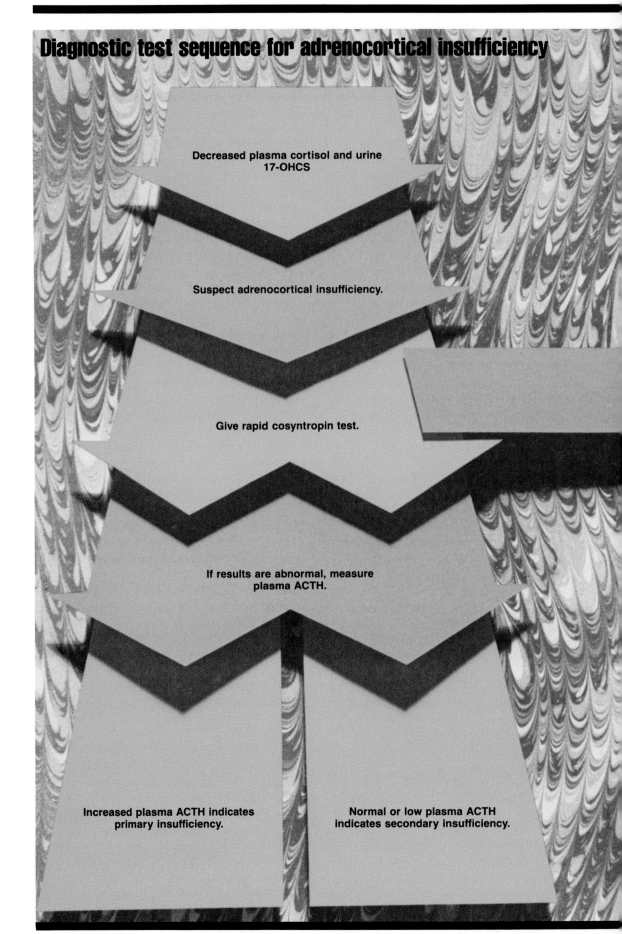

Decreased plasma cortisol and urine 17-OHCS

Suspect adrenocortical insufficiency.

Give rapid cosyntropin test.

If results are abnormal, measure plasma ACTH.

Increased plasma ACTH indicates primary insufficiency.

Normal or low plasma ACTH indicates secondary insufficiency.

creases, and 17-alpha-hydroxyprogesterone levels increase along with its metabolite, pregnanetriol.

Urine 17-KS may be low or absent in severe adrenal insufficiency. However, certain drugs may interfere with the test results' reliability.

Although less than 1% of the total cortisol secreted by the adrenals is excreted unchanged in the urine, measuring this amount can give useful information concerning hyposecretion or hypersecretion. Elevated levels are nearly always found in spontaneous Cushing's syndrome and during acute illness, pregnancy, and other physical stresses. Decreased levels, however, do not conclusively indicate adrenal insufficiency.

Urinary aldosterone levels may also be checked. An elevated aldosterone secretion rate, urinary aldosterone excretion rate, and plasma aldosterone concentrations indicate primary or secondary aldosteronism. Suppressed renin activity with a high aldosterone level indicates primary aldosteronism.

Stimulation tests: Useful screening
One screening test for adrenal deficiency is the rapid ACTH (cosyntropin) test. In this test, a baseline plasma cortisol level is obtained; then cosyntropin (synthetic 1-24 ACTH) is given I.V. or I.M. immediately. Blood samples for plasma cortisol evaluation are drawn again 30 and 60 minutes later. A positive response (rise in cortisol levels) rules out adrenocortical insufficiency, because ACTH normally elevates cortisol levels.

If cortisol levels fail to rise after the rapid ACTH test, the standard ACTH test is needed. More time-consuming than the cosyntropin test, the standard ACTH test usually involves obtaining a 24-hour urine specimen for 17-OHCS and giving cosyntropin intravenously for 8 hours over 3 consecutive days with concurrent 24-hour urine collections for 17-OHCS.

In primary adrenocortical insufficiency, urinary 17-OHCS levels fail to increase even with repeated stimulation. If the patient has adrenocortical insufficiency, he must be monitored closely during the test, because the test may further compromise his adrenal secretory capacity. A patient with secondary adrenocortical insufficiency shows a stepwise increment of urine steroid levels on successive days of stimulation, ending at about three times the base level on the third day. (See *Diagnostic test sequence for adrenocortical insufficiency*.)

Normal results rule out primary insufficiency.

To check for secondary insufficiency, give metyrapone test.

Abnormal results indicate secondary insufficiency.

Normal results rule out secondary insufficiency.

Diagnostic test sequence for Cushing's syndrome

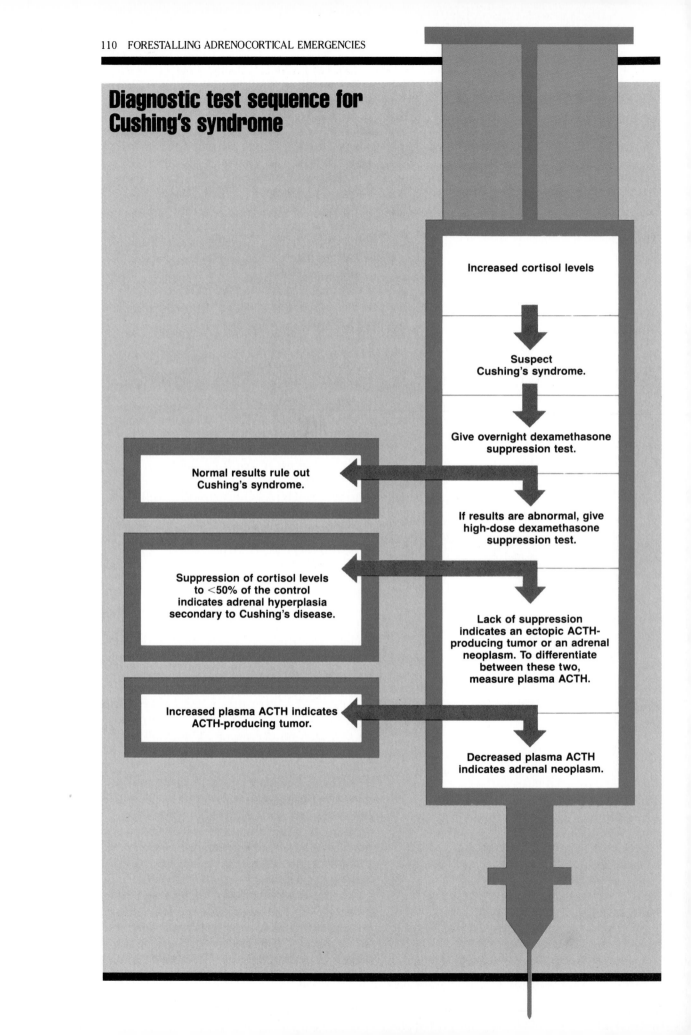

Increased cortisol levels

Suspect
Cushing's syndrome.

Give overnight dexamethasone
suppression test.

Normal results rule out
Cushing's syndrome.

If results are abnormal, give
high-dose dexamethasone
suppression test.

Suppression of cortisol levels
to <50% of the control
indicates adrenal hyperplasia
secondary to Cushing's disease.

Lack of suppression
indicates an ectopic ACTH-
producing tumor or an adrenal
neoplasm. To differentiate
between these two,
measure plasma ACTH.

Increased plasma ACTH indicates
ACTH-producing tumor.

Decreased plasma ACTH
indicates adrenal neoplasm.

In a patient with primary hyperaldosteronism, plasma aldosterone levels are elevated and plasma renin activity is low. Failure to increase plasma renin levels with sodium restriction and/or diuretics tends to confirm the diagnosis.

Suppression tests

If test results suggest adrenocortical hypersecretion, suppression tests are required. One screening method for preliminary evaluation of Cushing's syndrome is the overnight dexamethasone (Decadron) suppression test. Dexamethasone is given orally at midnight. The next morning blood is drawn to obtain a plasma cortisol level. If secretion is normal, this test suppresses plasma cortisol to below 5 mcg/dl. In Cushing's syndrome, the plasma cortisol level is not suppressed. However, stress and certain drugs such as diphenylhydantoin can interfere with results of this test.

A high-dose dexamethasone test may also be helpful. This usually involves a baseline 24-hour collection for 17-OHCS, followed by dexamethasone administration over 48 hours with simultaneous 24-hour urine collections for 17-OHCS. The 17-OHCS levels are suppressed to less than 50% of baseline values in Cushing's disease. (See *Diagnostic test sequence for Cushing's syndrome,* page 110.)

A mineralocorticoid suppression test may determine aldosterone abnormalities. Blood is drawn after infusing isotonic saline solution intravenously. In primary aldosteronism, volume expansion elicits no response because the renin-angiotensin system is already suppressed. Thus, plasma aldosterone concentration in adenoma or idiopathic hyperplasia will not be suppressed.

In the test known as the DOCA maneuver, the patient is maintained on a normal- or high-sodium intake; then desoxycorticosterone acetate is given over 3 to 5 days. High aldosterone levels that persist despite the DOCA maneuver indicate primary aldosteronism.

Special tests evaluate ACTH secretion

Certain laboratory tests can help assess responsiveness of the hypothalamic-pituitary-adrenal axis. Because insulin-induced hypoglycemia, arginine, vasopressin, and pyrogen all cause release of ACTH, their effects on glucocorticoid levels indicate ACTH response and thus determine the status of pituitary ACTH.

Metyrapone is also used to test ACTH responsiveness. This drug inhibits a hydroxylating enzyme, which eventually decreases cortisol blood levels, stimulating ACTH secretion. The increased ACTH stimulates the adrenal cortex to release cortisol. This test reliably evaluates the anterior pituitary's reserve capacity to release ACTH.

Radiographic tests detect tumors

Noninvasive procedures such as computerized tomography and ultrasonography of the adrenal glands are often used to localize well-developed tumors. Invasive tests, such as arteriography, venography, or nuclear scan techniques, may also be used to detect tumors.

Treating hyperfunction: Surgery, radiation, and drugs

Surgery, radiation, and drug therapy all have a place in the treatment of adrenal cortex hyperfunction.

Surgery may be indicated in adrenal gland hyperfunction. In adrenal-induced Cushing's syndrome and in primary aldosteronism, a unilateral adrenalectomy may be done; in many patients, the remaining gland regains normal function after several months. Steroid therapy is necessary in the interim. When bilateral adrenalectomy is necessary, patients need lifetime treatment with glucocorticoids and mineralocorticoids.

Cortisol hypersecretion caused by pituitary hypersecretion of ACTH is now often treated by transsphenoidal removal of a microadenoma. But, when diagnostic tests fail to locate the microadenoma because of its minute size or obscure location, hypophysectomy may be required. After hypophysectomy, the patient will need treatment with glucocorticoids.

If an ectopic tumor is causing the disorder, it is surgically removed. In congenital adrenal hyperplasia, surgery may be needed to correct genital abnormalities.

Radiation is used to treat bilateral hyperplasia or to help prevent postoperative Nelson's syndrome (progression of an ACTH-secreting adenoma, which may appear 2 to 3 years after bilateral adrenalectomy). Radiation may be applied internally or externally.

Internal radiation is applied through transsphenoidal implantation of radioactive pellets. Conventional external radiation is administered over several weeks. In some centers, another form of external radiation called alpha particle or proton beam radiation is used. Because proton beam radiation allows for a more sharpened focus, it doesn't damage surrounding structures.

Both forms of external radiation are not recommended for severe hyperplasia because of the lag time between treatment and remission and because the remission rate is less than 50%. And both internal and proton beam radiation may cause complications, such as ocular nerve palsy and hypopituitarism.

Drugs that interfere with adrenal hormone synthesis or ACTH production may be used to treat adrenal hyperfunction. When adrenal metastatic or residual disease remains, mitotane is most commonly used to treat hypercortisolism. This drug suppresses cortisol production and decreases plasma and urine steroid levels by destroying the mitochondria of cells within the two inner layers of the adrenal cortex—in effect performing a "medical adrenalectomy." The adrenal enzyme inhibitors metyrapone and aminoglutethimide are also used because they inhibit cortisol synthesis.

Other less commonly used drugs in adrenocortical hyperfunction include cyproheptadine and bromocriptine. Cyproheptadine, a serotonin antagonist, and bromocriptine, a dopamine agonist, interfere with ACTH secretion and are therefore effective only in treating pituitary Cushing's syndrome.

Primary aldosteronism may be treated with dietary sodium restriction and the aldosterone antagonist spironolactone. Triamterene may also be helpful. This distal potassium-sparing diuretic affects the renal tubule by inhibiting sodium reabsorption independent of aldosterone.

The treatment of choice in congenital adrenal hyperplasia is daily doses of glucocorticoids (dexamethasone, prednisone, or cortisone) to suppress pituitary ACTH secretion. Children with salt-wasting defects may need salt-deficit correction plus small doses of a potent mineralocorticoid such as 9-alpha-fluorohydrocortisone.

Hormone replacement for hypofunction
Treatment of adrenal gland hypofunction requires replacement of deficient hormones to meet the body's metabolic requirements.

In primary adrenocortical deficiency, replacing both glucocorticoids and mineralocorticoids is usually necessary. Cortisone is the major glucocorticoid drug used and is usually given in two daily doses to mimic the body's diurnal variation in cortisol secretion. Supplemental therapy controls electrolyte balance.

For mineralocorticoid replacement, the synthetic drug 9-alpha-fluorohydrocortisone is also given. The steroid dosages should be increased whenever the patient is under stress. Also, his salt intake should be increased during hot weather, exercise that results in sweating, or GI upsets.

Secondary adrenocortical insufficiency also requires glucocorticoid therapy. It doesn't usually require mineralocorticoid therapy because this condition doesn't affect aldosterone secretion.

In hypoaldosteronism, aldosterone secretion cannot be increased appropriately during severe salt restriction. However, treatment with potent mineralocorticoids, such as 9-alpha-fluorohydrocortisone, can reverse salt wasting and restore electrolyte balance.

Treating complications of hypofunction
Acute adrenal insufficiency poses a medical emergency and must be treated immediately. This crisis may follow infection, trauma, GI upsets, or any form of stress that requires an immediate increase of adrenocortical hormones in the patient with adrenocortical insufficiency; it may also follow abrupt withdrawal of corticosteroids from a patient with chronic insufficiency after prolonged replacement therapy. Symptoms of acute adrenal crisis may range from headaches to listlessness and lethargy, mental fatigue and physical weakness, nausea and vomiting, and intractable abdominal pain. If untreated, vascular collapse and shock may quickly follow. Treatment consists of rapidly elevating circulating glucocorticoids and immediately replacing the sodium and water deficit by infusing cortisone and saline solution as rapidly as possible.

Another acute crisis, adrenal hemorrhage, usually accompanies overwhelming septicemia (Waterhouse-Friderichsen syndrome), although it may occur with other disorders. (Septicemia usually results from meningococcemia.) Its fulminating onset—characterized by chills, headache, vertigo, vomiting, and prostration—is followed by a rash that progresses to extensive purpura. Circulatory collapse then follows, leading to death in 6 to 48 hours. Immediate treatment includes vigorous antibiotic therapy to control infection, intravenous vasopressors, and massive doses of steroids.

NURSING MANAGEMENT
Now that you can picture the systemic effects of cortisone, aldosterone, and androgens and understand the changes that follow hyposecretion or hypersecretion of these hormones,

CT scan showing adrenal adenoma

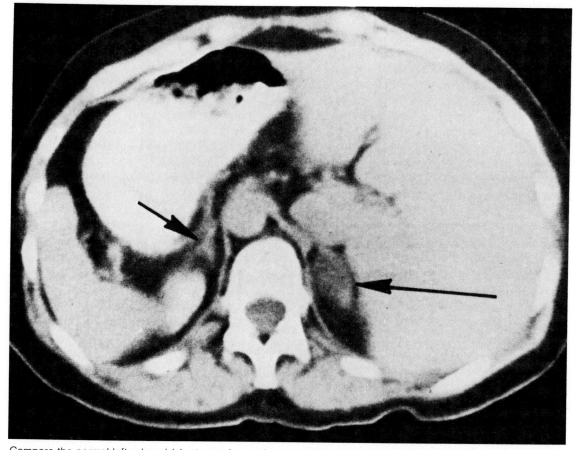

Compare the normal left adrenal (short arrow) near the stomach to the nonfunctioning right adrenal adenoma (long arrow) near the liver margin.

you're better able to take a detailed patient history and perform a thorough physical examination. Then, after collecting this subjective and objective data, you'll be ready to form nursing diagnoses, set care goals, and plan and evaluate your interventions.

Take detailed patient history

In your nursing history, try to find out how the patient is tolerating his hormonal imbalance, both physically and emotionally. For example, since cortisol and aldosterone hypersecretion as well as adrenocortical insufficiency bring on muscle weakness, you should ask how far the patient can walk without feeling tired. Ask him to tell you what daily activities seem to be too difficult or tiring.

Has he ever had osteoporosis, fractures, or back problems? These conditions could be due to wasting of the bone matrix in Cushing's syndrome.

Because cortisol hypersecretion can cause extreme emotional lability, observe the patient for signs of depression, irritability, or confusion. Also, does the patient suffer frequent

headaches? That could indicate primary aldosteronism.

Has the patient noticed any changes in his physical appearance? If so, have him describe them. Listen carefully for changes in verbal tones, pauses, sighs, hesitations, or even an abrupt change of subject—subtle clues that signal the patient's disturbed feelings concerning body image. Excess androgen production can cause masculinization in the female patient, making her feel embarrassed, angry, and concerned about her femininity. Ask about her menstrual cycle (oligomenorrhea or amenorrhea are common with adrenal dysfunction). Ask about frequency of urination and thirst. In aldosteronism, polydipsia usually follows polyuria because of impaired renal concentrating ability.

Ask if the patient bruises easily. Excessive secretion of cortisol, as you recall, causes capillary fragility so that small bumps or injuries may easily produce a widespread ecchymotic area.

Ask the patient about anorexia, nausea, vomiting, abdominal pain, and diarrhea. Such

GI disturbances are common in hypocortisolism. Has the patient lost weight over the past few weeks or months? Since the onset of adrenocortical insufficiency is slow and subtle, the patient may not know when his disease actually began, but he can tell when he began to notice the symptoms. Ask the patient if he experiences faintness, sweating, or dizziness when he skips meals.

Of course, if the patient has been admitted to the hospital with acute adrenal insufficiency and is severely compromised hemodynamically, your first priority must be to stabilize vital signs. Your nursing history can wait until the patient has responded to initial emergency therapy.

Be sure to get a family history, especially pertaining to adrenal disorders. Also be sure to get a psychosocial history and an accurate medical history (which may uncover, for example, overmedication with cortisol).

Perform the physical exam
Begin your physical examination by assessing vital signs. Remember that elevated blood pressure may indicate hyperaldosteronism or hypercortisolism, while low pressure or weak pulse may indicate hypocortisolism.

Observe the patient for hirsutism. A patient with cortisol hypersecretion may have a fine downy coat over his face and upper body. Excessive androgen production causes coarsening of body hair and can be accompanied by thinning or balding of scalp hair.

Notice the patient's weight distribution, because secretory dysfunction can affect it severely. Does he have a moon face, buffalo hump, or truncal obesity? Because of protein wasting and decreased muscle mass, the patient's arms and legs may be unusually thin.

Examine your patient's skin for characteristic signs of adrenal dysfunction, such as excessive bruising and petechiae. These signs occur because of capillary weakness resulting from protein loss and from loss of perivascular collagen support. Polycythemia may produce facial redness.

Adrenal cortex hyposecretion can cause pigmentation changes such as vitiligo, irregular patchy areas of depigmentation surrounded by highly pigmented skin. In cortisol hyposecretion, a compensatory mechanism increases MSH production, exaggerating skin pigmentation. An unusually persistent tanning following sun exposure darkens progressively to diffuse brown, tan, or bronze, especially on the hands, face, neck, arms, pressure points, recent scars, palm creases, and normally pigmented areas such as nipples and genitalia. Bluish black patches may appear on the buccal mucosa.

Look for striae, another common manifestation of cortisol hypersecretion. These wide purple bands usually appear on the breasts, abdomen, shoulders, and hips—areas where the underlying fat accumulation has stretched the weakened skin. Their unique coloring comes from polycythemia and skin fragility due to protein loss, which makes the capillaries quite visible. Roughened skin with acne may indicate androgen excess.

A patient with hypercortisolism is likely to look edematous and puffy because of sodium and water retention. However, a patient with aldosteronism may not show overt edema because of increased urine output (potassium excretion is accompanied by large amounts of water) and the renal escape mechanism.

Check the patient's arms and legs. A patient with hyperaldosteronism may experience episodic muscular weakness as well as tetany and paresthesia secondary to hypokalemia and alkalosis.

Observe the breasts of a patient with suspected congenital adrenal hyperplasia. Look for gynecomastia in a male, diminished breast size in a female. Assess the genitalia. Is development normal for the patient's age and sex? In a newborn girl, has excessive androgen secretion caused ambiguous genitalia? In an adult woman, assess for clitoral enlargement as well as for virilization (increased muscle mass and a deepened voice). Although virilizing symptoms may be difficult to detect in the adult male, assess for sexual precocity and short stature; review test results.

Be sure to review the results of all diagnostic tests. For example, serum electrolyte imbalance or abnormal X-ray findings can help you determine the cause of adrenocortical dysfunction. Also check for electrocardiographic abnormalities resulting from potassium disturbances.

Develop nursing diagnoses
Successful management of the patient with adrenocortical dysfunction depends on the nursing diagnoses you formulate and on the goals and nursing interventions you choose to help the patient's recovery. Use all available data—laboratory test results, patient history, and physical examination—to help formulate nursing diagnoses.

Potential adrenal crisis related to cortisol

and aldosterone insufficiency. To prevent this life-threatening crisis, you need to assess vital signs frequently and to assess level of consciousness and GI function. Pay close attention if the patient complains of headaches, which could be the first sign of impending adrenal crisis. Monitor laboratory studies (particularly electrolyte and hormone levels). A pattern of decreasing sodium and cortisol with increasing potassium signals potential problems. Report such findings promptly. Be sure the patient receives the drugs ordered. Keep him away from stressful situations, and take precautions to prevent infection.

Evaluate your interventions. Consider them successful if adrenal crisis was avoided, vital signs are normal, the patient is alert, GI function appears normal, laboratory values are within normal limits, stress was avoided, and follow-up of patient complaints leads to prompt and effective treatment.

Disturbance in self-concept related to hormonal imbalance. Your goals are to help the patient accept an altered body image and to encourage him to understand the differences between normal and abnormal function. To achieve these goals, explain the normal anatomy and physiology and relevant pathophysiology in terms the patient can understand. Encourage him to express his feelings. Offer support and show acceptance. Remind the patient that others with the same disorder have learned to live with it and that treatment may relieve some of its distressing effects. Assist with activities the patient can't manage himself. Enhance the patient's self-image by encouraging him to be more independent when he is ready.

Consider your interventions successful if the patient understands the pathophysiology of his illness, asks appropriate questions about it, and realistically accepts his altered body image.

Potential for injury related to loss of bone matrix and abnormal fat distribution. To help the patient avoid injury, be sure the floor in his room is kept clean, uncluttered, and dry. If the patient can walk, encourage the use of a walker or cane to improve balance. Instruct him always to use the handrails in the bathroom when getting on or off the toilet. Encourage the patient to wear properly fitted low-heeled shoes or closed slippers that provide stability.

You can be sure your teaching has been effective if the patient complies with your suggestions and avoids injury.

Impaired mobility related to excessive protein catabolism. You know the patient needs to be as physically active as possible but must avoid injury. Thus, you should plan appropriate rest periods following moderate exercise. Also, help the patient understand and accept his physical limitations.

Consider the patient's response to therapy positive if he allows sufficient rest between activity periods and realizes the limitations his disease imposes.

Knowledge deficit related to treatment of an adrenocortical disorder. Your goal is to ensure that the patient is aware of the treatment options available to him. To help him acquire this knowledge, explain the methods, rationale, and expected effects of surgery, radiation, drug therapy, and diet restrictions. Answer questions without giving false hope. Be sure the patient realizes that hormone replacement must continue for life, that dosages must be adjusted in times of stress, and that he will need to wear a "medical alert" identification bracelet.

Consider your interventions successful if the patient discusses treatment options and asks appropriate questions; if he or his family administers the drug properly and understands the dosage, effects, and side effects; and if he obtains and wears the medical alert bracelet.

Potential for bruising and skin trauma related to capillary and protein wasting. Your goals are to prevent petechial hemorrhage and maintain skin integrity. To achieve these goals, try to avoid excessive venipuncture. Apply firm pressure and observe the site frequently after necessary venipuncture. To prevent further skin trauma, use special hypoallergenic or paper tape when necessary after venipuncture. Avoid prolonged overinflation or repeated inflations of the blood pressure cuff. Also, tell the patient to avoid wearing constrictive clothing.

After effective teaching of appropriate skin care, the patient's skin should remain intact and it should be free of petechiae.

A last word

Good nursing care of the patient with an adrenal cortex dysfunction requires that you be particularly alert for subtle physical changes that can rapidly threaten the patient's life. Be especially understanding and supportive when this illness causes distressing changes in body image that threaten the patient's psyche.

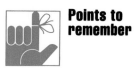

Points to remember

- Adrenal hypersecretion can result in Cushing's syndrome or disease, hyperaldosteronism, or virilization.
- Adrenocortical insufficiency, also known as Addison's disease, occurs in primary and secondary forms.
- A patient with adrenal insufficiency requires lifelong hormone replacement and should wear a medical alert bracelet.
- Acute adrenal insufficiency constitutes an adrenal crisis, a medical emergency requiring rapid glucocorticoid and saline solution administration.

9 RECOGNIZING PHEOCHROMOCYTOMA

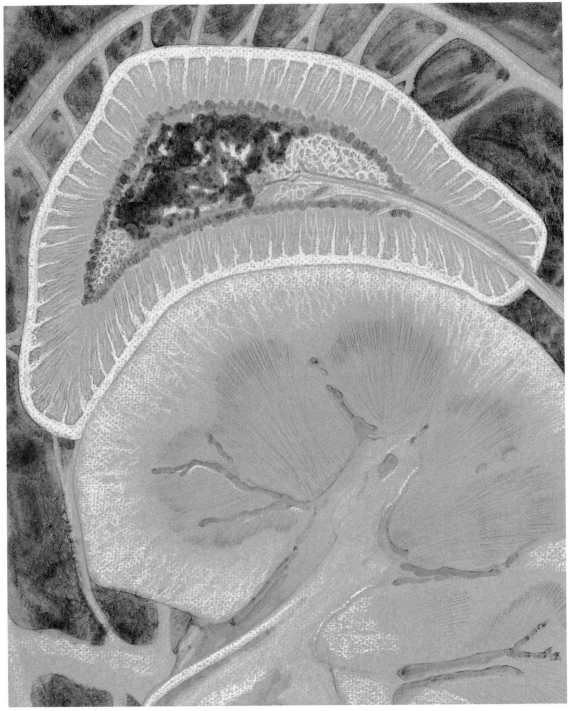

Pheochromocytoma of the adrenal medulla

Although the adrenal cortex and medulla are both parts of the same gland, their functions are vastly different. The cortex secretes steroid hormones essential for controlling fluid and electrolyte balance. The medulla, however, produces the catecholamines epinephrine and norepinephrine, which are normally secreted in small amounts to maintain blood vessel tone. The medulla normally secretes these hormones in large amounts only in times of physical or emotional stress.

Occasionally, though, the medulla secretes excessive amounts of catecholamines at inappropriate times, putting the body in an almost constant state of stress. This hypersecretion results from a rare, potentially fatal tumor of the adrenal medulla, called a pheochromocytoma, and can lead to spontaneous cerebrovascular accident or cardiovascular crisis if untreated. Unfortunately, signs and symptoms of pheochromocytoma are so diffuse that they're often attributed to other diseases, and many patients who could be cured by surgery are identified only after cardiovascular crisis.

But even though pheochromocytoma mimics other diseases, one sign is classic—paroxysmal attacks of hypertension, usually accompanied by headaches, diaphoresis, palpitations, and chest pain. And this is where your assessment skills come into play. Since you'll be taking the patient's vital signs and observing him closely, no one's in a better position than you to recognize a paroxysmal hypertensive attack. Obviously, then, to achieve accurate assessment and develop an appropriate care plan, you'll need to know as much about pheochromocytoma as possible—its other signs and symptoms, current diagnostic tests, and treatments. This knowledge will also help you provide effective patient teaching, because the more your patient knows about his disease, the less anxious he'll be.

What is pheochromocytoma?

A pheochromocytoma is a chromaffin-cell tumor that secretes an excess of epinephrine and norepinephrine. (See *The inside story,* page 118.) More than 95% of these tumors occur in the abdominal and pelvic cavities, with the majority being located in the adrenal medulla. Typically, the tumor is unilateral, well encapsulated, and benign, but it may be malignant in up to 10% of patients. For the tumor to be classified as malignant, metastasis must have occurred in areas where chromaffin tissue doesn't normally grow.

Pheochromocytoma may result from an inherited autosomal dominant trait and occurs frequently in association with multiple endocrine neoplasia (MEN-II). It also accompanies certain other diseases, such as neurofibromatosis. It affects all races and both sexes. Even though it's most common between ages 40 and 60, it does occur in children, who are more likely to have bilateral, multiple, or extraadrenal tumors. Pheochromocytoma may cause up to 1% of all cases of hypertension, although symptoms may persist for years before a confirming diagnosis is made.

In benign tumors (95%), prognosis after surgery is good—less than 5% mortality. However, in malignant tumors the 5-year survival rate is less than 50%.

PATHOPHYSIOLOGY

Although pheochromocytoma's cause is unknown, the tumor does evolve from chromaffin cells, which are widespread during fetal life. After birth, however, most chromaffin cells degenerate and disappear, and the majority of those which persist form the adrenal medulla. Consequently, more than 90% of these tumors occur in the adrenal medulla.

Normally, the medulla contains about 80% epinephrine and 20% norepinephrine stored in different types of chromaffin cells. However, pheochromocytoma alters this ratio and raises total catecholamine levels from the normal 0.10 to 0.75 mg/g of tissue to 8.51 to 9.12 mg/g of tissue.

What happens when the medulla secretes an excess of catecholamines? Norepinephrine and epinephrine adversely affect various organs by interacting with alpha and beta receptors in cell membranes. Norepinephrine excites mainly alpha receptors, while epinephrine excites both alpha and beta receptors.

Alpha-receptor stimulation by norepinephrine causes generalized arteriolar constriction and vasoconstriction of blood vessels within the skeletal muscle and myocardium. This, in turn, causes increased peripheral resistance and either persistent or paroxysmal hypertension, depending on the amount of catecholamines released by the tumor. Alpha-receptor stimulation also decreases blood flow to the intestines, impairing motility, and inhibits insulin secretion, causing carbohydrate intolerance. In addition, alpha stimulation activates the sweat glands, causing marked diaphoresis.

The inside story

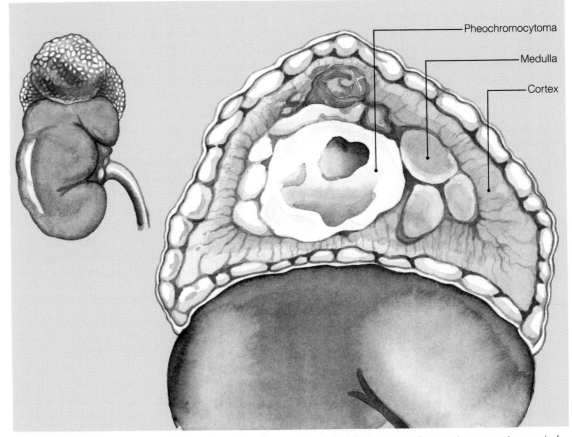

The medulla, the innermost part of the adrenal gland, synthesizes, stores, and secretes the catecholamines epinephrine and norepinephrine. Occasionally, though, it secretes too little or too much of these hormones. Al-though insufficient secretion produces no abnormal effects if the sympathetic nervous system is intact, excessive secretion can cause fatal complications. Typically, such hypersecretion results from a pheochromocytoma.

Beta-receptor stimulation by epinephrine causes bronchodilation, tachycardia, increased myocardial contractility, and peripheral vasodilation, resulting in hypotension. It promotes glycogenolysis and secretion of free fatty acids from adipose tissue. Also, it may relax the smooth muscle tone of the intestines, thereby interfering with normal digestion and causing nausea and vomiting. Lastly, beta-receptor stimulation by epinephrine increases the metabolic rate, ultimately leading to weight loss and heat intolerance.

MEDICAL MANAGEMENT

Diagnosis of pheochromocytoma relies on the patient history and symptoms but requires confirming laboratory studies. Often pheochromocytoma is diagnosed during pregnancy, when uterine pressure on the tumor induces more frequent attacks. (See *Pheochromocytoma in pregnancy,* page 119.) Effective treatment focuses on surgical removal of the tumor or long-term drug therapy to control symptoms.

Diagnostic tests

Although urine tests are the primary means of detecting pheochromocytoma, blood, pharmacologic, and radiologic tests may also provide valuable information to help confirm diagnosis.

Urine tests. In suspected pheochromocytoma, the complete diagnostic workup of catecholamine secretion includes measurement of urine catecholamines and the metabolites metanephrine, normetanephrine, homovanillic acid (HVA), and vanillylmandelic acid (VMA). The specimen of choice for these tests is a 24-hour urine specimen, since catecholamine secretion fluctuates diurnally and in response to pain, exercise, temperature changes, emotional stress, and other factors. Also, these tests require abstention from drugs, such as guaifenesin and salicylates; from vitamins; and from foods high in vanillin, such as chocolate and bananas, to prevent false-positive results. (Chlorophyll in breath mints also interferes with catecholamine test results.)

Elevated urine catecholamine levels following a hypertensive attack usually indicate pheochromocytoma. With the exception of HVA, catecholamine metabolites may also increase at this time. Abnormally high levels of HVA, however, rule out pheochromocytoma, because this tumor mainly secretes epinephrine, whose primary metabolite is VMA, not HVA.

Plasma tests. Compared with urine tests, plasma catecholamine tests are difficult to perform and expensive—but under carefully controlled conditions, these tests can be quite accurate. They require the same dietary and drug restrictions as the urine tests but may also require insertion of an indwelling venous catheter at least 45 minutes before sample collection, since the stress of venipuncture itself may sharply raise catecholamine levels. Also, the patient must be relaxed and recumbent for at least 30 minutes before sample collection, since postural changes raise catecholamine levels.

Pharmacologic tests. Occasionally, pharmacologic agents are used in diagnosing pheochromocytoma, but their accuracy and safety are questionable. Administration of glucagon, tyramine, and histamine may cause hypertension and increased catecholamine production in patients with pheochromocytoma. And very small doses of phentolamine, an alpha-adrenergic blocking agent, may produce profound hypotension in patients with this tumor.

Radiologic tests. Although hormonal tests detect most endocrine tumors, radiologic tests are being used more frequently to locate tumors before surgery. Both computerized axial tomography scan and ultrasonography reliably detect tumors. In contrast, X-rays and intravenous pyelography have limited value. Arteriography, venography, and other invasive tests are controversial, since the contrast material injected during these tests may promote catecholamine secretion and precipitate a severe hypertensive attack. Catheterization of the inferior or superior vena cava to determine concentrations of catecholamines in the blood at different levels is restricted to tumors that cannot otherwise be located. This difficult procedure must be performed by a radiologist skilled in this technique.

Treatment: Surgery or drugs
Pheochromocytoma requires either surgery or long-term drug therapy.

Surgery. Pheochromocytomectomy—the surgical removal of a pheochromocytoma—

offers a 95% recovery rate for patients with benign tumors. Before surgery, alpha-adrenergic blocking agents are given to help prevent intraoperative hypertensive episodes. During surgery, anesthetics, such as nitrous oxide, are used to prevent or control dysrhythmia. However, halogenated hydrocarbons are contraindicated because these anesthetics sensitize the myocardium to catecholamines, thereby causing life-threatening dysrhythmias.

The pheochromocytoma should be removed with the capsule intact and with minimal manipulation to decrease the risk of releasing additional catecholamines during surgery. During surgery, the patient's central venous pressure, intraarterial blood pressure, and electrocardiogram are monitored. If hypertensive episodes occur, they're usually treated with phentolamine or nitroprusside. Tachycardia and dysrhythmia require propranolol or lidocaine. Hypotension, which almost always follows excision of this tumor, usually requires blood- or plasma-volume expanders.

Surgical stress often causes hypertension during the first postoperative day. Persistent hypertension, however, can indicate hypervolemia, renal or arterial damage, or the presence of other tumors.

Drug therapy. Unfortunately, long-term drug therapy is the only treatment available for patients with inoperable pheochromocytoma, because this tumor is resistant to radiotherapy and chemotherapy. For these patients, alpha-adrenergic blocking agents are the treatment of choice. These drugs reduce blood pressure by inhibiting the peripheral vasoconstricting effects of catecholamines. For example, phentolamine, a short-acting alpha adrenergic blocker administered I.V., controls severe hypertensive episodes. Phenoxybenzamine, a longer-acting alpha adrenergic blocker, prevents or controls hypertension.

Metyrosine, an enzyme inhibitor that inhibits catecholamine production, may be used for long-term treatment. Beta blockers, such as propranolol and nadolol may also be used in patients receiving alpha blockers to treat catecholamine-induced tachycardia. But these may cause paroxysmal hypertension or even congestive heart failure in patients with previous inadequate blockade of alpha receptors.

NURSING MANAGEMENT
In pheochromocytoma, nursing management begins with a detailed patient history and physical examination. After collecting this

Pheochromocytoma in pregnancy
Pheochromocytoma may be first detected during pregnancy when uterine pressure on the tumor provokes increasingly frequent attacks of hypertension. Unfortunately, though, the tumor is often misdiagnosed as toxemia, eclampsia, or a ruptured uterus at delivery.

Pheochromocytoma is associated with 50% maternal mortality and an only slightly lower fetal mortality—the result of cerebrovascular accident, acute pulmonary edema, hypoxia, or dysrhythmia. The risk of spontaneous abortion is high. Although phenoxybenzamine controls symptoms until the fetus matures enough to be delivered by cesarean section, the drug's effects on the fetus have not yet been determined.

Assessment findings in pheochromocytoma

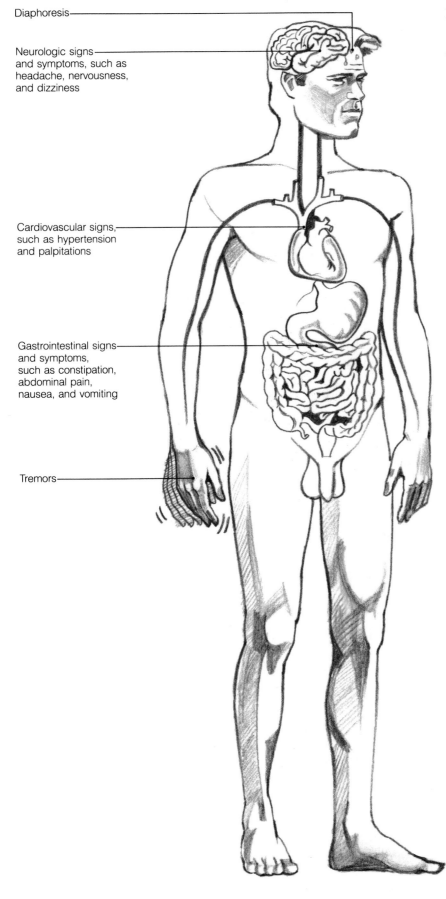

Diaphoresis

Neurologic signs
and symptoms, such as
headache, nervousness,
and dizziness

Cardiovascular signs,
such as hypertension
and palpitations

Gastrointestinal signs
and symptoms,
such as constipation,
abdominal pain,
nausea, and vomiting

Tremors

subjective and objective data, you'll be ready to form nursing diagnoses, set care goals, and plan and evaluate your intervention.

Collect subjective data

With the pathophysiology and medical management of pheochromocytoma in mind, you'll be especially alert if the patient reports sweating or symptoms like "anxiety attack," palpitations, or headaches. If the patient describes these symptoms to you, include these questions in your history:

• How often do you have anxiety attacks? Do they occur without warning, or can you feel one coming on? Do position or temperature changes, exercise, laughing, urination, consumption of coffee, or smoking precipitate an attack or make it worse?

• Do you experience headaches with the anxiety attacks? How often do you have headaches? Where do you feel their pain?

• Do you perspire excessively only during an anxiety attack or at other times, too?

• Have you ever had high blood pressure? If so, has it been a persistent problem? Also, be sure to ask about low blood pressure.

• Have you experienced heart palpitations? Have you ever felt chest pain during palpitations? Where do you feel it? Is it actually pain, or is it more like a tightness?

• Have you lost weight recently? How much? When did you first notice loss of weight? Keep in mind that some patients with pheochromocytoma do not lose weight.

• Does hot weather bother you a great deal?

After discussing these symptoms with the patient, complete the history. Ask about previous hospitalizations, drug use, a history of skin pallor or tumors, and any recurrent familial diseases.

Collect objective data

Start the physical examination by checking the patient's blood pressure, pulse, and respirations, and then record your findings to serve as a baseline. Note any hypertension or tachycardia. Also, check for orthostatic hypotension, which may be a sign in some patients. Weigh the patient and note if he's unusually thin. Then check the patient's overall appearance. Is he pale or flushed? Diaphoretic? Does he appear nervous or apprehensive?

Next, check the eyes for hemorrhages and infarcts, since hypertension can cause blood vessel damage in the retina. Also examine the pupils for dilation, caused by excess norepinephrine.

Last, check the patient's extremities for tremors. If your examination reveals this symptom, describe these as accurately as possible.

Unfortunately, if the patient isn't experiencing a paroxysmal attack of hypertension, the physical examination may show no significant abnormalities. Keep in mind that palpation of the abdomen over the adrenal gland can induce an acute attack. Refrain from using this assessment technique to avoid inducing a possible hypertensive crisis.

Formulate nursing diagnoses
With the information you've gleaned from the history and physical exam, you're now prepared to formulate nursing diagnoses, set goals, and plan interventions. Of course, your nursing diagnoses will reflect the needs of each patient, but typically they'll include the following:

Potential for hypertensive crisis because of release of catecholamines. Your goal is to reduce the risk of hypertensive crisis by minimizing internal and external stressors. To accomplish this, monitor vital signs closely, especially if the patient's condition changes. Provide a quiet, restful environment and give prescribed drugs as ordered. Advise the patient to refrain from smoking, consumption of coffee, sudden position changes, and excessive activity.

Potential for incapacitating headaches because of release of catecholamines. Your goal is to help prevent headaches by promoting rest, comfort, and freedom from pain. To accomplish this, position the patient comfortably, provide a quiet, restful environment, and advise the patient against excessive activity. In addition, administer analgesic drugs, as ordered.

Heat intolerance because of increased metabolism. Your goals are to provide a comfortable environment and to explain the reasons for heat intolerance. To accomplish these goals, maintain a cool room temperature during a hypertensive attack and provide the patient with additional blankets and gowns to prevent chills during periods of diaphoresis. Ensure that the patient bathes frequently, and explain the metabolic effects of catecholamine secretion.

Knowledge deficit about pheochromocytoma and adrenalectomy. Your goal is to help the patient understand his disease; diagnostic tests and his participation in some, such as the 24-hour urine collection; and the need for surgery and its anticipated results. To accomplish this, explain the normal functions of the catecholamines, the mechanisms of abnormal catecholamine production and the effects of their increased secretion, the factors that may precipitate an attack, and the effects of drugs used for treating his condition. Also, explain pheochromocytomectomy, its possible complications and their treatment, and the characteristically high cure rate. Encourage the patient's questions and alleviate his anxiety by providing appropriate, accurate information about his condition.

Poor nutrition because of increased metabolic rate. Your goal is to promote weight gain by increasing the patient's caloric intake. To accomplish this, provide small, frequent meals that are high in vitamins, minerals, and calories. Encourage the patient to choose his favorite foods, and provide high-calorie between-meal snacks. Also explain the cause of his weight loss and the importance of gaining weight.

Evaluate your care plan
If your care plan is working, you'll notice several changes in your patient.
• He'll experience fewer or no paroxysmal attacks of hypertension because you've removed the precipitating factors—environmental stress, caffeine, cigarettes, excessive activity, and so on.
• He'll report fewer incapacitating headaches—the result of his lowered stress and activity level.
• He'll be more comfortable and perspire less profusely because you've maintained a cool room temperature. He'll also understand the reason for diaphoresis.
• The patient will gain weight from the high-calorie diet.

Most important, the patient will understand pheochromocytoma—what causes his attacks and what surgery and recovery involve. He'll also ask questions and feel comfortable about discussing his disease.

The nursing challenge
Signs and symptoms of pheochromocytoma are diffuse and baffling—seemingly, the patient could have any number of diseases. But once you understand the pathophysiology of pheochromocytoma, the confusion surrounding this disease disappears. Then you'll be ready to put your assessment skills into practice—and these skills can help make possible early diagnosis and a complete cure.

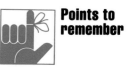

Points to remember

• Pheochromocytoma is a tumor of the adrenal medulla that secretes excessive amounts of the catecholamines epinephrine and norepinephrine. Usually unilateral, the tumor may be malignant in 10% of patients.
• Early diagnosis of pheochromocytoma is critical since the tumor can be fatal. However, the cure rate with surgery is high.
• Signs and symptoms of pheochromocytoma vary with the predominant catecholamine. The most common ones include persistent or paroxysmal hypertension, headache, palpitations, diaphoresis, and chest pain.

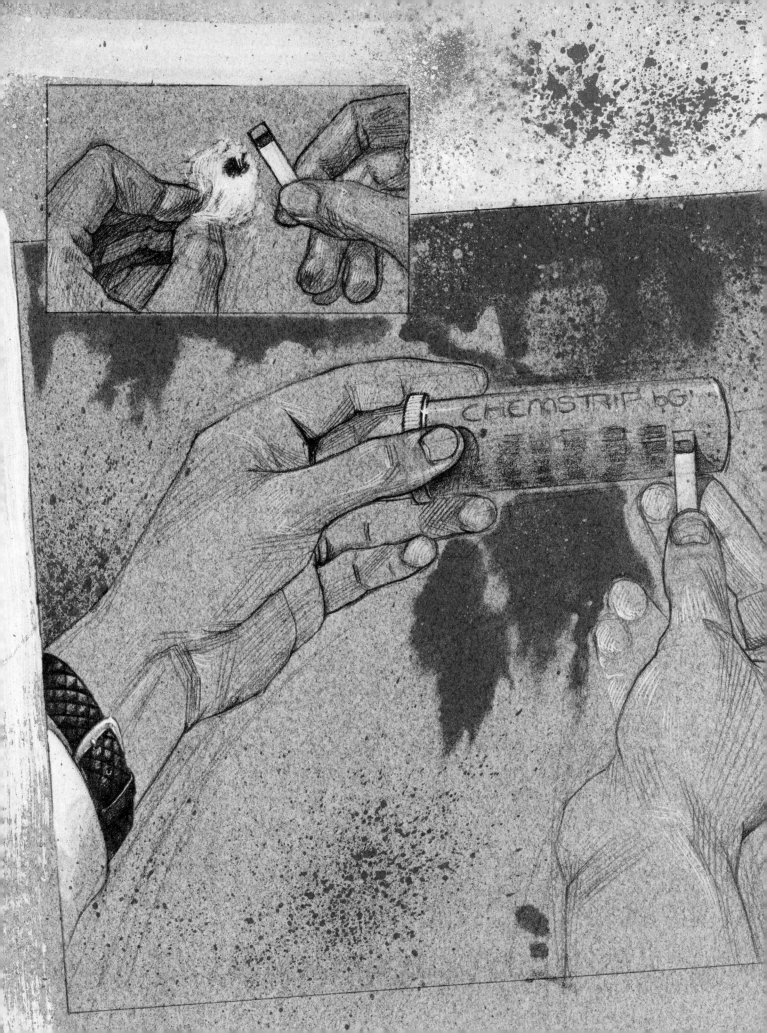

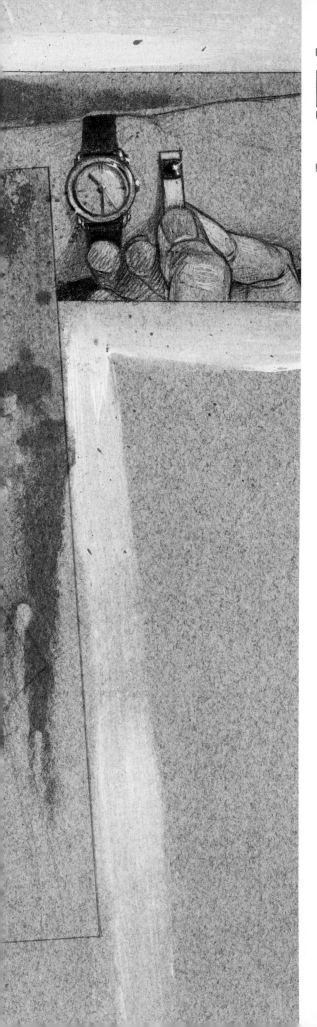

DISORDERS OF
THE PANCREAS

10 DEALING WITH DIABETES MELLITUS

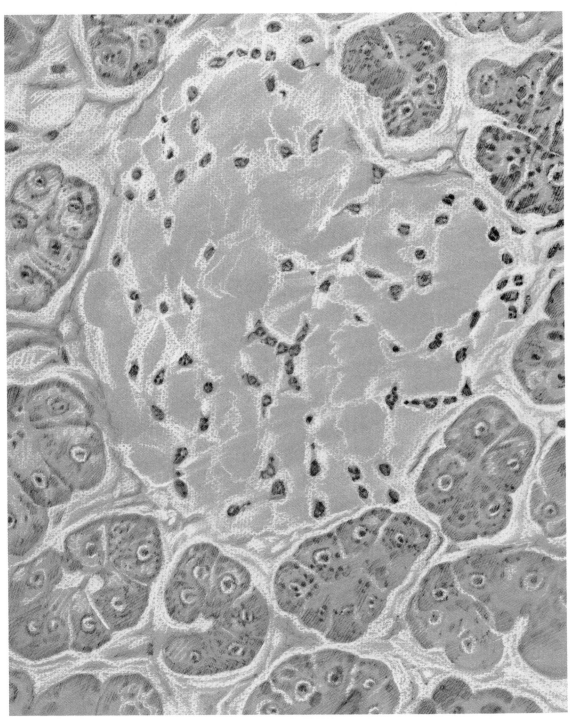

Hyalinization of pancreatic tissue in diabetes

Diabetes mellitus is the most common endocrine disorder. According to the American Diabetes Association (ADA), this disease afflicts more than 10 million persons and during the coming year will be diagnosed in an estimated 600,000 more. Diabetes is the third largest cause of death by disease in the United States, after heart disease and cancer. In addition, the ADA says, diabetes more than doubles the risk of coronary heart disease and stroke, is associated with an almost 40-fold higher amputation rate, accounts for nearly 20% of all patients with end-stage renal disease entering dialysis, and causes most new blindness.

Whether you work in a hospital, newborn nursery, nursing home, or community agency, you'll meet diabetic patients. And because this disease has such widespread systemic effects, you'll have to consider diabetes carefully even when it isn't the patient's chief complaint. To manage patients with diabetes successfully, you must understand and know how to deal with its diverse implications. For example, you must know how to manage insulin replacement, how to monitor the effects of therapy, how to promote optimum control of hyperglycemia to prevent acute complications, how to teach and monitor nutrition to help the patient maintain an optimum nutritional state, how to monitor progression of the disease, and how to deal with chronic complications.

Patient education is the key to successful management. Usually, patients with diabetes must administer their own replacement dosages of insulin. Because compliance with the treatment regimen is so important, careful teaching is your primary obligation. Many diabetic patients are elderly; typically, they may miss medical appointments, forget to take prescribed medication, and fail to adhere to dietary restrictions. Although you can't guarantee total compliance with treatment, you can improve it by helping patients understand diabetes and correct the underlying reasons for noncompliance. To meet these goals, you must thoroughly understand the pathophysiology and medical management of diabetes.

What is diabetes mellitus?

Diabetes mellitus is a chronic systemic disease. It represents a syndrome of insulin deficiency that is intimately bound up with a variety of hereditary and environmental factors. Its chief manifestations include alterations in metabolism of carbohydrates, fats, and proteins and in the structure and function of nerves and blood vessels. Early signs and symptoms of this disease stem from metabolic disorders (such as hyperglycemia); later complications stem from vascular disorders (such as microvascular disease involving the kidneys and retina) and neuropathies.

Since the 1930s, researchers have taken two major approaches to the origin of diabetic complications. One school of thought holds that complications are genetically predetermined and, therefore, inevitable and unalterable. The other approach maintains that complications are related to elevated blood glucose levels and other abnormal metabolic effects of this disease; therefore, they can be controlled or prevented by "tight" physiologic control of the disease. Since accumulating evidence supports the second view, the approach to how diabetic patients are managed is beginning to change from an attitude of permissiveness to one of restraint.

Not a single disease

Clearly, diabetes is not a single disease but a cluster of disorders related by abnormal glucose metabolism. To coordinate research efforts, in 1979 the National Diabetes Data Group (NDDG) of the National Institutes of Health established a classification system for diabetes mellitus and other categories of glucose intolerance. The NDDG divides diabetes mellitus into several different types:

Insulin-dependent diabetes mellitus. IDDM or Type I, formerly known as ketosis-prone or juvenile diabetes, may be genetic, environmental, or acquired. Most Type I patients are young, but this disease may strike at any age. It's apparently associated with certain histocompatibility antigens, with some viruses, and with abnormal antibodies that attack the patient's own islet cells. This form of diabetes may result from a combination of two or more of these etiologic factors. For example, a genetically predisposed patient may contract a viral infection that destroys beta cells in the islets of Langerhans, or an abnormal genetic code may instruct the immune system to attack the beta cells.

Environmental influences, such as toxic chemicals, have also been shown to induce Type I diabetes. In one instance, an accidental injection of the rodenticide Vacor induced a ketosis-prone form of diabetes. Certain drugs, such as the antineoplastic streptozocin, used to combat islet cell tumors of the pancreas,

Classifying diabetes

In 1979, the National Diabetes Data Group of the National Institutes of Health proposed new categories of diabetes mellitus and other glucose intolerance–related conditions.

NDDG class	Former terms
Diabetes mellitus	
• Type I. Insulin-dependent diabetes mellitus (IDDM)	• Juvenile diabetes, juvenile-onset diabetes, ketosis-prone diabetes, unstable or brittle diabetes

• Type II. Non-insulin-dependent diabetes mellitus (NIDDM)
  Nonobese NIDDM
  Obese NIDDM (includes families with autosomal dominant inheritance)
	• Adult-onset diabetes
	• Maturity-onset diabetes
	• Ketosis-resistant diabetes, stable diabetes

• Other types, including diabetes mellitus associated with certain conditions and syndromes: pancreatic disease; hormonal; drug- or chemical-induced; certain genetic syndromes; insulin receptor abnormalities	• Secondary diabetes
Impaired glucose tolerance (IGT)	
• Nonobese IGT	• Asymptomatic diabetes
• Obese IGT	• Chemical diabetes
• IGT associated with certain conditions and syndromes: pancreatic disease; hormonal; drug- or chemical-induced; insulin receptor abnormalities; certain genetic syndromes	• Latent diabetes, borderline diabetes, subclinical diabetes
Gestational diabetes	
• Occurs only during pregnancy	• Gestational diabetes
Statistical risk classes	
• Previous abnormality of glucose tolerance: patients now have normal glucose tolerance but previously had diabetic hyperglycemia or impaired glucose tolerance, either spontaneously or in response to a known stimulus; includes former gestational and obese diabetics and others who have had transient hyperglycemia	• Subclinical diabetes, prediabetes, latent diabetes
• Potential abnormality of glucose tolerance: includes persons who have never had abnormal glucose tolerance but who are at increased statistical risk for diabetes because of age, weight, race, or family history	• Prediabetes, potential diabetes

may have diabetogenic side effects.

Non-insulin-dependent diabetes mellitus. NIDDM or Type II, formerly known as ketosis-resistant or adult-onset diabetes, accounts for about 80% of all diabetic patients. This type is thought to be hereditary. Type II patients rarely develop ketosis, and most are obese and over age 40. So far, the etiologic factors involved in Type I have not been found to contribute to development of Type II diabetes.

Diabetes associated with certain conditions and symptoms. Also known as secondary diabetes, this type is accompanied by conditions known or suspected to have caused the disease, such as certain genetic syndromes, action of various drugs or chemical agents, malnourishment, or pancreatic disease.

Impaired glucose tolerance. IGT occurs in patients who have normal fasting blood glucose levels, but who develop two or more glucose levels above 200 mg/dl in oral glucose tolerance testing. It is sometimes also called "chemical," "latent," or "borderline diabetes." These terms are now considered obsolete.

Gestational diabetes. This type develops during pregnancy and makes such women more susceptible to perinatal complications. Why the disease develops in some pregnancies and not in others is still unknown.

Because some persons have a history of past abnormal glucose tolerance or have a potential for it in the future, the new classification includes two statistical risk groups. Called *previous abnormality of glucose tolerance* and *potential abnormality of glucose tolerance,* these two risk groups may actually represent stages in the development of diabetes mellitus.

PATHOPHYSIOLOGY

Diabetes mellitus is a syndrome that embraces many etiologies and abnormalities that share *hyperglycemia* as a common characteristic. Diabetic symptoms may result from insulin deficiency or from insulin resistance that renders insulin ineffective. The causative abnormality may be in beta cells in the islets of Langerhans, in the circulation (prereceptor abnormality), in the cell membrane (receptor abnormality), or in the target cells (postreceptor defect). Type I (IDDM) is usually a defect of insulin secretion in a dead or dying beta cell. Type II (NIDDM) may result from a defect occurring at any point in insulin secretion, circulation, or peripheral action.

Insulin is the key

Insulin, a hormone secreted by beta cells in the pancreas, regulates blood glucose levels. It's also the primary hormone controlling the storage and metabolism of carbohydrates, proteins, and fats. (See *How insulin affects metabolism.*) In diabetes mellitus, impaired carbohydrate metabolism coexists with impaired protein and fat metabolism.

After a meal, minimal insulin deficiency leads to elevated blood glucose levels because not enough of the hormone is available to enable cells to utilize the extra glucose. Severe insulin deficiency has the same effect but also causes excessive mobilization of endogenous fuels (glucose, amino acids, and free fatty acids) when the patient isn't eating (fasting state). An acute insulin deficiency may lead to *diabetic ketoacidosis (DKA)* by altering carbohydrate, fat, and protein metabolic pathways. Without corrective measures, DKA progresses to diabetic coma and death. The metabolic consequences of acute insulin deficiency are summarized in the diagram, *Consequences of insulin deficiency* on pages 128 and 129.

Other hormones involved. Excessive levels of glucagon, cortisol, catecholamines, and growth hormones frequently accompany insulin deficiency. These substances counteract the insulin and thus promote increasing hyperglycemia. Because of hypoinsulinemia,

glucagon is not suppressed by hyperglycemia in either Type I or Type II diabetes. If the insulin deficiency is not corrected, chronic hyperglycemia and hyperlipidemia follow.

In contrast to Type I, beta cells in Type II diabetes (NIDDM) do not disappear; they may produce insulin, but at a sluggish rate. In addition to delayed insulin secretion, some subsets of NIDDM manifest insulin resistance in target tissues (muscle, liver, and adipose tissue).

Obesity and insulin resistance. To understand insulin resistance, it's important to recognize that insulin binds first to receptors on the cell plasma membrane. Insulin resistance can be categorized as occurring before the hormone-receptor interaction (prereceptor), during the interaction (receptor), or after the interaction (postreceptor).

Obesity is the best-known factor associated with insulin resistance because most Type II diabetics are obese. Insulin resistance is a heterogeneous disorder not directly related to the degree of obesity. In obese NIDDM patients with mild hyperinsulinemic resistance, the resistance is primarily due to a deficiency of insulin receptors on the plasma membrane. In obese NIDDM patients who have marked resistance, the receptor deficiency is accompanied by a postreceptor defect. However, the deficiency of receptors appears to be the major cause of such diabetes. Fortunately, weight reduction reverses this receptor deficiency and usually normalizes the patient's insulin response.

Glycosylation and vascular complications. Research has established that hyperglycemia and its attendant metabolic abnormalities cause glucose to combine with numerous proteins in the body (glycosylation) and to cause capillary basement membrane thickening (CBMT). Glycoproteins are a normal component of capillary basement membranes. Hyperglycemia causes excessive glycosylation of these proteins, resulting in thickening and functional impairment of the capillary basement membrane.

Vascular complications can be categorized as small vessel disease, or *microangiopathy,* and large vessel disease, or *macroangiopathy.*

Microangiopathy resulting from CBMT involves small arteries and arterioles throughout the body but commonly manifests itself in diabetics as retinal and renal disease. Clinical evidence of eye disease (retinal hemorrhage, detachment, and other changes) may appear in patients who have had diabetes

How insulin affects metabolism

The body stores and metabolizes ingested nutrients largely through insulin's control. Insulin acts on the three major fuels—carbohydrates, proteins, and fats—and acts on them chiefly in the liver, in muscle, and in adipose tissue. In each of these tissues, anticatabolic as well as anabolic effects of insulin act to reinforce each other, as shown here. Metabolic dysfunction in diabetes reflects the degree of absolute or relative deficiency of insulin.

Anticatabolic effects decrease

Liver
Glycogenolysis
Gluconeogenesis
Ketogenesis

Adipose tissue
Lipolysis

Muscle
Protein catabolism
Amino acid output

Anabolic effects increase

Liver
Glycogen synthesis
Fatty acid synthesis

Adipose tissue
Glycerol synthesis
Fatty acid synthesis

Muscle
Amino acid uptake
Protein synthesis
Glycogen synthesis

Consequences of insulin deficiency

Insulin, essential to metabolism, affects all three metabolic
pathways—carbohydrates, fats, and proteins. Besides controlling
glucose utilization, insulin enhances fat storage and protein
synthesis. The total impact of insulin is pervasive and complex.

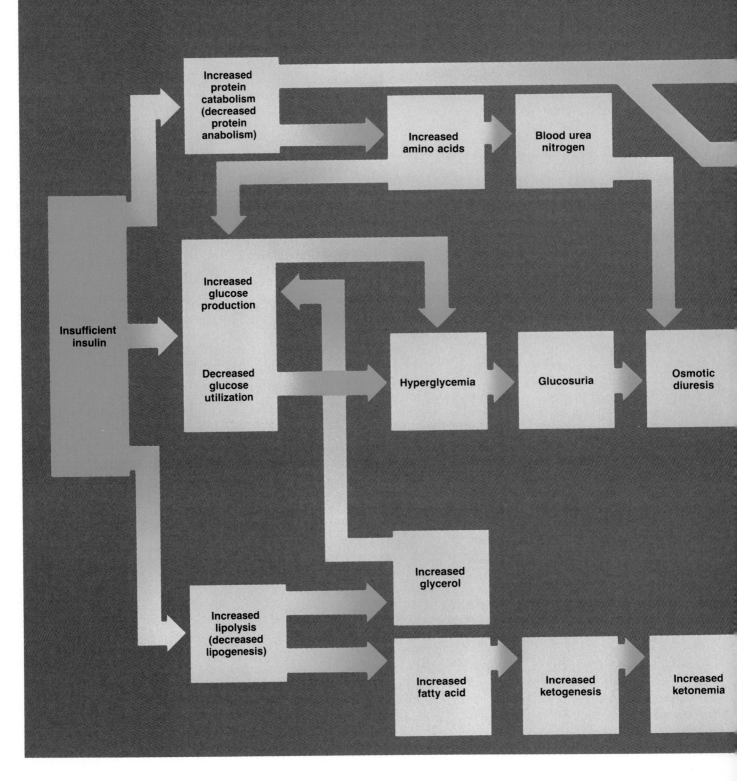

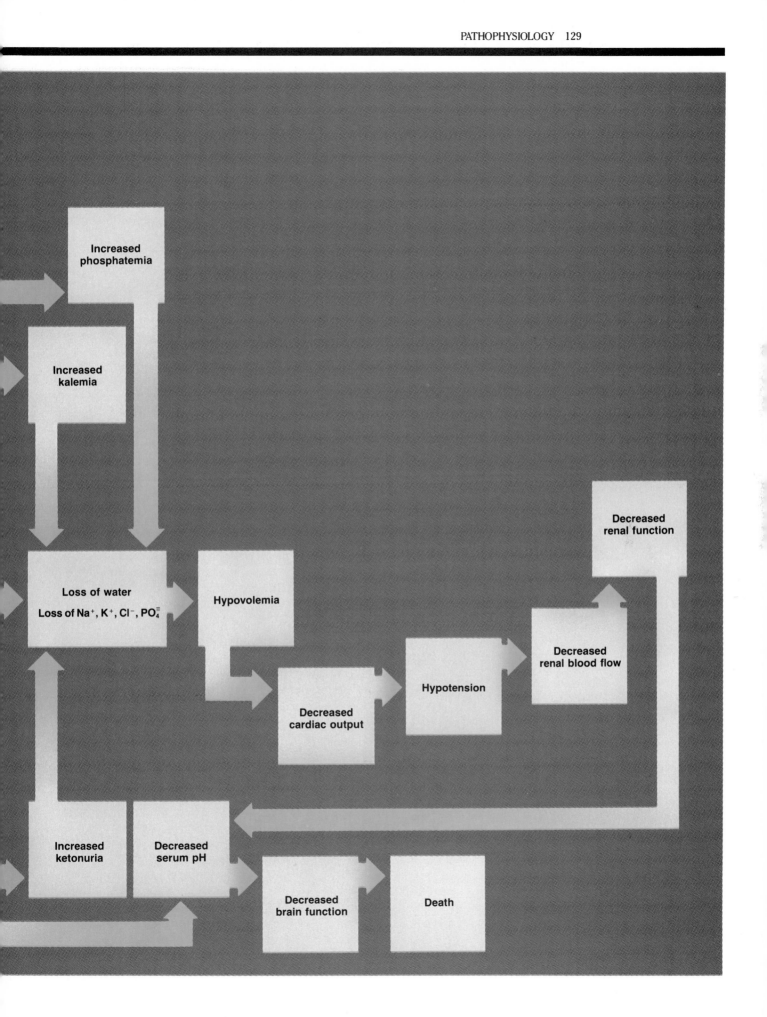

for 8 to 12 years; if untreated, it can progress rapidly to blindness. Renal microangiopathy leads to progressive proteinuria, loss of renal function, and, eventually, renal failure.

Macroangiopathy may involve any large vessel, causing such disorders as peripheral vascular disease, cerebral vascular disease, coronary artery disease, and hypertension, which occur primarily as a result of atherosclerosis. In diabetics, these disorders appear at an earlier age and progress more rapidly if blood glucose levels are uncontrolled. No complications appear before puberty, no matter what the level of control, except in some forms of mononeuropathy.

Diabetic neuropathy. Marked by axonal degeneration and myelin loss, this neuropathy may result from the effects of glycosylation-related CBMT or from hyperglycemia-caused deposition of sorbitol in nerve cells. It may involve sensory or motor nerves or both and may also involve the autonomic nervous system. Neuropathy most commonly begins as sensory loss in the extremities, resulting in foot injury or pressure ulcers, which may progress to infection, osteomyelitis of the foot bones, and gangrene, often leading to amputation. Diabetic autonomic neuropathy may cause abnormalities in almost every body system.

MEDICAL MANAGEMENT
Although medical management varies according to the form of diabetes—whether Type I or Type II—the overall goals are to control blood glucose levels and to reach and maintain appropriate body weight through diet therapy alone, diet therapy with oral hypoglycemics, or insulin replacement with dietary management.

Diagnosis: Type I or Type II?
Most cases of diabetes mellitus are easily diagnosed. This is especially true in acute manifestations of Type I: when a child presents with coma and a blood glucose level of 400 mg/dl, there's no question of the diagnosis. However, verifying early or mild Type II diabetes may be more difficult.

The patient with Type II diabetes may have few overt symptoms. Most Type II patients are overweight and may have mild symptoms (nocturia, monilial vaginitis and vulvitis, weakness, lethargy) but little else. The physical examination may reveal fasting hyperglycemia in an otherwise healthy patient. Frequently, the diabetes appears as a triad—

hyperglycemia, obesity, and hypertension—in relatively asymptomatic patients. Occasionally, a Type II patient may present in coma with severe hyperglycemia but no ketosis—a state known as *hyperglycemic hyperosmolar nonketotic coma* (HHNC). In this condition, blood glucose may reach levels of 1,500 to 3,000 mg/dl; such coma results from dehydration rather than acidosis.

Of course, hyperglycemia does not in itself confirm diabetes. A careful drug history and physical exam should distinguish true diabetes mellitus from drug reactions that also raise blood glucose (from, for example, Dilantin or adrenocortical steroids) and from other disorders (such as Cushing's syndrome, acromegaly) that produce mild to moderate hyperglycemia.

It's important to remember that severe stress or trauma may suppress insulin release in Type II and increase gluconeogenesis by the liver in both Types I and II. The extra glucose fuels anaerobic metabolism carried on by muscles and healing tissues. Since this metabolism takes place without sufficient insulin, the resulting hyperglycemia represents functional diabetes. This diabetic effect is commonly present in severe trauma, myocardial infarction, stroke, burns, pneumonia, peritonitis, and septicemia.

In the severely traumatized patient with preexisting diabetes, the carbohydrate abnormality tends to be more severe and more obvious. If such a patient is given parenteral glucose, the hyperglycemia resulting from his relative or absolute lack of insulin may worsen, and he may undergo HHNC. However, if he's less severely injured, he may have glucose intolerance due to less severely depressed insulin release.

Treating Type II diabetes
Therapy for Type II diabetic patients centers on diet modification and an exercise program. Oral hypoglycemics and insulin may also be required in some cases.

Recent changes in dietary therapy include lowering the patient's intake of saturated fats, substituting polyunsaturated fatty acids to delay the onset of atherosclerosis, and adding fiber to reduce postprandial hyperglycemia.

Oral hypoglycemics help. If high blood glucose levels persist despite good compliance in diet and exercise, oral hypoglycemic agents are also indicated. Four such agents, all sulfonylureas, are currently in use:

• *Tolbutamide (Orinase)* is a short-acting oral

Staging diabetic retinopathy

A major complication of diabetes—and the most common cause of new blindness—retinopathy may be one of the first signs of the underlying disease, or it could develop many years after other diabetic symptoms occur. Retinopathy chiefly involves the retinal capillaries. Over time, the capillary walls weaken and develop microaneurysms. These may hemorrhage into the retinal tissue, frequently causing blindness from exudation into the macular region. Although the course of retinopathy is variable, a rough scheme of staging is used for diagnostic purposes. The eyegrounds below represent stages of retinopathy as they would appear through an ophthalmoscope. Treatment of retinopathy varies with the degree of the disorder.

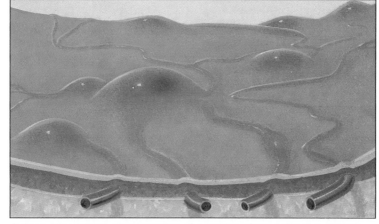

A three-dimensional reconstruction of a portion of the retina in a diabetic patient, revealing the capillary network with clusters of aneurysms, which occur chiefly in the macular region.

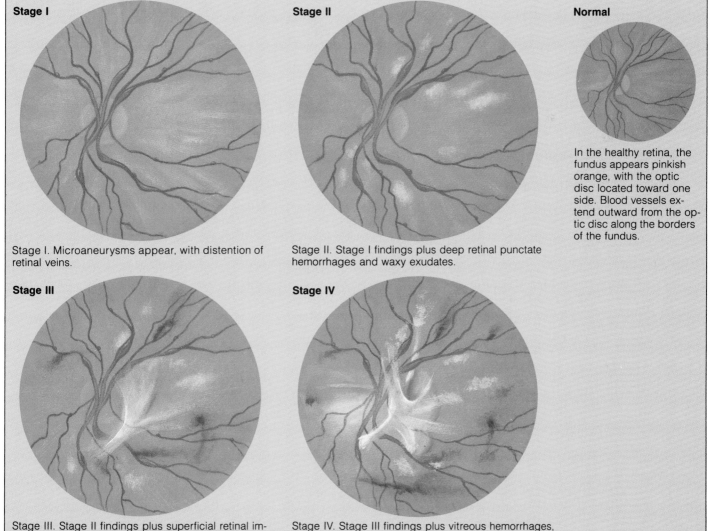

Stage I

Stage II

Normal

In the healthy retina, the fundus appears pinkish orange, with the optic disc located toward one side. Blood vessels extend outward from the optic disc along the borders of the fundus.

Stage I. Microaneurysms appear, with distention of retinal veins.

Stage II. Stage I findings plus deep retinal punctate hemorrhages and waxy exudates.

Stage III

Stage IV

Stage III. Stage II findings plus superficial retinal images, dilatation of existing capillary networks, neovascularization, preretinal hemorrhages, and fibrosis of the retinal surface.

Stage IV. Stage III findings plus vitreous hemorrhages, proliferating retinopathy with its sequelae—rubeosis iridis diabetica, retinal detachment, secondary glaucoma, and loss of useful vision.

agent that may be used to encourage insulin secretion in patients who have elevated basal insulin secretion but cannot produce sufficient insulin to deal with their food intake. However, tolbutamide is a weak sulfonylurea agent that may require high dosage (up to 4 times daily) to be effective.

• *Chlorpropamide (Diabinese)* is a longer-acting oral agent given to patients who have low basal insulin secretion but can produce some bolus insulin. It may exert a cumulative effect because of its long duration of action and can produce profound and long-lasting hypoglycemia. This agent need only be given once daily.

• *Tolazamide (Tolinase) and acetohexamide (Dymelor)* are intermediate-acting agents and are best used to enhance both basal and postprandial insulin secretion.

A second generation of more potent sulfonylurea hypoglycemics are currently used in Europe. Two of these, glyburide and glipizide, are used in some institutions in the United States. While not differing greatly in action from other oral agents, they are effective in smaller doses and thus show fewer toxic or other side effects.

Some dietary-compliant Type II patients who fail to respond to oral hypoglycemics require insulin therapy to correct hyperglycemia. Some Type II patients with severe hyperglycemia may need a short course of insulin therapy to control symptoms (such as polyuria or nocturia). Patients may also need temporary insulin therapy during periods of stress. Such patients should be treated only with highly purified insulin to avoid buildup of insulin antibodies.

Regular exercise important. Exercise is as important as insulin and diet in treating diabetes. It may lower blood glucose levels, help maintain normal cholesterol levels, and, by increasing circulation, help the blood vessels to perform more effectively. Many of these effects increase the body's ability to accept glucose, and, in some patients, may reduce the therapeutic dose of insulin.

The successful exercise program must be *consistent*—part of a daily routine. The program should be tailored to the patient's physical ability—based on a complete physical examination, with exercise EKG, to determine physical capacity.

Treating Type I diabetes

A patient with Type I diabetes may present in DKA with coma, severe dehydration, and acidosis, or in mild ketosis with hyperglycemia and without dehydration or acidosis. According to the National Diabetes Data Group, hyperglycemia that manifests fasting blood glucose levels above 140 mg/dl on two consecutive occasions confirms the diagnosis of Type I diabetes. (Since the patient's fasting plasma glucose levels usually exceed 200 mg/dl, a confirming glucose tolerance test is rarely needed.) Serum electrolyte tests usually show somewhat depressed serum sodium and chloride levels; normal, elevated, or depressed serum potassium levels; and reduced serum bicarbonate levels.

Insulin-dependent diabetic patients must receive daily injections of insulin to control their blood glucose levels. Most such patients use crystalline (regular) and NPH or Lente Insulin preparations. Insulin purity has been steadily improving over the last 10 years to reduce the risk of autoimmune reactions, which can lead to allergies, lipodystrophy, and insulin resistance. Two new preparations, in the form of exact replicates of human insulin, have recently been developed. One is made by converting pork insulin to the amino acid sequence of human insulin; the other is made by using recombinant DNA technology to induce *Escherichia coli* bacteria to manufacture insulin. The latter is known as biosynthetic human insulin, or Humulin; it's available in regular or NPH form. A third preparation, an analogue of human insulin, is being tested in university settings. These human insulin analogues should further reduce the risk of an allergic response.

Which insulin is best? Since individual patients' responses to insulin vary widely, therapy must be decided by trial and error. Certain controllable features, such as smoking, stress levels, and exercise, may contribute significantly to this variability. The duration of action for an intermediate preparation such as NPH may be 12 hours in one patient and 18 hours in another; its effects may peak as early as 4 hours after administration or as late as 16 hours afterward.

When adjusting the dosage, it's best to use the same quantity of insulin for several days before stepping it up or down; generally, dosage should not change more than 5 or 6 units per step. However, if the patient becomes moderately to severely hypoglycemic, the insulin dose should be decreased immediately, unless hypoglycemia is known to be nonrecurrent, as in unexpected, excessive exercise. A newly diagnosed diabetic patient should start his insulin treatments with instruction in diet, self-testing of blood or urine, and insulin administration.

Minimum insulin therapy required for physiologic management is a two-dose, split-mixed insulin schedule. If this doesn't ensure euglycemia most of the time or if there is evidence that the patient needs flexibility in his life-style, three or more doses are recommended.

The Somogyi effect. Some patients who take insulin experience a hypoglycemic reaction, only to undergo rebound hyperglycemia, which appears in the next glucose test. Increasing insulin dosage only aggravates this cycle. Too much insulin decreases the glucose level and stimulates secretion of epinephrine, glucagon, adrenal corticosteroids, and growth hormone—all in the body's attempt to oppose excessive insulin action. Epinephrine causes glycogenolysis in the liver; the corticosteroids stimulate gluconeogenesis. These compensatory physiologic effects stimulate the cycle of rebound hyperglycemia, known as the Somogyi effect. If the doctor mistakes this rebound for a worsening of blood glucose control, he may increase the insulin dosage, which only aggravates the cycle. Paradoxically, decreasing the insulin dosage or increasing food intake in such patients eliminates the hyperglycemia and stabilizes the patient's condition.

Management strategies

The goal of minimizing the long-term complications of Type I diabetes is being approached from two fronts: improvements in insulin delivery and more accurate monitoring of blood glucose levels. One insulin injection per day won't achieve the continuous 24-hour normalization of blood glucose and lipids thought to be most desirable. To achieve this, two to four injections of insulin may be taken before meals and at bedtime; some patients may require intermediate insulin, along with regular insulin given at dinner or at bedtime, to control occurrence of nocturnal hyperglycemia.

Insulin pumps. To avoid multiple insulin injections, small infusion pumps have been devised to meter precise insulin doses into the bloodstream at precise intervals. The *closed-loop* pump system, such as the Biostator artificial pancreas, can detect and respond to changing glucose levels like a functioning pancreas. Used only in hospitals, this system withdraws blood and infuses insulin intrave-

nously at the same time. The other system is an *open-loop* pump that does not respond to changes in blood glucose levels. Known as a continuous subcutaneous insulin infusion pump, this battery-driven unit fits on the patient's belt. It delivers a continuous small basal dose and large bolus doses before meals, via a subcutaneous needle. The patient usually sets the infusion rate himself.

Pancreas transplants. Ideally, a successful pancreas transplant would most efficiently supply adequate insulin replacement. Although numerous transplants have been performed, the recipient must take immunosuppressive drugs to prevent rejection of the transplant. Pure islet cell transplants, envisioned for the near future, may not require immunosuppressive drugs.

Insulin in pregnancy and surgery. Diabetic patients undergoing surgery or delivery should receive regular insulin I.V., instead of subcutaneous insulin, to ensure that a known quantity of the hormone reaches the bloodstream. Insulin can be given before anesthesia, and dextrose 5% or 10% in water should be infused during the procedure. Blood glucose and ketone levels should be monitored frequently and additional insulin given as needed. Plasma glucose levels should be monitored hourly, or preferably more frequently, during prolonged procedures for all Type I diabetics.

New methods monitor glucose. Until recently, urine testing was the only way a diabetic patient could monitor his own blood glucose levels at home. But the urine test is an indirect and inaccurate method that is affected by changes in the renal threshold. What's more, urine tests do not detect hypoglycemia itself. However, for patients with normal renal thresholds, first-voided urine glucose tests give helpful information about control over a period of time. Urine testing for ketones (such as Acetest) is a must if the Type I diabetic is ill, uncontrolled, or pregnant. (See *Diabetic ketoacidosis,* page 138.)

New blood glucose monitoring products allow the diabetic patient to test his blood glucose levels accurately. These new products are easy to use, are more reliable than urine testing, and help the patient to better understand his disorder. To perform this test, the patient simply pricks his finger with a sterile lancet to obtain a drop of blood, moistens a test strip with the blood, and obtains the glucose level by comparing the strip to a standard color scale or reading it with a colorimeter. Since the lancet, used alone, may

Getting a drop of blood

A simple procedure, obtaining a drop of capillary blood is essential for proper blood glucose monitoring. When teaching this procedure to your patient to use in self-monitoring blood glucose, stress that it allows him to see how diet, exercise, and drug therapy affect his glucose levels and that he'll thereby gain a fundamental understanding of the relationship of therapy to control.

You can get a drop of blood for testing two ways: manually or with a mechanical bloodletting device. Regardless of which method you prefer, the patient should know how to do both in case one method fails.

The equipment and supplies you'll need include lancets, mechanical bloodletting devices (with platforms), and alcohol wipes.

Obtaining blood manually

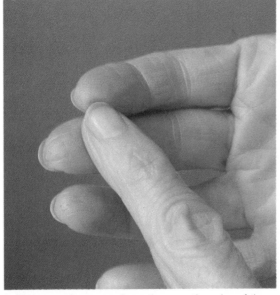

1. Choose a site on any fingertip, *near the edge* of the fingertip. Avoid using a site on the pad of the patient's finger, where nerves and blood vessels are concentrated.

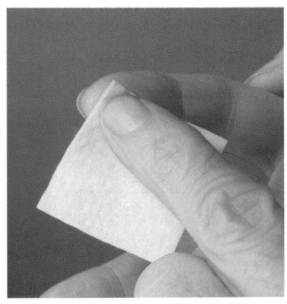

2. Wipe the chosen fingertip with alcohol. (Omit this step if the patient has washed his hands first.) Let the alcohol evaporate, and fan the finger in the air to hasten drying. Wet alcohol may interact with the reagent strip to produce a false-high reading.

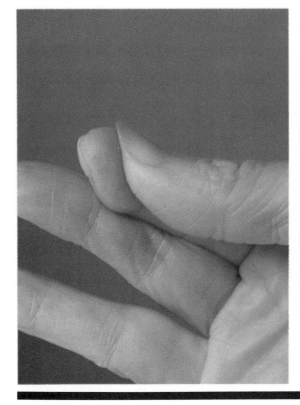

3. Instruct the patient to squeeze his fingertip with the thumb of the same hand to well up blood at the puncture site. Tell him to keep his thumb pressed against the fingertip.

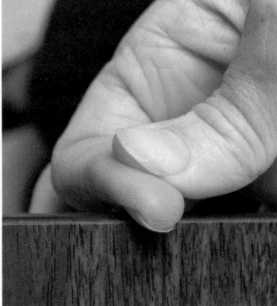

4. Have him place his fingertip against a firm surface, such as the edge of a table or counter. This will prevent him from instinctively moving away from the lancet. Explain that, by stabilizing his finger, he'll need less force to puncture the skin.

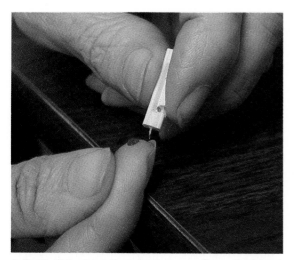

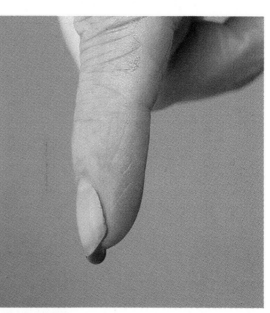

6. Milk his finger gently until you get a hanging drop of blood that looks large enough to cover the reagent area of the test strip. Be patient; keep trying to milk the finger before you make a second puncture, otherwise the patient may find himself bleeding from several puncture sites.

5. Twist off the lancet's protective cap. Grasp the lancet and quickly pierce the skin at the site you've chosen, as shown. Remove the patient's thumb from his fingertip to release pressure and permit blood flow.

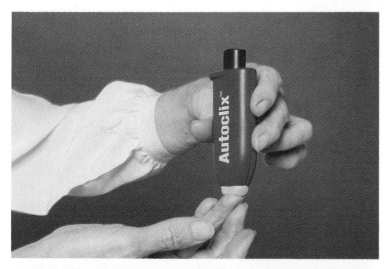

Obtaining blood mechanically

As described previously, choose a puncture site, instruct the patient to wash his hands or clean the site with alcohol, then squeeze his fingertip. Now:

1. To use the Autoclix, first depress its plunger to insert a new Monolet lancet. Remove the lancet's protective cap. Then position the lancet at the puncture site and gently press the Autoclix to release the lancet into the skin.

The Autoclix is designed so the lancet doesn't show. Its platforms come in three depths to accommodate different skin thicknesses.

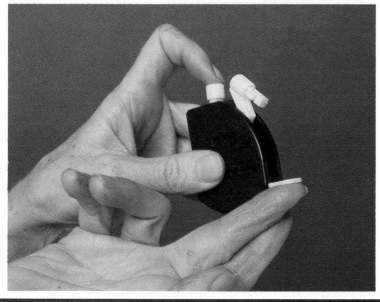

2. To use the Autolet, first put on a new platform, then insert a new Monolet and remove its protective top. Position the platform on the puncture site. The patient should see his skin through the hole in the platform. Now press the button that operates the arm containing the lancet.

Monitoring blood glucose

Three types of reagent strips are commonly used for testing blood glucose visually: Chemstrip bG (Bio-Dynamics), Visidex (Ames), and Dextrostix (Ames). Visidex essentially replaces Dextrostix for visual testing. Dextrostix is used more often when testing blood glucose with a meter, so it's not shown here.

Using Chemstrip bG

1. Remove a Chemstrip from its vial and tightly replace the vial's cap. Carefully lift the Chemstrip to the drop of blood. Note that the Chemstrip has a shiny, slippery surface; the blood will roll off if you don't place it on the strip correctly.

Let the blood completely cover the reagent area without rubbing or smearing it. If the blood smears, start again with a new reagent strip.

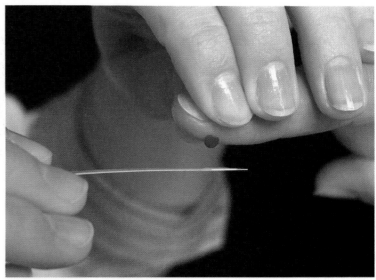

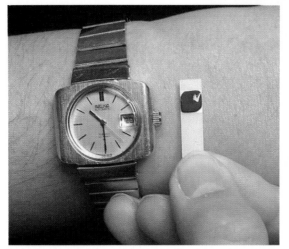

2. As you put the drop of blood on the reagent area, look at your watch or clock. Time exactly 60 seconds. Be sure to keep the strip level.

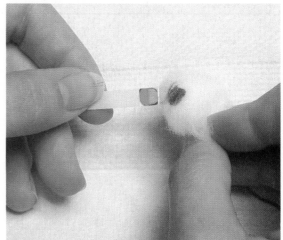

3. After 60 seconds, use a clean, dry cotton ball to gently wipe all the blood off the reagent area. Wipe a total of three times, each time using a clean side of the cotton ball. Then wait another 60 seconds.

4. Now determine blood glucose value by comparing the colors that have appeared on the reagent area with the two-colored blocks (on the 2-minute row) on the Chemstrip vial. Example: If both colors match the block labeled 80, the approximate value is 80 mg/dl.

If the colors fall between two blocks, take the average of the two numbers. Example: If colors fall between blocks labeled 180 and 240, the approximate blood glucose value is 210. If the reading exceeds 240 mg/dl, wait another 60 seconds. Then compare the reagent area with the blocks on the 3-minute row.

Write the date, time, and your initials on the reagent strip and store it in a tightly sealed, empty Chemstrip vial. The colors on the reagent area are stable for up to a week.

Record the blood glucose reading.

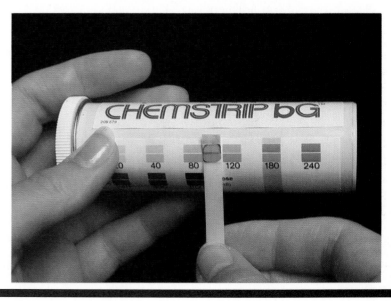

Using Visidex

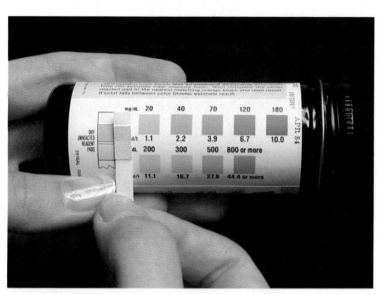

1. Remove a Visidex from its bottle and tightly replace the bottle's cap. Compare the yellow Visidex reagent pads (there are two) with the "dry, unreacted reagent pads" block on the label's color chart, as shown. If the reagent pads don't match, discard that strip and use one from a new bottle. Discoloration means the reagent has deteriorated and won't give you an accurate test result.

Lift the Visidex to a large, hanging drop of blood. Let the blood completely cover both reagent pads without smearing. Time exactly 60 seconds, keeping the strip level.

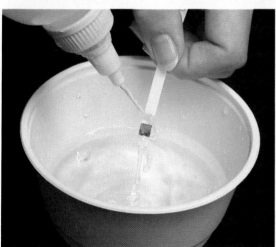

2. After 60 seconds, flush the blood from the pads for no more than 3 seconds, using a steady stream of water from either a wash bottle or faucet.

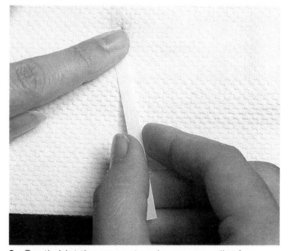

3. Gently blot the reagent pads once on a lint-free paper towel. Don't wipe or rub.

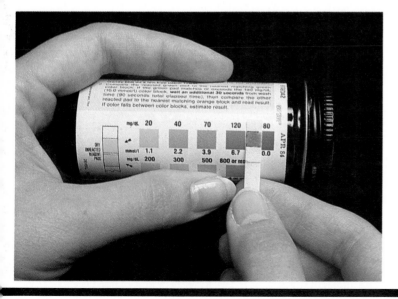

4. One reagent pad will have turned green. Immediately compare it to the green blocks on the Visidex bottle label. If that pad is darker than the darkest green block (180 mg/dl), wait another 30 seconds for the lower pad to turn orange. Then compare the orange reagent pad to the orange blocks on the label.

If the color on the reagent pad falls between two color blocks, take the average of those two values to get your result. Then record the blood glucose reading, along with all pertinent information.

(Note: A newer version of this test, Visidex II, has become available. It's a "dry" system, like Chemstrip bG.)

cause pain, self-testing should be done with an automatic bloodletting device, such as the Autoclix or Autolet. (See *Getting a drop of blood,* pages 134 and 135; *Monitoring blood glucose,* pages 136 and 137; and *Using a blood glucose meter,* page 139.)

Glycosylated hemoglobin test. A relatively new tool, this test measures three minor hemoglobins—Hgb A_{1a}, A_{1b}, and A_{1c}—which are variants of Hgb A formed by glycosylation. This is an irreversible process in which glucose adheres to a hemoglobin molecule. Since glycosylation occurs at a constant rate during the 120-day life span of an erythrocyte, glycosylated hemoglobin levels reflect the average blood glucose level over the past 2 to 3 months and thus can be used to evaluate the long-term effectiveness of diabetes therapy. This test requires far fewer venipunctures and is more accurate over time. The test may help prevent serious complications by alerting the doctor and patient to the need for changing the diabetic treatment regimen.

Glycohemoglobin levels reliably indicate the degree of diabetic control. Typically, a glycohemoglobin level of 7.5% or lower (normal: 3.5% to 6.2%) is rated as "good" control; a level of 7.6% to 8.9% is "fair"; and a level of 9.0% or more is "poor."

COMPLICATIONS OF DIABETES
Controlling blood glucose levels with diet and drugs is the key to medical management. No less important, however, is the management of acute and chronic complications of this disease. The acute complications, if identified correctly, are reversible with treatment; the chronic complications account for most of the morbidity and mortality.

Acute complications
Diabetic patients are vulnerable to three types of metabolically induced coma. (The term "coma" as used here denotes a diabetic crisis accompanied by unconsciousness or altered mentation.) The three states are hypoglycemia, DKA, and HHNC. (See *Comparing DKA, HHNC, and hypoglycemia,* page 140.)

Hypoglycemia ("insulin shock"). This occurs when blood glucose falls below levels required to sustain homeostasis. It can result from too much insulin, too little food, or excessive physical activity. Its onset varies with the type of insulin administered, injection site, and time of last meal. Hypoglycemia may occur 1 to 3 hours after a dose of regular insulin, 4 to 18 hours after NPH or Lente In-

sulin, and 18 to 30 hours or more after Protamine Zinc or Ultralente Insulin. Although hypoglycemic episodes may occur at any time, most occur before meals. Hypoglycemia may cause permanent neurologic damage. It may also impair diabetic control, since release of counterregulatory hormones results in rebound hyperglycemia, occasionally accompanied by mild ketosis. Recurrent hypoglycemia can be caused by the onset of pregnancy, renal failure, exercise, failure to decrease an insulin dose after recovery from an illness, or lipohypertrophy.

If the hypoglycemic patient is conscious, treatment begins with administration of simple carbohydrate-containing foods (such as orange juice or candy) by mouth. In the hospital or emergency department, the comatose patient should receive 50% glucose by I.V. push. The patient should regain consciousness within minutes. If he fails to regain consciousness, or if his blood glucose level hasn't risen above 60 mg/dl, another dose may be administered, according to your hospital's protocol. Most patients respond to a push of 10 to 25 g of glucose.

At home, family members are taught to administer glucagon (0.5 mg up to age 3, and 1 mg over age 3, or according to hospital protocol). Once the patient regains consciousness, usually in 15 to 20 minutes, simple sugar-containing solutions may be given until nausea, if any, subsides.

Diabetic ketoacidosis. This condition results from too little insulin. Insulin deficiency in blood and tissue sets off a chain of metabolic events. The first effect of insulin deficiency is that glucose cannot enter cells and so accumulates in the blood. When accumulated glucose exceeds the renal threshold, it spills into the urine. The excess urine glucose becomes an osmotic diuretic; thirst and dehydration follow.

At the same time, fats are broken down to supply energy to glucose-starved cells. But since the fats break down faster than they can be used (because insulin isn't there to suppress lipase enzymes), ketones, end products of fat metabolism, form in the liver, accumulate in the bloodstream, and enhance acidosis.

The body tries to buffer the increasing acidosis, but renal acid excretion and bicarbonate ion conservation mechanisms are now insufficient. The lungs (which excrete carbonic acid by venting carbon dioxide) try to compensate for this by going into the rapid Kussmaul's respirations characteristic of DKA.

Using a blood glucose meter

Several models of blood meters are currently available for self-testing blood glucose from fingerstick samples. They're divided into "wet" and "dry" types: a "wet" meter requires that blood be rinsed off the test strip before it's inserted into the meter; a "dry" meter requires blotting it off the strip before insertion. Instructions on how to use a typical "wet" meter system are given here.

Before using the Glucometer, you may need to complete its calibration and control procedures. Calibration checks only the accuracy of the meter. The control procedure checks the accuracy of the whole system. Follow the manufacturer's directions for calibrating your particular unit.

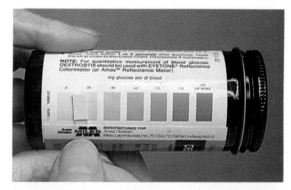

Testing blood glucose

1. Remove a Dextrostix from its bottle and tightly replace the cap. Compare the Dextrostix with the "0" block on the color chart. If the reagent pad color doesn't closely match or is discolored, discard that strip and choose one from a new bottle.

2. Obtain a large, hanging drop of blood. Turn on the Glucometer and press the TIME button. Quickly apply the drop of blood to the reagent pad. You have 4 seconds. Completely cover the pad without smearing.

3. You should have the blood on the pad by the time the buzzer sounds and you see a "60" on the digital display. This signals the beginning of the 60-second count. Hold the Dextrostix strip level during the count.

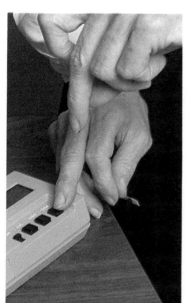

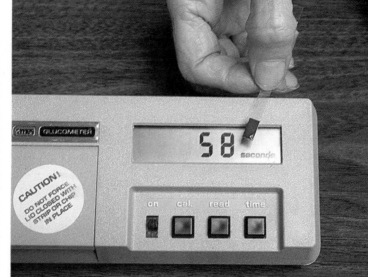

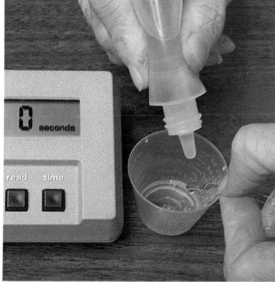

4. When the buzzer sounds again (and "0" shows up on the digital display), flush the blood from the pad for 1 to 2 seconds, using a stream of water from a wash bottle. Don't wash it under a faucet.

Gently blot the pad on a lint-free paper towel; don't wipe or rub it.

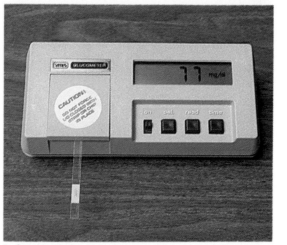

5. Quickly lift the test chamber lid and insert the strip as far as it will go into the strip guide, with the reagent pad facing down. Close the test chamber lid and press the READ button. Record your results.

Comparing DKA, HHNC, and hypoglycemia

Factor	Diabetic ketoacidosis	HHNC	Hypoglycemia
Type of diabetic	Insulin-dependent (Type I)	Non-insulin-dependent (Type II); nondiabetic person	Insulin-dependent
Signs and symptoms	History of nausea, vomiting, warm and dry skin, flushed appearance, dry mucous membranes, soft eyeballs, Kussmaul's respirations or tachypnea, abdominal pain, alterations in level of consciousness, hypotension, tachycardia, acetone breath	Same as in DKA except without Kussmaul's respirations or acetone breath	Nausea, hunger, malaise, cool and moist skin or diaphoresis, pallor, bradycardia, bradypnea, visual disturbances, alterations in level of consciousness: memory loss, confusion, hallucinations, generalized or focal seizures, status epilepticus, primitive movements (sucking, smacking lips, picking or grasping, Babinski's reflex) may be present
Precipitating factor	Undiagnosed diabetes; neglect of treatment; infection; cardiovascular disorder; other physical or emotional stress	Undiagnosed diabetes; infection or other stress; drugs (Dilantin, thiazide diuretics, mannitol steroids); dialysis; total parenteral nutrition; acute pancreatitis; central nervous system disorders; major burns treated with high concentrations of sugar	Delayed or omitted meal; insulin overdose; excessive exercise without alterations in food and/or insulin
Onset of symptoms	Slow (hours to days)	Slow (hours to days)	Rapid (minutes to hours)
Laboratory findings: Blood glucose Serum sodium Serum potassium Blood urea nitrogen Serum ketones White blood cell Hematocrit Urine glucose Urine ketones Arterial blood gases	 Usually less than 800 mg/dl Normal or decreased Normal or elevated at first, then decreased Elevated Elevated Elevated Elevated Elevated Elevated Metabolic acidosis with compensatory respiratory alkalosis	 Over 800 mg/dl Elevated, normal, or low Same as DKA Elevated Normal Elevated Elevated Elevated Normal Normal or slight metabolic acidosis	 60 mg/100 ml or less Normal Normal Normal Normal Normal or elevated Normal Normal Normal Normal or slight respiratory acidosis
Treatment	Insulin; I.V. fluids, such as normal or possibly half-normal saline solution; potassium* when urine output is adequate; sodium bicarbonate if pH is less than 7.0	Insulin; I.V. fluids, such as half-normal or normal saline solution; potassium when urine output is adequate	Candy; glucose paste; orange juice if awake; dextrose 50% I.V. push; 5% to 10% D/W I.V. drip; glucagon; epinephrine

*Potassium phosphate rather than potassium chloride may be used since patients may have hypophosphatemia.

When this mechanism fails to correct metabolic acidosis, the blood pH drops and ketoacidosis accelerates.

Protein stores also break down to provide energy to glucose-deprived cells. The liver, intervening, breaks amino acids into glucose and nitrogen. But without insulin the glucose remains unavailable to cells and increases in the blood, intensifying glycosuria and osmotic diuresis. Blood urea nitrogen (BUN) levels may rise as urea formation outstrips excretion. And protein breakdown brings marked loss of intracellular potassium, though circulating potassium may be low, normal, or even high. As blood glucose levels rise, ketones rise, too. This brings on osmotic diuresis, which stimulates release of *more* stress hormones. Unless the cycle of ketosis, acidosis, tissue breakdown, more ketosis, and more acidosis is broken by proper treatment, DKA results in coma and death.

Most often, infection, stress, and rapid growth are the precipitating factors in the onset of DKA. A careful history and physical examination are important in guiding diagnostic studies and treatment. DKA must be suspected in any diabetic patient with altered sensorium. Confirming this diagnosis requires that certain other disorders with some similar effects—such as hypoglycemic coma, lactic acidosis, alcoholic ketoacidosis, and drug intoxication—be ruled out.

Initial studies usually include a rough estimate of blood glucose levels using reagent strips (for example, Chemstrip or Visidex) and of urine ketones; further studies sometimes employed for differential diagnosis include serum acetone dilutions, blood glucose determination, serum electrolytes (sodium, chloride, potassium, and carbon dioxide), urinalysis, BUN, serum calcium and phosphorus, arterial blood gases (ABGs), complete blood count, EKG, chest X-ray, and blood/urine/stool cultures.

Successful treatment of DKA requires normalization of cellular metabolism through insulin administration, replacement of fluid and electrolytes to correct deficits, and treatment of the underlying cause. Thus, it requires frequent checks of blood glucose, ketones, electrolytes, and arterial blood gases during therapy.

Hyperglycemic hyperosmolar nonketotic coma. This condition is basically DKA without ketoacidosis; in HHNC the patient has enough insulin to inhibit lipolysis. The condition is a life-threatening emergency with a high mortality rate.

Although HHNC can occur in any diabetic patient, it usually occurs in Type II patients, rarely in children. Severe osmotic diuresis is present, with water loss exceeding electrolyte loss. Blood glucose levels may be 800 to 1,000 mg/dl or higher. The increasingly high plasma osmolality increases dehydration, which leads to neurologic symptoms; hemoconcentration may cause thromboses. Polyuria, polydipsia, and polyphagia appear at onset, but later on progressive dehydration, volume contraction, and coma interfere with normal CNS stimulation of the thirst mechanism.

Intravascular volume expansion is the treatment of choice for HHNC. As in DKA, electrolytes must be replaced, but smaller insulin doses are needed. Fluid therapy is monitored with a central venous pressure line. If the underlying cause of HHNC is known, it must be eliminated or treated. Among the known causal factors of HHNC are: drug therapy with thiazides, I.V. phenytoin, high-dosage corticosteroids, and propranolol, which impair glucose removal or insulin secretion; dialysis, which infuses large amounts of glucose; and infection.

Chronic complications

Diabetic patients may develop additional chronic complications long after the onset of overt hyperglycemia. These lead to considerable morbidity and premature mortality. Major complications include diabetic retinopathy, nephropathy, neuropathy, and circulatory abnormalities. These are managed as in a nondiabetic patient, except that blood glucose levels must be normalized as much as possible. (See *Staging diabetic retinopathy,* page 131.)

In every form of diabetes mellitus, it's most important to strive to maintain normal blood glucose levels 24 hours a day every day. Balancing dietary intake, insulin or oral agents, and exercise to keep serum glucose and lipid levels normal can delay and perhaps prevent the vascular and neurologic complications of diabetes.

Complications during pregnancy

Without meticulous control of diabetes throughout pregnancy, the fetus and mother may suffer numerous adverse consequences. Poor diabetic control causes hyperglycemia, with a transfer of glucose to the fetus. This causes fetal hyperinsulinemia, resulting in excessive fat deposition and an abnormally large neonate. Other serious diabetic effects include spontaneous abortion, congenital defects, premature delivery, intrauterine death, hypocalcemia, and jaundice.

Ideally, control of diabetes should begin at least 3 to 4 months before beginning the pregnancy and continue through to delivery. Even mild gestational diabetes will require two to three doses of insulin per day. As the pregnancy advances, the patient's insulin demand may rise to four times the baseline level and often requires four doses or an insulin pump. In such patients, daily blood glucose self-monitoring is required to allow dosage adjustments.

In pregnant patients, blood glucose levels must be kept lower than normal, with fasting values at 60 to 90 mg/dl and postprandial levels below 120 mg/dl. An insulin pump or multiple daily injections provides optimal control. With meticulous control, the prognosis for a diabetic pregnancy is usually good. The birth defect rate is reduced, and pregnancy can be carried to term with vaginal delivery of normal neonates.

NURSING MANAGEMENT

Since it may affect nearly every body system, diabetes presents many nursing challenges. In addition to its own widespread systemic effects, diabetes can interfere with resolution of other clinical problems, such as postoperative

Testing urine with reagent strips

Available products

Chemstrip uG
Chemstrip uGK (tests both glucose and ketones)
Clinistix
Clinitest
Diastix
Keto-Diastix (tests both glucose and ketones)
Tes-Tape
Acetest (tests ketones)

Note: To test urine with a 2- or 5-drop Clinitest tablet test, collect urine in a clean receptacle. Using the dropper, place 2 or 5 drops of urine in a test tube. Rinse the dropper and add 10 drops of water. Drop a tablet into the test tube. Watch it *during boiling and for 15 seconds after boiling stops*. Then shake the tube gently and match the color chart.

If you use Acetest tablets to check urine ketones, place 1 drop of urine on one tablet and wait 30 seconds before reading results.

Reagent strip tests (such as Tes-Tape, Chemstrip uG, Clinistix, and Diastix) test the urine for glucose. Strips such as Keto-Diastix and Chemstrip uGK test the urine for ketones as well as glucose. You may find ketones in the patient's urine if he is losing weight, is sick, or has very high blood glucose levels.

1. Remove a reagent strip from the bottle and close the cap tightly to protect strips from humidity and light. (With Tes-Tape, tear off about 1½" [3.8 cm].) Hold the strip at the end without reagent pads, making sure that the printing is facing up. Don't touch the reagent pads.

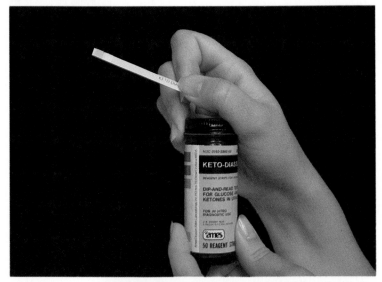

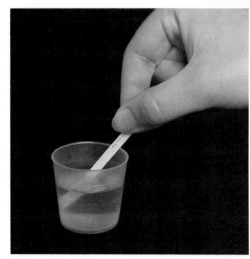

2. Dip the strip into the urine specimen for at least 2 seconds. The reagent pads must be thoroughly wet.

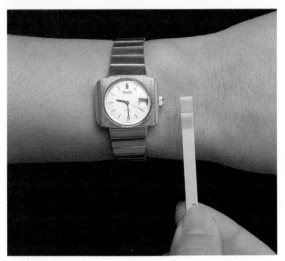

3. Then, remove the strip, tap it against the side of the container to remove excess urine, and begin timing the strip.

4. When the required time has elapsed, compare the color change on the reagent pad to the color chart on the container, and record the results.

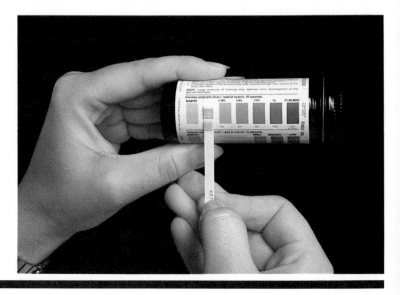

wound healing or steroid administration in rheumatoid arthritis. Clearly, the physical problems related to diabetes are as difficult to manage as they are numerous and complex. But managing psychological support is no less important. You should be ready to deal with a patient who's fearful of the disease and its treatment and worried about its long-range effects. Appropriate teaching and counseling are essential to an effective care plan. As always, these rest on accurate assessment.

Accurate assessment critical

To plan effective care, it's important to determine what the patient knows and does about his condition and what, if any, treatment he's had up to this point. During the initial patient interview, find out his *chief complaint.* The Type I diabetic usually mentions the classic symptoms of diabetes mellitus—polyuria, polydipsia, polyphagia, and (if the disorder is undiagnosed or out of control) weight loss. Sometimes these symptoms develop so rapidly that the patient is seen in an emergency setting. If such a patient is unconscious, obtain information as soon as possible from the person who brought him in for emergency treatment.

The Type II diabetic patient complains of vague symptoms involving almost any part of his body. An undiagnosed Type II patient usually seeks care for a seemingly unrelated problem, such as vision changes or fatigue; female patients frequently complain of vaginal itching and/or discharge.

Sometimes Type II diabetes is diagnosed in a patient who has sought preventive health care and has no chief complaint; a routine physical may disclose elevated blood glucose levels or glycosuria as the first sign of diabetes.

Getting a history

When you've determined the patient's chief complaint, obtain a chronologic history of all symptoms from their onset to the present. Review each body system to discover previously unsuspected problems. If you can't get a history from the patient himself, a family member or friend may prove helpful. You may be able to interview the patient more thoroughly after his condition improves.

The Type I diabetic patient usually describes his symptoms as acute, of abrupt and recent onset, while the Type II diabetic patient usually presents a vague and gradual onset, over months or years.

If your patient's been previously diagnosed as diabetic, his history may reveal his level of understanding of the disorder, the kinds of problems he's encountered, and, not least important, how well or how poorly he's managed his diabetes in the past. Question him about his medications; this may help identify drugs (such as steroids) affecting the degree of diabetic control.

Since diabetes may also affect growth and development, review your patient's developmental history, especially if he's a child.

Ask the adult patient about other diabetics in his family to be aware of possible familial tendencies. Try to elicit any recent history of physical or emotional stress, infection, trauma, divorce, or bereavement. When assessing a child, try to evaluate his interaction with siblings and parents.

Finally, because diabetes affects carbohydrate metabolism, assess the patient's nutritional status. This usually includes a description of 3 days' food intake, assessment of components from each of the four basic food groups, and the presence of any previous nutritional problems.

The physical examination

A careful physical examination may disclose early warning signs of diabetes long before such conclusive symptoms as weight loss, polydipsia, polyuria, polyphagia, and hyperglycemia appear. Early signs commonly involve the skin, in the form of shin spots, recurrent infections, or resistant fungal infections. (See *Potential diabetic physical findings,* page 144.)

Formulate nursing diagnoses

Drawing on the information you've gathered from the patient interview, medical history, and physical examination, you're ready to formulate nursing diagnoses that clearly define the patient's problems and allow you to plan appropriate goals and interventions. Keep in mind that you may not identify all of the patient's problems at once. Some problems, such as sexual dysfunction, may surface only after you've established a rapport with the patient and gained his trust. Typically, your nursing diagnoses reflect the following physiologic and psychological consequences of diabetes and the need for patient teaching about adequate self-management of the disease.

Potential for DKA related to metabolic disturbance. Your goals in this diagnosis are to identify the factors that precipitated DKA, to

Potential diabetic physical findings

Cardiovascular
Hypotension/hypertension
Tachycardia, other
   cardiac dysrhythmias
Hypovolemia; dehydration
Pulses normal, absent, or
   altered (bounding,
   weak, thready)

Respiratory
Abnormal breath sounds
   (decreased)
Rate and rhythm (hyper-
   pneic, labored)
Possible dyspnea
Possible fruity odor on
   breath

Renal
Urinary output: polyuria,
   anuria, or oliguria
Glucose or acetone in
   urine
Altered specific gravity
Evidence of infection
   (cloudy, malodorous
   urine)

Central nervous system
Headache
Drowsiness
Nervousness
Depression
Anxiety
Stupor
Coma

Sensorimotor
Depressed muscular tone
Depressed reflexes
Blurred vision
Altered response to
   stimuli

Skin, head, and neck
Skin lesions
Skin appears dry, flaky, or
   shiny (necrobiosis
   lipoidica diabeticorum)
Hair loss
Thickened toenails
Brown spots on skin of
   lower extremities ("shin
   spots")
Enlarged lymph nodes
   (infection)
Localized irritation or
   inflammation at
   injection sites, skin
   folds, between toes
Generalized rash
Hypertrophy or atrophy at
   injection sites
Presence of xanthomas
   (yellowish pustules)

educate the patient about the causes, signs, and early management of this hazardous complication, and to establish and maintain normal blood glucose levels and normal fluid and electrolyte balance.

To achieve these goals, assess your patient for changes associated with symptoms of diabetes. A flushed face, blurry vision, diminished deep tendon reflexes, paresthesia, abdominal pain, nausea, and vomiting indicate acidosis. Watch for dry skin with poor turgor, eyeballs that feel soft, and rising pulse rate with falling blood pressure. Drowsiness and stupor eventually progress to coma; the breath smells fruity and respirations are intermittent, with dyspnea interspersed with Kussmaul's respirations.

Monitor closely the patient's vital signs, level of alertness, urine volume, and cardiac status.

As ordered, check laboratory results (usually every hour): BUN, ABGs, serum glucose, serum ketones, and serum electrolytes. Administer I.V. fluids, insulin, and electrolyte supplements as needed.

Correct fluid volume deficit with rapid infusions of I.V. isotonic or hypotonic saline solution. The large fluid volume rehydrates the patient, dilutes hypertonic extracellular fluid, and encourages renal excretion of glucose. (In patients with cardiac or renal disease, volume status can be monitored with a central venous catheter.) When the plasma glucose level falls below 250 mg/dl, change the I.V. fluid from saline solution to 5% glucose in water to prevent both hypoglycemia and cerebral edema that may accompany a rapid insulin-induced drop in blood glucose levels.

As fluids are replaced, check urine volume, blood glucose levels, and urine ketones every hour. Potassium phosphate (rather than potassium chloride) may be added to the I.V. fluid, as ordered, to correct potassium deficit.

If the patient is incontinent, insert an indwelling catheter to accurately monitor urine output. When he's alert enough to control voiding, remove the catheter to reduce the risk of infection.

Correct hyperglycemia by giving low doses of regular insulin by continuous I.V. drip.

When the patient can take solid food, give subcutaneous insulin every 6 hours to gradually move him up to his preketosis meal pattern and insulin dosage. It may take several days to stabilize his blood glucose level with food, insulin, and activity.

Before discharge, assess your patient's knowledge of his treatment regimen. Answer

his questions as completely as you can.

Consider your interventions effective when DKA is resolved, as evidenced by maintenance of euglycemia and a normal fluid and electrolyte balance.

Potential for HHNC related to metabolic disturbance. Your goals are to enable the patient to learn about the signs and early management of HHNC, to establish and maintain normal blood glucose levels, and to maintain a normal fluid and electrolyte balance. To achieve these goals, assess the patient for signs of HHNC: polyuria, polydipsia, polyphagia, and weight loss.

Blood pressure falls; the urine becomes more concentrated; and tachycardia, fever, and thirst develop. The patient's skin and mucosae become dry. His tongue appears leathery, his eyeballs shrunken and soft under finger pressure.

Laboratory results reveal higher blood glucose levels than in DKA, but without ketonuria or ketonemia. Serum osmolality, hematocrit, hemoglobin, and BUN levels will be elevated because of dehydration.

In severe HHNC, the patient may experience confusion, lethargy, weakness, paralysis, and seizures. If left untreated, death usually results from coma. Provide care as for DKA; since this patient is not ketotic, give less insulin but more fluid to combat extreme hyperosmolality.

Consider your interventions effective when your patient demonstrates resolution of HHNC, as evidenced by euglycemia and a normal fluid and electrolyte balance.

Potential for hypoglycemia related to insulin excess. After you reach this diagnosis, your goals are to enable the patient to recognize signs of impending hypoglycemia, to administer treatment, and to help the patient prevent hypoglycemia in the future.

To achieve these goals, assess your patient for signs of hypoglycemia, such as personality changes, nervousness, hunger, nausea, excessive perspiration, lethargy, and double vision. Without treatment, convulsions and coma ensue.

Patients who receive intermediate and long-acting insulins may develop hypoglycemia at night, may experience nightmares or sleepwalking, or may cry out in their sleep. Check the patient hourly at night for signs of hypoglycemia by feeling his skin for moisture; if in doubt, by shining a light on the sleeping patient's eyes. If he's merely asleep, he'll shut both eyes tightly to the light (the "squint challenge reflex"); if he's comatose, he won't respond at all.

If hypoglycemia occurs, give carbohydrates. If the patient is alert and can swallow, give a rapidly absorbable carbohydrate (such as fruit juice, candy, or a carbonated beverage containing sugar). The amount you give should equal 5 to 10 g of quick-absorbing carbohydrate (about 4 oz of orange juice, for example). In some patients, 1 to 2 teaspoons of honey or sugar in a small amount of water may give a better response than orange juice. As the patient improves, give supplemental, slowly metabolized carbohydrates to restore liver glycogen and prevent recurring hypoglycemia.

If your patient is unresponsive and can't swallow, notify the doctor and, if permitted by your hospital, prepare to administer glucagon. By mobilizing liver glycogen stores, glucagon can arouse a comatose patient to the point where he can accept food.

If the patient fails to respond to treatment after 20 minutes, he should be given intravenous glucose or another dose of glucagon. When the patient regains consciousness, he should then be given complex carbohydrates to replenish glycogen stores and ward off further hypoglycemia.

When the patient recovers from hypoglycemia, try to determine what caused it. Consider too much insulin, too little food, or, if the patient's receiving physical therapy, possible overexertion of the injected extremity.

Before discharge, teach the patient and his family to recognize the signs of hypoglycemia, and instruct them about treatment and preventive measures. Tell the patient that he risks the recurrence of hypoglycemia by excessive use of alcohol or from certain drugs, such as aspirin, propranolol, or sulfonamides.

Consider your interventions effective if the patient is free of hypoglycemia, shows understanding of the signs of impending hypoglycemia, and knows what to do about them.

Anxiety related to being diagnosed as diabetic. Your goal is to reduce anxiety by teaching the patient about diabetes, its treatment, and its management. Assess the patient for signs of anxiety, such as uneasiness, apprehensiveness, withdrawal, a sense of dread, or hyperactivity. Encourage him to verbalize his beliefs about diabetes and his apprehensions about the changes required by treatments (daily injections, diet restrictions). Spend time with the patient to explain the disease and its treatment and management. Reassure him

that someone will be available to answer further questions. Provide him with printed information that he can take home and use.

Your interventions will be successful if the patient can deal effectively with diabetes and its management.

Knowledge deficit related to diabetes management. Your goals are to enable the patient to understand the relation between good diabetes management and health, to understand the diabetic treatment regimen, and to become aware of the degree of diabetic control being achieved.

Your patient's knowledge requirements vary with the type of treatment. Instruct him about the pathophysiology of the disease and the signs and symptoms of hypoglycemia and hyperglycemia. Provide dietary guidelines and explain how physical activity affects treatment. Instruct the patient about urine testing (see *Testing urine with reagent strips,* page 142), foot care, hygiene, sick day rules, treatment of minor injuries (see *Caring for your skin and feet,* page 147), identification for the diabetic, and how and when to seek appropriate medical advice.

If the patient's treatment includes an oral hypoglycemic agent, instruct him about it and explain how it counteracts hyperglycemia. If treatment includes insulin, instruct him about insulin administration, prevention of hypoglycemia and hyperglycemia, and blood glucose self-testing (see *How to give yourself an insulin injection,* page 148; and *Monitoring blood glucose,* pages 136 and 137.) Whenever possible, provide group teaching as well as individual instruction to give your patient valuable emotional support. Individual instruction allows you to refine your nursing care plan and deal effectively with the patient's emotional problems. When teaching the patient and his family, let them proceed at their own pace, and encourage their questions. At discharge, provide written instructions and refer the patient to a community health nurse, a nurse practitioner, or a local clinic for follow-up care and teaching.

Consider your interventions successful when your patient understands the relation between diabetes and health, understands the component parts of prescribed treatment, demonstrates appropriate management techniques, and strives for optimal control of his condition.

Altered nutrition exceeding body requirements related to metabolic disturbance. Your goals are to help the patient lose excess weight and maintain optimum weight, maintain proper nutrition, and control diabetes as his weight changes.

Assess your patient's present diet. Look for imbalances in carbohydrate, protein, and fat distribution. Ask about snacking; does he tend to go on "binges"? Determine the patient's daily caloric intake. Obtain a reducing diet order from the doctor, and request diet instructions from the dietitian.

Explain to the insulin-dependent diabetic patient that close medical supervision is needed because insulin must be decreased as his weight decreases. Help him understand the relation between excess weight and diabetes. This often strongly motivates a patient to lose weight. Alert him to situations that may tempt him to overeat or reduce his physical activity.

Consider your interventions effective when the patient can lose weight and keep it at an optimum level.

Ineffective coping related to diabetes and its complications. After reaching this diagnosis, your goals are to help the patient become aware of his feelings and how they influence compliance with diabetic treatment, attain better coping strategies, and establish realistic goals for living.

To achieve your goals, invite the patient to express his feelings about the treatment. Help him to explore different ways of handling stress. Tailor the diabetic treatment regimen to the patient's life-style and ethnic group. Provide accurate information that will dispel misconceptions. Inform him of diabetic clubs or support groups that will allow him to share concerns, problems, and ideas with others in similar situations. If appropriate, encourage him to seek psychological counseling and therapy as needed to learn better ways to deal with the stress of living with a chronic illness.

Consider your interventions successful if the patient establishes realistic goals for daily living and can follow his treatment regimen.

Potential for injury related to small and large vessel disease and neuropathy. After you reach this diagnosis, your goals are to prevent patient injury and to promote tissue perfusion.

To achieve these goals, assess the patient's skin for general condition, breaks or lesions, evidence of infection, or such abnormalities as lipodystrophy at injection sites. Check the legs for clues to circulatory status. Cold feet, thickened toenails, thin and shiny atrophic skin on the legs, and absence of hair on the toes and lower legs may indicate vascular insufficiency.

Teach the patient to care for minor injuries to his feet and legs. Fresh skin breaks should be thoroughly washed with soap and warm water, then dried and kept covered to prevent infection. Check with the patient's doctor for the preferred antiseptic since some are known to promote skin breaks from excessive skin drying. If the wound fails to heal, arrange for prompt treatment. Periodically review foot care procedures with the patient.

Consider your interventions successful when the patient performs effective preventive skin and foot care and avoids injury.

Pain related to neuropathy. Your goal is to minimize the pain of diabetic neuropathy. To achieve this goal, assess the patient for signs of neuropathic pain: aching or burning sensations felt in the extremities, usually at night.

Encourage the patient to walk, which may help relieve the pain. In some patients, the slightest stimulus to their feet causes pain; provide foot cradles for such patients to prevent contact with the bedclothes. Maintain a euglycemic state to reduce neuropathic pain, which is most often associated with increased blood glucose levels.

Consider your interventions successful if the patient is comfortable and free from pain.

Altered bowel and bladder elimination related to neuropathy. Your goals are to help the patient maintain adequate elimination patterns, prevent urinary tract infections, and maintain his self-esteem.

To achieve these goals, assess the patient for bowel and bladder dysfunction. He may experience alternating periods of constipation and diarrhea, nocturnal fecal incontinence, infrequent voiding, weak stream or dribbling, and symptoms of urinary tract infection.

Provide psychological support to the patient by ensuring his privacy to minimize embarrassment. Encourage him to talk about his feelings and answer his questions as completely as you can.

As ordered, administer prescribed drugs: Lomotil or codeine phosphate for diarrhea; metoclopramide (Reglan) for gastroparesis; tetracycline or neomycin to prevent excessive bacterial growth in the atonic bowel; Urecholine for bladder paralysis; and various antibiotics for urinary tract infections. Instruct the patient about the importance of close follow-up care during long-term use of these drugs.

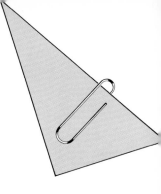

PATIENT-TEACHING AID

Caring for your skin and feet

Dear _____

Skin and foot care are important parts of your self-care plan. Dry skin is a common problem; it causes cracks in the skin that allow bacteria to lodge in crevices, resulting in infection. Minor foot injuries may have severe consequences because of poor circulation or peripheral nerve damage. You can help avoid such complications by practicing good preventive care, especially by maintaining good control of your blood glucose. Poor control encourages and complicates skin disorders.

Skin care
• Keep your skin clean and dry, especially in the skin folds; fungal infections are especially apt to begin in warm, moist areas, such as the armpits, the groin, and under the breasts.
• When you bathe, avoid very hot water and, if you have dry skin, avoid bubble baths; wash with superfatted soaps, such as Dove, Basis, Alpha Keri, and Oilatum. After bathing, you may also need to apply an oil-in-water skin preparation, such as Lubriderm or Keri Lotion. Also, avoid dry air in your home; use a humidifier if necessary.
• Don't use harsh medications on your skin. Use mild shampoos and avoid "feminine hygiene" sprays as well as scented soaps. Typically, you

don't need to use hypoallergenic makeup or special shampoos, deodorants, nail polishes, or acne medications. (Acne is not more common or virulent in patients with diabetes.) If you have special skin problems, see a dermatologist.

Foot care
• Wash your feet daily. Dry them carefully, especially between the toes.
• Inspect your feet daily, including the toe webs, for blisters, cuts, redness, and scratches.
• Never put your feet into hot water. Always check the water temperature first with your elbow before putting your feet in. This will prevent burns from water that is too hot. Soak your feet for 5 to 10 minutes.
• Apply oil or lotion to your feet immediately after washing and drying. This will seal in the water, prevent dryness, and keep your skin soft. If you have sweaty feet, use a mild foot powder. Put it between your toes, in your socks, and in your shoes.
• If your feet feel cold in bed, wear socks to sleep. Don't use hot water bottles or heating pads; if you have any loss of sensation, you can burn your feet without realizing it.
• Don't use chemical lotions or ointments for corns, calluses, or

warts; these products are often too harsh for a diabetic patient's skin. Don't try to remove corns and calluses yourself.
• Before putting on shoes, check them for foreign objects, torn linings, and protruding nails.
• Buy socks, stockings, and shoes that fit well. Don't buy shoes that will have to be "broken in" to be comfortable. Wear even well-fitting new shoes for short periods of time at first.
• Always wear leather shoes, which allow some air to circulate to your feet. Plastic shoes can cause your feet to perspire and can lead to fungal infections, blisters, and rashes.
• Don't wear hosiery that's been mended or has seams, because bumpy areas can put pressure on your feet. Change socks every day.
• Don't wear constricting garters or rubber bands on your legs.
• Never walk in bare feet. When walking in your home at night, turn on a light to avoid bumping your feet.
• Cut toenails straight across, unless they're flanked by deep skin folds.
• See your doctor and podiatrist regularly. Inform each new doctor that you are a diabetic.
• Consult your doctor at the first sign of inflammation or infection.

If the patient has a bladder dysfunction, establish a regular 2-hour voiding schedule to avoid problems that may arise from urine stasis. Encourage him to drink an appropriate amount of fluid each day (if not contraindicated) to promote adequate flushing of the renal system. Manage urinary tract infections and renal failure as you would in any patient with these problems.

Consider your interventions successful if the patient has adequate elimination and no

urinary tract infection and if he maintains a positive self-image.

Potential for sensory loss related to retinopathy. Your goal is to help the visually impaired patient maintain independence and self-esteem. To achieve this goal, offer encouragement and psychological support; help the patient achieve a positive attitude that focuses on his abilities, not on his losses. Encourage independence by allowing him to do as much for himself as he can do safely.

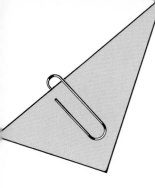

PATIENT-TEACHING AID

How to give yourself an insulin injection

Dear _____

This aid is meant to supplement, not replace, instructions from your nurse. Use it as a written reminder of what the nurse has taught you.

1. Before beginning the procedure, wash your hands thoroughly. Then remove the insulin from the refrigerator. Warm it until it's reached room temperature. Then mix it by rolling the vial between your palms. Check the expiration date, and read the label to make sure the medication's the correct strength and type, and made by the same manufacturer. *Important: Never shake the vial.* Cleanse the rubber stopper on top of the vial with an alcohol swab.

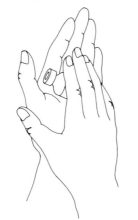

2. Select a proper site, remembering what you learned from the nurse about site selection. Pull the skin taut, and use an alcohol swab or a cotton ball soaked in alcohol to clean it in a circular motion.

3. Take the cover off the needle and put it aside temporarily. Hold the syringe like a pencil. Inject an equal amount of air into the vial before you draw up the insulin. This way, you avoid creating a vacuum in the vial and make withdrawing your insulin easier. *Note:* If you see air bubbles in the syringe after filling it with insulin, tap the syringe lightly to remove them.

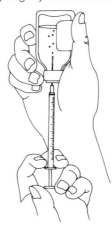

4. Now pinch the skin at the cleansed site between your thumb and forefinger, and quickly plunge the needle into the fat fold. Hold the needle at a 45° angle if the fat fold is less than 1″ (2.5 cm) and at a 90° angle if it is greater than 1″. As you hold the syringe with one hand, pull back on the plunger slightly with your other hand to check for blood backflow. If blood appears in the syringe, discard everything and start again. If no blood appears, inject the insulin slowly.

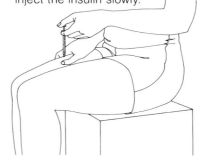

5. Place an alcohol swab over the site, and press lightly with it after you withdraw the needle. Snap the needle off the syringe, and dispose of the needle and syringe properly. Chart where you made your injection.

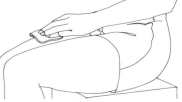

6. Don't use the same injection site more than once every 2 months. It's important to "rotate sites" to prevent changes in the fatty tissue that can interfere with insulin absorption.

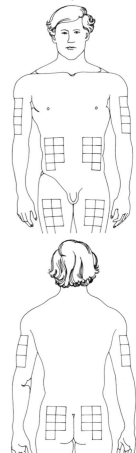

Alert the patient and his family to potential everyday safety hazards.

Help the patient adjust to techniques of insulin injection and urine collection. For example, other family members, neighbors, or a community health nurse can help with the urine testing, read the color standards (audible devices are also available), administer the insulin, or help with physical care. Acquaint your patient with available self-help devices; for example, magnifiers that make the insulin syringe easier to read and dosage monitors that withdraw the exact amount of insulin. *Aids for the Blind,* a publication available from the American Foundation for the Blind, offers other suggestions for blind or visually impaired diabetic patients.

Teach the visually impaired patient how to administer his own insulin. He should inject it by placing the needle at the skin surface and pushing it in rather than holding it above the skin and thrusting it in.

A 7-day supply of insulin can be withdrawn into separate insulin syringes by a community health nurse or other sighted person and placed in the patient's refrigerator. Insulin deteriorates slightly during such storage, and maintaining sterility may be a problem. Also, the patient must roll the syringe in his hand before administration to mix and warm the solution.

If necessary, your patient may be able to use the "yeast method" to estimate urine glucose levels. In this test, the patient adds ¼ teaspoonful of baker's yeast to a large test tube containing 12 ml of urine. He then fits a rubber fingercot over the mouth of the tube, making sure it's completely deflated, and shakes the tube vigorously. If glucose is present, it will interact with the yeast to form carbon dioxide, which inflates the fingercot. When performed at room temperature, this test may indicate glucose concentrations as low as 0.25% in 20 to 30 minutes. A fingercot that fails to inflate indicates little or no glucose; a partially inflated fingercot suggests a medium amount of glucose; and a taut, fully inflated fingercot indicates a large amount of glucose. This test method can provide reassurance and a sense of independence for the blind patient.

Remember: Because of the elevated renal threshold older patients may have, blood glucose testing is the method of choice, plus urine ketone testing for Type I patients who are ill or have blood glucose levels higher than 250 mg/dl.

Consider your interventions successful when your patient can care for himself, as shown by his ability to inject insulin and test his urine for glucose.

Sexual dysfunction related to neuropathy. Your goal is to help your patient regain sexual self-confidence and satisfaction within the limits imposed by physiologic impairment. To achieve this, encourage the patient to verbalize his feelings, and provide accurate answers to his questions.

Explain that hormonal therapy is of no help if neuropathy is involved. He may ask about penile prostheses; an open, honest discussion of these aids may encourage him to seek professional counseling.

Consider your interventions successful if your patient understands his problem and obtains appropriate medical assistance to help him and his partner achieve a more satisfactory sex life.

Altered parenting related to diagnosis of diabetes in the child. Your goals are to help parents maintain a healthy relationship with their child and to help them understand their role in managing their child's diabetic regimen.

To achieve these goals, assist the parents in supporting the growing child with empathy, understanding, and discipline. Involve the parents in your teaching plan for the child's care. Encourage the parents to join a support group or to talk to other parents of diabetic children.

Consider your interventions successful when the parents have established a relaxed and working relationship with their diabetic child.

Looking to the future
Although diabetes continues to afflict large numbers of people, current research has provided some hope for the future. It has illuminated the complexity of this disorder and its complications and has led to practical ways to arrest, reverse, or even prevent at least some of the consequences. Precise serum radioimmunoassay techniques have expanded our knowledge of how insulin and glucagon are produced, activated, and inactivated. The development of human insulin has guaranteed an unlimited supply of the hormone. Perhaps, in the future, implants of beta cells or an implanted artificial pancreas may be used to maintain good blood glucose control, eliminating daily insulin injections. Until then, managing this complex disease will continue to challenge all of your nursing skills.

Points to remember

• Diabetes mellitus, which affects nearly every body system, is now the third leading cause of death by disease in the United States.
• The etiology of Type I diabetes is thought to involve genes, viruses, and autoimmunity. The etiology of Type II is thought to be predominantly hereditary.
• Hyperglycemia and hyperlipidemia can cause vascular disease, such as microangiopathy and macroangiopathy.
• Home blood glucose monitoring and Hgb A_{1c} testing illustrate the advances made in monitoring blood glucose levels. Concurrently, new developments have occurred in insulin therapy, such as biosynthetic human insulin and insulin infusion pumps.
• You must understand thoroughly the differences between the three diabetic comas—DKA, HHNC, and hypoglycemic coma—to effectively and accurately plan your patient's care.
• Thorough assessment and patient education are crucial to ensure compliance with the diabetic treatment regimen.

11 CORRECTING HYPOGLYCEMIA

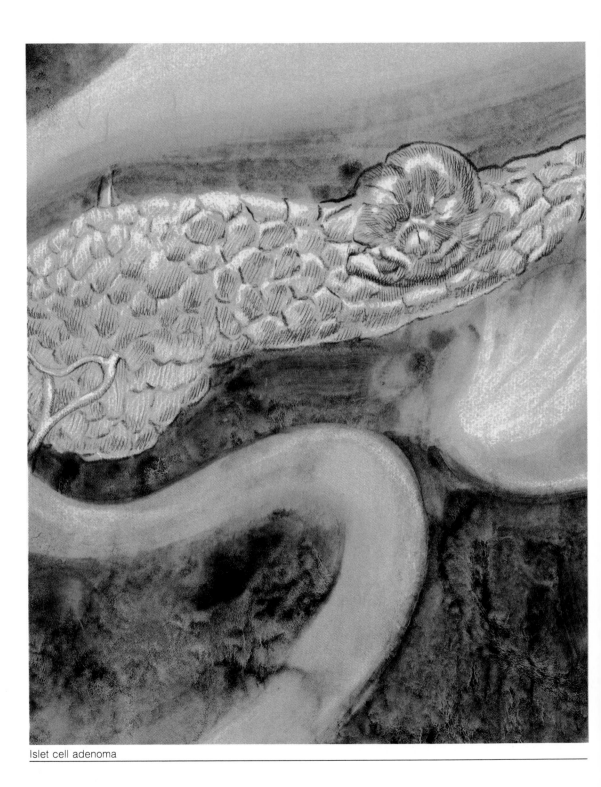

Islet cell adenoma

f you've worked with diabetic patients, you're no doubt familiar with hypoglycemia as a common reaction to excessive insulin effect. But how well do you know hypoglycemia as a separate disease? Though it's a specific endocrine imbalance, its symptoms are often vague.

Broadly defined as a drop in blood glucose levels to below 50 mg/dl, hypoglycemia may occur at higher glucose levels, and symptoms often depend on how quickly the patient's glucose levels drop. If not corrected, severe hypoglycemia may result in coma and irreversible brain damage. Milder forms of this imbalance cause faintness, weakness, hunger, anxiety symptoms and palpitations. To help your patients cope with hypoglycemia effectively, you must first understand how it arises and how to recognize it.

PATHOPHYSIOLOGY

Normally, glucose is the body's chief energy source. The body burns available glucose and stores the rest as glycogen in the liver and muscle tissues. When the body's glucose level drops, the liver converts glycogen back to glucose (glycogenolysis) or makes new glucose from noncarbohydrates, such as amino acids or fatty acids (gluconeogenesis).

How does this happen? Through the action of four hormones: glucagon, secreted by the pancreas; epinephrine, secreted by the adrenal medulla; growth hormone, secreted by the pituitary gland; and cortisol, secreted by the adrenal glands. (See *Hormonal responses to hypoglycemia,* page 152.) These hormones assist in glycogenolysis and gluconeogenesis and encourage utilization of fatty acids instead of glucose as fuel by most body tissues. This allows available glucose to nourish the brain, which must utilize glucose directly. If glucose levels continue to drop, starvation ketosis can occur, resulting in cerebral hypoxia and edema.

Hypoglycemia occurs when glucose is used too rapidly; when the glucose release rate lags behind tissue demands; or when excessive insulin enters the bloodstream. The disorder is classified two ways: *reactive* and *fasting.*

Reactive hypoglycemia

Reactive hypoglycemia may take several forms. In a diabetic patient, it may result from administration of too much insulin or—less commonly—too much oral hypoglycemia medication. In a mildly diabetic patient (or one in the early stages of diabetes mellitus),

reactive hypoglycemia may result from delayed and excessive insulin production after carbohydrate ingestion. Similarly, a nondiabetic patient may suffer reactive hypoglycemia from a sharp increase in insulin output after a meal. Sometimes called *postprandial hypoglycemia,* this type of reactive hypoglycemia usually disappears when the patient eats something sweet. In some patients, reactive hypoglycemia may have no known cause (idiopathic reactive) or may result from hyperalimentation due to gastric dumping syndrome and from impaired glucose tolerance.

Idiopathic reactive hypoglycemia produces symptoms about 2 to 5 hours after eating, but the reason for this is unclear. In some patients, insulin levels rise; in others, intestinal glucose absorption increases. This often puzzling disorder is sometimes dubbed "nonhypoglycemia," because of its vague symptoms and difficult diagnosis.

Nonspecific symptoms suggesting epinephrine release (such as sweating, tremor, rapid heartbeat, dizziness, and confusion) arise and subside spontaneously in 15 to 20 minutes. The syndrome is easily mistaken for an actual pathologic state unless the patient's blood glucose level is measured while he is experiencing symptoms. (See *Idiopathic reactive hypoglycemia,* page 156.)

Hyperalimentation hypoglycemia occurs in patients who've had gastric surgery, such as gastrectomy, gastrojejunostomy, vagotomy, or pyloroplasty. In this type of hypoglycemia, the gastric contents are ejected into the intestines and thus into the bloodstream shortly after digestion, causing a dumping syndrome. Hypoglycemic symptoms occur within several minutes to 2 hours after food ingestion.

Impaired glucose tolerance occurs approximately 3 to 5 hours after ingestion of carbohydrates. It's characteristically manifested by early hyperglycemia, followed by a delayed rise in insulin levels that causes a marked decrease in blood glucose. Signs and symptoms include tachycardia, sweating, weakness, anxiety, hunger, poor concentration, and occasionally visual difficulty. This type of hypoglycemia sometimes leads to diabetes.

Fasting hypoglycemia

Fasting hypoglycemia usually results from an excess of insulin or insulinlike substance or from a decrease in counterregulatory hormones. Fasting hypoglycemia can be *exogenous,* resulting from such external factors as alcohol or other drug ingestion, or *endoge-*

Hormonal responses to hypoglycemia

Hormone	Secretion	Action	Effects
Glucagon	Rapid	Rapid	Increases hepatic glycogenolysis and gluconeogenesis
Epinephrine	Rapid	Rapid	Inhibits glucose utilization by muscle; increases hepatic gluconeogenesis; stimulates glucagon secretion; inhibits insulin secretion
Cortisol	Delayed	Probably immediate	Increases hepatic gluconeogenesis; inhibits glucose utilization by muscle; alters insulin actions in target organs
Growth hormone	Delayed	Delayed	Inhibits glucose utilization by muscle; may increase hepatic gluconeogenesis; alters inside actions in target organs

nous, resulting from organic problems.

Endogenous hypoglycemia may result from tumors or liver disease. Insulinomas, small islet cell tumors in the pancreas, secrete excessive amounts of insulin, which inhibits hepatic glucose production. They are generally benign (in 90% of patients). Extrapancreatic tumors, though uncommon, can also cause hypoglycemia by increasing glucose utilization and inhibiting glucose output. Such tumors occur primarily in the mesenchyma, liver, adrenal cortex, gastrointestinal system, and lymphatic system. They may be benign or malignant. Among nonendocrine causes of fasting hypoglycemia are severe liver diseases, including hepatitis, cancer, cirrhosis, and liver congestion associated with congestive heart failure. All of these conditions reduce the uptake and release of glycogen from the liver. (See *Two paths to hypoglycemia,* page 153.) Some endocrine causes include destruction of pancreatic islet cells; adrenocortical insufficiency, which contributes to hypoglycemia by reducing the production of cortisol and cortisone needed for gluconeogenesis; and pituitary insufficiency, which reduces ACTH and GH levels.

Generally slow in onset, fasting hypoglycemia produces CNS symptoms similar to those in reactive hypoglycemia; however, they are more severe, and if uncorrected may lead to convulsions, hemiplegia, coma, and manic or psychotic behavior. (See *Signs and symptoms of hypoglycemia,* page 154.) The patient with fasting hypoglycemia experiences distressing hunger during prolonged periods of fasting, such as in the middle of the night; he can ease his symptoms by eating.

Fasting hypoglycemia and drug reactions
Fasting hypoglycemia results most commonly from insulin reactions but may also follow ingestion of oral hypoglycemics, such as sulfonylureas (see also Chapter 10, *Dealing with Diabetes Mellitus*), and ingestion of drugs that potentiate the effects of oral hypoglycemics, such as salicylates and ethanol.

Ethanol-induced hypoglycemia is probably the most underdiagnosed type of hypoglycemia. It is most dangerous in the fasting state because ethanol interferes with hepatic gluconeogenesis. The reactions, which can be mistaken for inebriation, can progress to hypothermia, convulsions, and coma. Hypoglycemia is rarely fatal, but when it is, ethanol ingestion is usually involved. Chronic alcoholics are most vulnerable to this type of hypoglycemia; so are small children, victims of starvation, and decompensated diabetics.

MEDICAL MANAGEMENT
Since the causes of hypoglycemia are many and often unrelated, identifying them may be as difficult as it is necessary. Successful medical management depends not only on accurate diagnosis of hypoglycemia, but also on diagnosis of the kind of hypoglycemia present. Before deciding what kind of diagnostic workup to order, the doctor must discover by careful questioning, whether the patient's symptoms are related to eating or fasting.

Getting a handle on glucose
A general diagnosis of hypoglycemia stems from a determination of blood glucose below 40 mg/dl (50 mg/dl for plasma or serum) for reactive hypoglycemia, and below 50 mg/dl

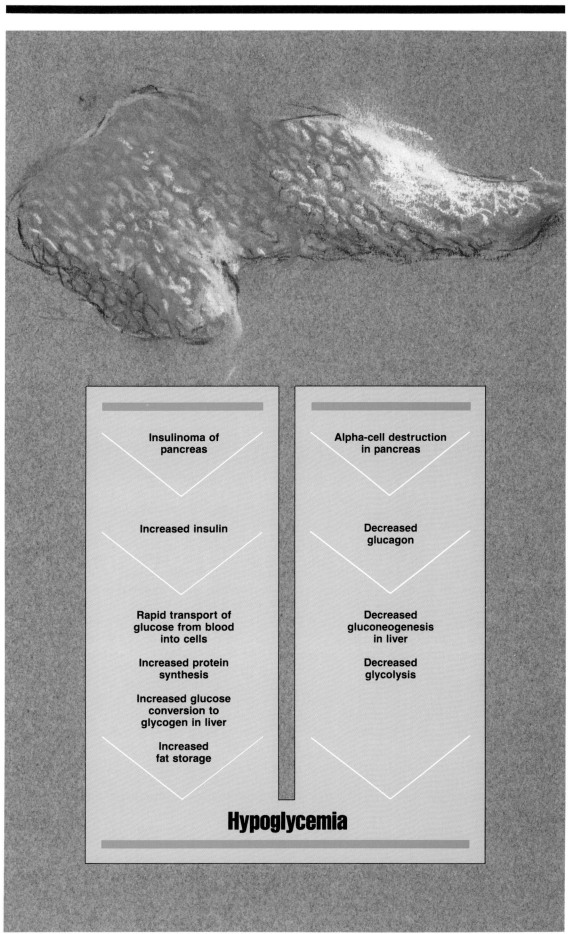

Two paths to hypoglycemia

Insulin and glucagon, which both originate in the islets of Langerhans in the pancreas, exert opposite physiologic effects: insulin decreases blood glucose and glucagon increases it. Too much insulin causes hypoglycemia; too little glucagon may cause it also.

Insulinoma of pancreas

Increased insulin

Rapid transport of glucose from blood into cells

Increased protein synthesis

Increased glucose conversion to glycogen in liver

Increased fat storage

Alpha-cell destruction in pancreas

Decreased glucagon

Decreased gluconeogenesis in liver

Decreased glycolysis

Hypoglycemia

Signs and symptoms of hypoglycemia

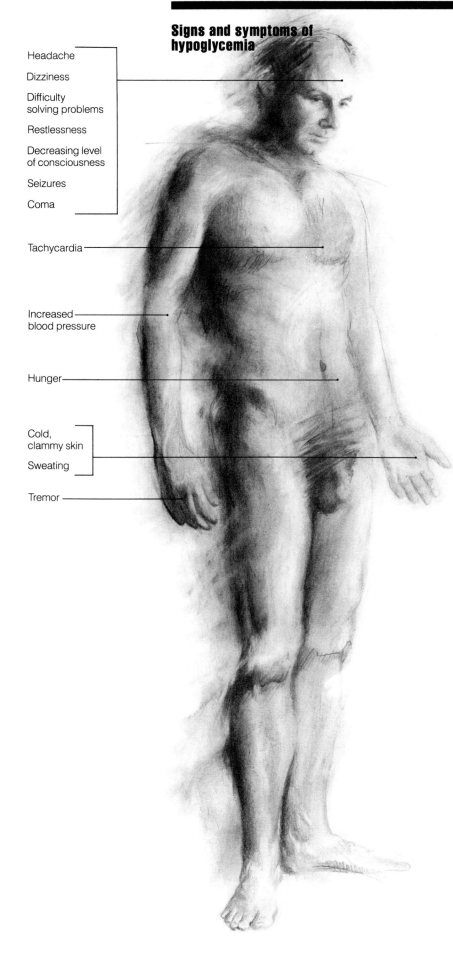

Headache

Dizziness

Difficulty solving problems

Restlessness

Decreasing level of consciousness

Seizures

Coma

Tachycardia

Increased blood pressure

Hunger

Cold, clammy skin

Sweating

Tremor

(60 mg/dl for plasma or serum) for fasting hypoglycemia. (Remember that glucose concentrations in plasma or serum are 10% to 15% higher than in whole blood.)

Fasting blood glucose. The best test to confirm fed or fasting hypoglycemia is to withhold the patient's food for 24 to 72 hours, while closely monitoring his blood glucose levels. Most patients with fasting hypoglycemia show abnormally low glucose levels after 24 hours; all show it after 72 hours. During the fast, glucose levels are checked every 6 hours at first, then more often as the fast continues. In addition, glucose and insulin levels should be checked while the patient is experiencing symptoms. Postfast plasma levels below 50 mg/dl in men and below 35 mg/dl in women strongly suggest organic fasting hypoglycemia.

Insulin/glucose ratio

The ratio of overnight fasting plasma glucose to fasting insulin levels may be studied to rule out beta cell insulinoma, an important cause of fasting hypoglycemia. In such patients, abnormally high insulin levels persist in the presence of low glucose levels during a 3-day fast. Insulin is measured in radioassay measurements as immunoreactive insulin in µU/ml, and glucose in mg/100 dl. The insulin/glucose ratio should be checked every 2 to 4 hours while the patient is awake and every 4 to 6 hours during his sleep. Although an insulin/glucose ratio below 2.5 usually indicates insulinoma, a consistent rise in the I/G ratio is the primary diagnostic feature. Such tumors may be surgically removed or treated with chemotherapy.

Glucose tolerance test. Although not completely accurate, the oral glucose tolerance test is most commonly used to investigate reactive hypoglycemia. The patient ingests a challenge dose of glucose, and blood samples are drawn every 30 minutes for 5 hours. To obtain a conclusive diagnosis, blood should be drawn while the patient experiences symptoms. The interval between carbohydrate ingestion and onset of symptoms helps distinguish the type of reactive hypoglycemia he's experiencing. (See *Idiopathic reactive hypoglycemia,* page 156.)

Other diagnostic tools. Other specialized tests may be needed to pinpoint the cause of hypoglycemia, especially of the fasting type. To differentiate endogenous or organic fasting hypoglycemia from exogenous or drug-induced hypoglycemia, the circulating C-peptide level is measured. During insulin production in the beta cells, insulin and C-peptide are cleaved from proinsulin and stored in the beta cells before secretion. The C-peptides have proved useful as indicators of beta-cell function. In organic hypoglycemia, the C-peptide level is high, suggesting endogenous oversecretion/overproduction; but in insulin-induced hypoglycemia, the C-peptide level remains normal because the circulating insulin was administered exogenously.

Difficult diagnoses may require still other specialized tests, such as liver function tests; adrenal and pituitary gland function tests (levodopa, adrenocorticotropic hormone, thyrotropin-releasing factor); and intravenous pyelography, ultrasound, or computer scanning to detect extrapancreatic tumors.

Treating hypoglycemia

Treating reactive hypoglycemia depends mainly on modifying the diet to provide less carbohydrate, more protein, and a fair amount of fat. Low carbohydrate intake helps prevent rebound hypoglycemia, while the high protein component provides energy by a slower breakdown than carbohydrates. This diet, taken in frequent, smaller meals, helps prevent the cycle of glucose overload followed by rebound hypoglycemia. In patients with severe reactive hypoglycemia, anticholinergics may help by slowing down gastric emptying.

Treatment of fasting hypoglycemia is directed at the underlying cause. For example, hypoglycemia that results from tumors generally requires surgery. If surgery is not feasible, drug therapy with streptozocin or oral diazoxide may be used. Ethanol-induced hypoglycemia requires alcohol withdrawal and good dietary control. Adrenal insufficiency or other endocrine causes require hormonal replacement therapy.

An acute episode of hypoglycemia can be treated with I.V. glucose or oral feedings. Drugs that increase glucose, such as glucagon, are ineffective against hepatic or tumor-induced hypoglycemia.

NURSING MANAGEMENT

Managing the hypoglycemic patient requires knowledge, astute judgment and an open-minded approach. Since hypoglycemia appears in many forms with varying severity, you must be able to adapt your care to each patient's individual needs.

Take a detailed patient history

In the initial interview, ask the patient to describe his symptoms, including his chief complaint. Observe him for signs of sweating or tremors. Ask if he feels anxious, hungry, weak, or confused. Ask how often his symptoms occur and what, if anything, precipitates them. Be sure to find out, as precisely as possible, when they occur in relation to meals (to determine fasting or reactive hypoglycemia). Ask if he's had hypoglycemia in the past, whether he thinks he has it now, and how much he knows about it.

Ask the patient if he has or had any chronic diseases related to hypoglycemia, such as diabetes or liver or kidney disease. Find out if he's taking any medications. Remember that some drugs, like aspirin, potentiate the effect of hypoglycemic drugs.

Investigate possible causes of stress. Many people mistakenly attribute conditions such as depression, chronic fatigue, allergies, and alcoholism to hypoglycemia. If the patient hasn't been officially diagnosed as hypoglycemic, remember that his symptoms could be unrelated to this disorder. Ask the patient about personal relationships with family and friends that could be causing him stress. (However, don't be too quick to dismiss his symptoms as psychosomatic.)

Conduct a physical exam

Thorough neurologic assessment is the most important part of the physical examination, because repeated fasting hypoglycemic attacks can permanently affect neurologic function. Since the hormonal response to low blood glucose depends on the sympathetic and parasympathetic nervous systems, any neurologic impairment has the potential to either exacerbate symptoms of low blood glucose or to minimize them.

Neuroglycopenic symptoms result from disturbances that spread from the brain's higher centers to its more primitive areas. These symptoms progress from mild intellectual disturbances and hunger to coma and brain stem dysfunction. If the hypoglycemia is not corrected, it can lead to irreversible brain damage characterized by focal and diffuse brain syndromes. However, the extent of permanent brain damage can't be assessed immediately, since some of the changes may be reversible.

Take the patient's vital signs on admission, and use these values as baseline data for successive vital sign checks. When hypoglycemia occurs rapidly, you'll notice sharp increases in blood pressure and heart rate.

Idiopathic reactive hypoglycemia

These curves reflect blood glucose and blood insulin responses in 44 patients with idiopathic reactive hypoglycemia. The responses are compared with a series of normal controls (shaded areas). Short dashes above and below points indicate the range of individual responses, plotted at 30-minute intervals.

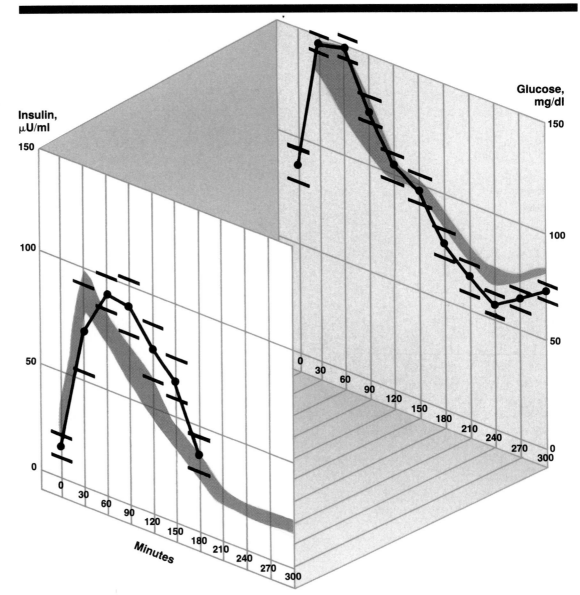

Be sure to review the patient's laboratory data to complete your assessment.

Formulate nursing diagnoses

After you've collected information from the patient's history and physical exam, you're ready to formulate your nursing diagnoses, set goals, and plan interventions. Your diagnoses may change as the patient's condition progresses.

Alteration in cerebral function related to inadequate blood glucose. After making this diagnosis, your goals are to correct glucose imbalance, protect the patient from injury, and help his family understand his disorder.

To meet these goals, administer quick-acting carbohydrates or the prescribed drug to raise the patient's glucose level. Keep emergency glucose at the patient's bedside, and safeguard his immediate environment by providing padded side rails and restraints, in case he experiences convulsions. Explain to his family that hypoglycemia can cause manifestations ranging in severity from mild confusion to coma. Let them ask you questions and encourage them to express their feelings. Suggest that the patient wear identification such as MedicAlert, and explain the importance of this to the patient and his family.

Evaluate your interventions. You'll know you've achieved your goals when the patient's glucose imbalance is corrected; cerebral function improves; he avoids personal injury; and his family understands and asks pertinent questions about his condition.

Potential nutritional deficit related to inadequate blood glucose. To correct this problem, you'll need to help the patient maintain a diet that meets cellular glucose needs; to help him stay rested and calm to maintain euglycemia; and to help him avoid complications such as coma.

Enlist a dietitian's help to formulate a sensible diet plan for the patient based on past and present eating habits, food preferences, and special dietary needs. Find out about the patient's life-style and eating habits outside the home. Explain that he may require six small meals a day with increased fiber content, to avoid rebound hypoglycemia. If the patient has hyperalimentation hypoglycemia, stress that he should eat slowly, utilizing smaller and more frequent meals, to reduce the speed of gastric emptying into the intestines. Discourage alcohol consumption by explaining that alcohol potentiates hypoglycemia. Try to assess the importance of alcohol in his life-style and suggest nonalcoholic substitutes. This is especially important if your patient is a chronic alcoholic, a decompensated diabetic, or is taking insulin or oral hypoglycemics. Assess his sensorimotor status and watch for signs of complications such as altered mentation or seizures.

Evaluate your interventions. You'll know you've achieved your goals for a patient with this diagnosis if he appears rested and relaxed and maintains a good nutritional state; if he adheres to dietary changes during hospitalization and after discharge; and if he avoids or severely limits his use of alcohol.

Knowledge deficit about hypoglycemia. Your goals in this diagnosis are to increase the patient's understanding of his condition through factual information and emotional support, and to teach him about self-care and prepare him for hospital discharge.

Provide detailed information about the patient's condition and its treatment. Teach him anticipatory problem-solving by role-playing possible situations he could encounter at home or work. For example, you might ask him what he would do if he started sweating, trembling, and had a headache when at a business lunch with his boss. By anticipating such situations, you can help the patient define appropriate actions and boost his self-confidence. At the same time, you'll be testing his knowledge of how to handle hypoglycemic reactions. Teach the patient and his family appropriate skills, such as home blood glucose monitoring and glucagon and insulin administration, using demonstration/return demonstration methods.

If the patient experiences a hypoglycemic reaction while he's in the hospital, use the episode to reinforce to him what the warning signs of a reaction will be. Stress the fact that his family and others at work or school also know how to administer a glucose source (or medication such as glucagon or epinephrine given subcutaneously) if he needs it, and be sure he knows which drugs to avoid. Help the patient and his family verbalize their feelings and concerns.

Evaluate your interventions. You'll know you've been successful if the patient and his family can explain hypoglycemia, describe its home treatment and ask appropriate questions; if the patient can demonstrate learned skills; if he describes appropriate actions in role-playing situations; and if he begins to verbalize feelings about his disorder and its effects on his life-style.

Noncompliance related to knowledge deficit or denial of disease. After reaching this diagnosis, your goals are to improve the patient's adherence to his prescribed treatment; to prevent self-injury that could result from noncompliance; and to increase his understanding and his family's understanding of his disorder and its treatment.

Explain to the patient the physiology of his disorder, its signs and symptoms, and the rationale for treatment. Use hypoglycemic episodes as learning situations, to correlate signs and symptoms with treatment. Try to explore the reasons for any noncompliance and denial. Enlist his family's support. Discuss possible job modifications with the patient, making sure he understands the importance of making a co-worker aware of the treatment for hypoglycemia. Give the patient and his family information about community support groups.

Evaluate your interventions. You will have succeeded if the patient begins to correctly discuss his condition and required treatment; if he admits he has hypoglycemia; if he discusses life-style changes necessary for controlling his condition, during and after hospitalization; if he begins to ask pertinent questions; and if he remains euglycemic.

Guidance is good therapy

As with diabetes mellitus, a big part of your treatment plan for a hypoglycemic patient consists of careful teaching of the patient and his family. Including the patient and his family in planning care is also necessary and helpful. By fostering their inner resources, you can help everyone cope with this disorder more effectively. With increased confidence and self-respect, your patient will start to feel like a person who happens to have hypoglycemia but is learning how to control it.

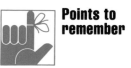

Points to remember

• Hypoglycemia can be a symptom of a disease or a separate health problem.
• When the body's supply of glucose becomes low, it can use other substrates, such as fat and protein, as energy sources.
• Hypoglycemia can be classified as endogenous, due to an internal dysfunction, or as exogenous, due to an external factor or abuse. If it occurs after food ingestion, it's known as reactive hypoglycemia; if it occurs in the absence of food, it's called fasting hypoglycemia.
• Fasting hypoglycemia is usually distinguished from the reactive type with a fasting blood glucose test. Other diagnostic tools include the oral glucose tolerance test, and studies of insulin/glucose levels and C-peptide levels.
• A thorough neurologic examination should be performed on patients with suspected hypoglycemia, since repeated fasting hypoglycemia can affect neurologic function.

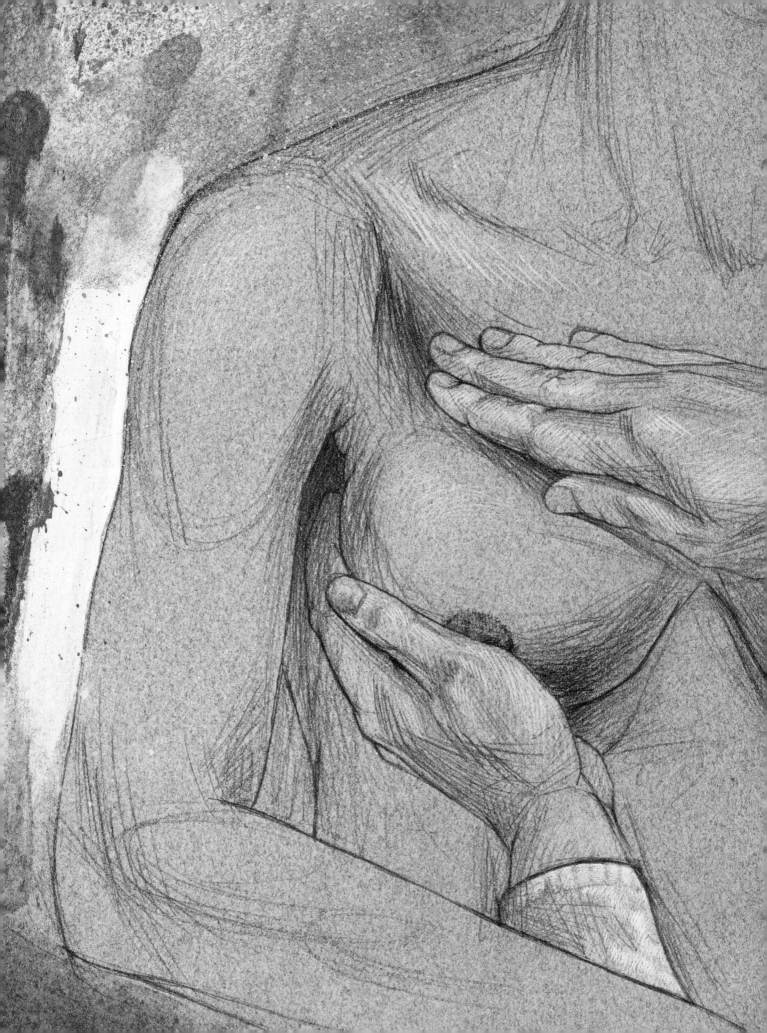

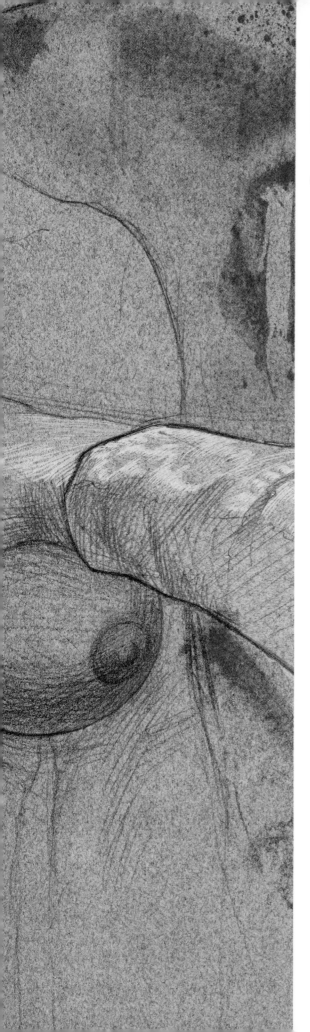

DISORDERS OF THE GONADS

12 COPING WITH FEMALE GONADAL DISORDERS

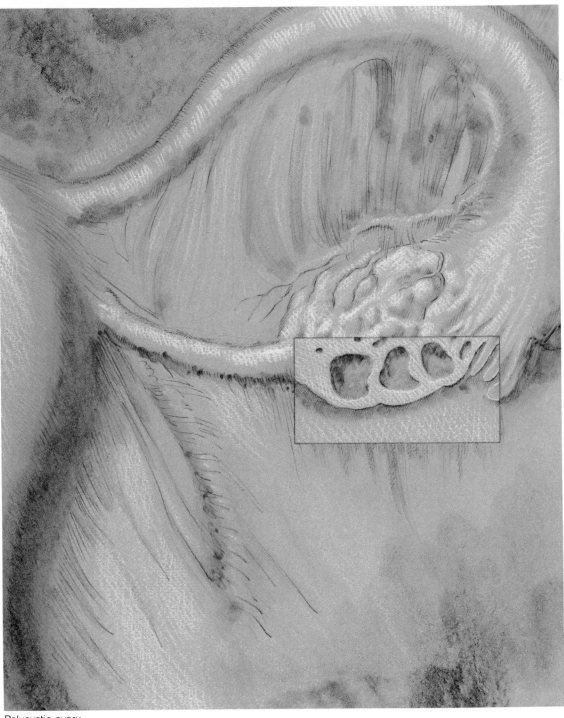

Polycystic ovary

Endocrine disorders of the ovary and breast are commonly recognized at puberty, when sex steroid hormone secretion and tissue response change drastically to establish childbearing potential with development of female secondary sex characteristics and a menstrual cycle. Because sex steroid hormones influence so many tissues, their abnormal secretion causes varying troublesome effects. Any disruption of a complete and timely expression of normal hormonal change may threaten both gonadal function and self-image—the perception and expression of sexuality.

Few disorders affect a woman's self-image as profoundly as these. Yet some may go unrecognized (for example, ovarian hypofunction in early childhood), unreported, and untreated because of ignorance or embarrassment (as in hirsutism or any menstrual abnormality). Except for choriocarcinoma and carcinoid tumors, these disorders are not in themselves life-threatening. Their prognoses are often expressed in terms of effects on sexuality and childbearing. Typically, they improve with early diagnosis and treatment.

To help women deal with the physical and psychological implications of gonadal disorders, you'll need to understand their pathophysiology, characteristic signs and symptoms, and medical management.

PATHOPHYSIOLOGY

The ovaries are essential for secretion and regulation of hormones associated with female gonadal development. (For more information, see *Understanding the link between hormones and menstruation,* page 162, and *Hormones control breast development,* page 163.) These ovarian hormones include estrogen, progesterone, and smaller amounts of androgens. Hypersecretion or hyposecretion of these hormones and ovarian dysfunction produce disorders with varied effects, depending on reproductive age.

Ovarian hyperfunction

Before menarche, increased levels of estrogen cause proliferation and growth of the cells of the uterus, vagina, and fallopian tubes, and development of female secondary sex characteristics. If these changes occur before ages 7 or 8, the result is precocious puberty (isosexual precocity). Heterosexual precocity (virilization) may result from excessive production of androgens by the ovaries, but it's usually related to an adrenal gland disorder.

During the reproductive years, excessive levels of estrogens or androgens, or both, can cause amenorrhea (the absence of menses). Hypersecretion of estrogen may prevent the normal decline in estrogen levels that stimulates a rise in follicle-stimulating hormone (FSH). Elevated androgen levels can exaggerate this effect through extraglandular conversion (peripheral conversion of androgens to estrogen), which can also increase estrogen levels. Also, elevated androgen levels may cause virilization.

After menopause, hypersecretion of estrogen can produce breast engorgement and tenderness, increased vaginal secretion, and bleeding. Hypersecretion of androgens produces virilization.

Ovarian hypofunction

During fetal development, ovarian hypofunction causes abnormal gonadal growth and genital differentiation; it's often associated with genetic abnormalities.

Before menarche, ovarian hormone secretion is normally low; consequently, ovarian hypofunction becomes easier to recognize at menarche (normally, between ages 9 to 16).

After menarche, abnormal ovarian function causes menstrual disorders and infertility. For example, diminished estrogen levels at midcycle prevent the luteinizing hormone (LH) surge. Anovulation results, accompanied by menorrhagia (excessive menstrual bleeding), metrorrhagia (intermenstrual bleeding), or both, with long periods of amenorrhea in between. These disorders, called anovulatory dysfunctional uterine bleeding, are common at both extremes of female reproductive life. Ovarian hypofunction, which results from inadequate gonadotropic stimulation from the hypothalamic-pituitary unit, may also cause amenorrhea. Regardless of the cause, hyposecretion of ovarian hormones disrupts the normal ovarian cycle.

In menopause, the ovaries stop producing estrogen and progesterone, and the menses cease, usually about age 50. In premature menopause, an abnormal condition, permanent amenorrhea occurs before age 40.

Ovarian tumors and dysfunction

Rarely, bizarre dysfunction results from ovarian neoplasms. For example, choriocarcinoma, a malignant tumor of the ovary, secretes human chorionic gonadotropin (HCG) and may induce precocious puberty in a female who is near puberty. Struma ovarii, generally a be-

Endocrine disorders of the ovary and breast

Ovarian hyperfunction
Primary
Feminizing tumors
Masculinizing tumors
Secondary
True precocious puberty
Persistent follicle cyst
Corpus luteum cyst
Polycystic ovaries (Stein-Leventhal syndrome) and hyperthecosis of the ovary

Ovarian hypofunction
Primary
Gonadal dysgenesis (Turner's syndrome)
Autoimmune disorders with anti-steroid-producing cell antibodies
Iatrogenic hypofunction
Resistant ovary syndrome
Menopause, premature or physiologic
Secondary
Hypothalamic disorders
Pituitary disorders
Anovulatory bleeding
Inadequate luteal phase

Ovarian dysfunction
Choriocarcinoma
Struma ovarii
Carcinoid tumors

Breast disorders
Galactorrhea
Breast aplasia
Macromastia
Fibrocystic breast disease

Understanding the link between hormones and menstruation

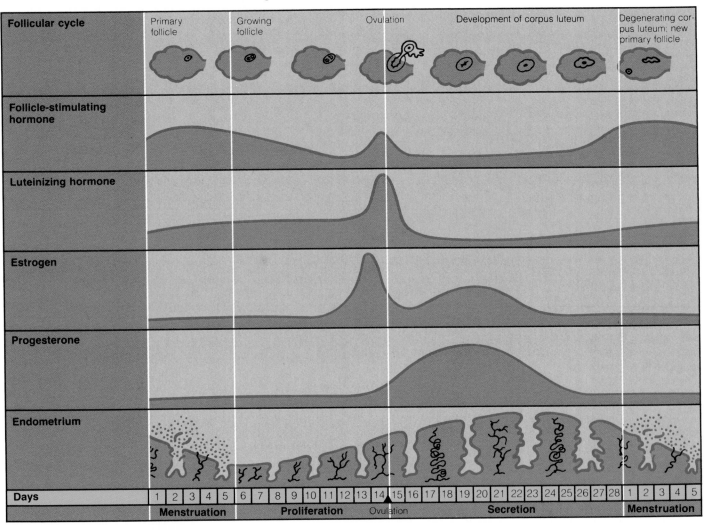

During childhood, small amounts of ovarian estrogen inhibit production of gonadotropic hormones secreted by the pituitary. During puberty, inhibitory effects decline, thus stimulating production of gonadotropic hormones (luteinizing hormone [LH] and follicle-stimulating hormone [FSH]) and ovarian hormones (estrogen, progesterone, and androgens).

At this time, the female sexual cycle, or menstrual cycle, begins—a rhythmic pattern of changes that occur in the ovaries, in sexual organs, and in hormone secretion. The average cycle is 28 days, but it may range from 20 to 45 days.

Follicular growth and ovulation
The cycle begins with the onset of the menses, when low levels of estrogen and progesterone trigger a rise in FSH levels and, soon after, LH levels. Increasing levels of FSH and LH stimulate development of a primary follicle, which secretes estrogen. As a result, the endometrium thickens, and increased estrogen causes a midcycle surge in LH and a lesser surge in FSH. Stimulated by LH and FSH, the follicle swells, estrogen levels fall, and progesterone levels rise. Then ovulation occurs.

Postovulation
Following expulsion of the ovum, the remaining granulosa cells undergo physical and chemical change (luteinization) to form the corpus luteum, which secretes large amounts of progesterone and estrogen. Progesterone causes swelling and secretory development of the endometrium. Also, increased estrogen and progesterone cause decreased FSH and LH secretion. If fertilization does not occur, the corpus luteum degenerates, reducing levels of estrogen and progesterone. Menstruation occurs and the cycle repeats.

When the cycle stops
Between ages 40 and 50, menstrual cycles may become irregular, anovulation may occur, and estrogen and progesterone levels diminish. The number of primordial follicles falls to zero, and LH and FSH levels rise since estrogen no longer inhibits their production. Progesterone production becomes essentially nonexistent. This period, the female climacteric, extends from the start of irregular cycles to their final cessation.

Hormones control breast development

Human mammary glands overlay the pectoral muscles. Each gland contains approximately 20 lobes, which are divided into lobules and alveoli. Ducts extend from the lobes through breast tissue and converge in the nipple. Fatty tissue and suspensory ligaments (Cooper's ligaments) surround the gland.

Changing hormone levels

During a woman's lifetime, changing hormone levels change the physiology of the breast.

During childhood, the ovaries are virtually inactive; therefore, the necessary hormones are not available to cause breast development.

At puberty, gonadotropin-releasing hormone from the hypothalamus stimulates pituitary secretion of luteinizing and follicle-stimulating hormones. These hormones prompt ovarian production of estrogen and progesterone that, along with other hormones, activate breast development.

During the menstrual cycle, estrogen causes some breast proliferation, and progesterone causes alveolar secretory activity. Following a period of involution, the cycle repeats.

During pregnancy, several hormones, including estrogen, progesterone, growth hormone, thyroxine, prolactin, adrenal glucocorticoids, human placental lactogen, and insulin, induce extensive breast development. Profound hormonal changes result in growth and branching of the ducts and in alveolar budding and secretory changes. Postpartum secretion of prolactin and oxytocin are essential for lactation. Oxytocin causes expression of milk from the alveoli into the ducts.

At menopause, loss of ovarian hormone activity causes breast atrophy.

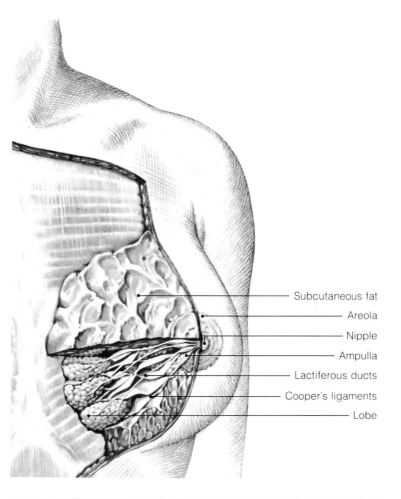

- Subcutaneous fat
- Areola
- Nipple
- Ampulla
- Lactiferous ducts
- Cooper's ligaments
- Lobe

Development of the duct system

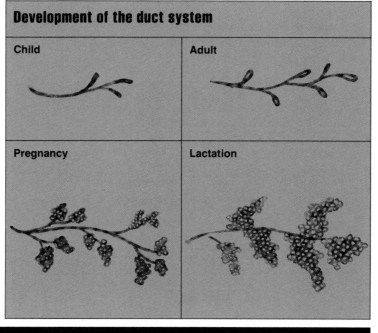

Child

Adult

Pregnancy

Lactation

nign neoplasm, may secrete thyroid hormone at any age. This tumor may secrete levels of thyroid hormone high enough to induce thyrotoxicosis. Carcinoid tumors are sometimes found in dermoid cysts containing residual embryonic epithelium (often intestinal or bronchial). Carcinoid tumors may cause carcinoid flush, cyanosis, and diarrhea; rarely, they may metastasize.

Breast disorders

The mammary glands begin to develop early in embryonic life. The ducts, glands, and supporting fibrous, connective, and adipose tissues are present at birth and grow substantially at puberty, but they may not complete development until pregnancy. At any life stage, abnormal hormone levels adversely affect the structure and function of the breast.

In normal breast development, estrogen secreted by the ovaries stimulates the growth, division, and elongation of the tubular duct system and maturation of the nipples. Progesterone, also secreted by the ovary, is required for alveolar growth. Other hormones that influence breast development and function include growth hormone, adrenal glucocorticoids, insulin, and prolactin.

Prolactin, a pituitary hormone, is required for lactation. In the nonpregnant woman, the hypothalamus secretes prolactin inhibitory factor (PIF), which inhibits pituitary release of prolactin into the blood. During pregnancy, the pituitary gland secretes prolactin; however, its lactogenic effects are suppressed by increased levels of estrogen and progesterone. After delivery, as estrogen and progesterone levels decline, prolactin's lactogenic effects establish normal lactation. Growth hormone and adrenal glucocorticoids are also essential for lactation.

Nonpuerperal lactation (galactorrhea) occurs in both men and women. Galactorrhea may be drug-induced, or it may result from lesions of the hypothalamus or pituitary, breast trauma, hypothyroidism, ectopic prolactin production, or unknown causes. In patients with galactorrhea, increased prolactin levels indicate disruption of prolactin's negative feedback control.

Hypersecretion of hormones at an early age causes precocious breast development. If breast tissue is oversensitive to normal amounts of hormone stimulation, the result is macromastia (abnormally enlarged female breasts). Hormonal hyposecretion, or perhaps breast insensitivity to hormonal stimulation,

results in hypoplasia or aplasia of the breasts—delayed or absent maturation.

Recurring breast changes preceding menstruation may cause fibrocystic breast disease or chronic cystic mastitis. Normally, cyclic menstrual changes stimulate tissue proliferation (through the effects of estrogen) and alveolar secretory activity (through the effects of progesterone), followed by involution. In some women, inflammatory breast changes associated with tenderness, engorgement, and increasing nodularity precede each menstrual period. More common in nulliparous women, this condition may subside after childbearing and lactation. In later reproductive life, continued recurrent stimulation and involution of the breasts with each menstrual cycle may cause diffuse and nodular fibrosis and cyst formation—chronic cystic mastitis.

MEDICAL MANAGEMENT

Various hormonal influences complicate diagnosis of female gonadal disorders. Diagnosis relies on laboratory measurements of hormone levels and on certain other tests. Test results are correlated with age-related fluctuations in hormone secretion to help confirm diagnosis of female gonadal disorders. Characteristically, the first test ordered is often a measurement of HCG to determine if the patient is pregnant or has a menstrual disorder.

Tests for hormonal imbalance

Laboratory studies reveal hormonal imbalance through analysis of blood or urine for hormone levels.

Estrogen. Elevated serum estrogen levels indicate ovarian hyperfunction associated with feminizing ovarian tumors, precocious puberty, or amenorrhea. Diminished levels, indicating hypofunction, suggest hypothalamic-pituitary failure or ovarian dysfunction. Elevated urinary estrogen levels indicate ovarian hyperfunction; diminished levels indicate hypofunction. Progesterone levels rise during pregnancy but may also rise because of an adrenal tumor.

Testosterone. Elevated levels of testosterone (usually secreted in small amounts in females) may suggest masculinizing ovarian tumors, polycystic ovaries, or adrenal gland disorders. (See also *Wedge resection in polycystic ovaries.*)

Gonadotropic hormones. Studies of blood levels of gonadotropic hormones—FSH and LH—also help distinguish female gonadal disorders. Increased levels indicate primary gonadal failure: Their continued secretion indicates inadequate response by the ovaries. Increased levels also occur in true precocious puberty (complete isosexual precocity). Decreased gonadotropic hormone levels suggest hypothalamic-pituitary failure.

Prolactin. Elevated prolactin levels occur in galactorrhea, amenorrhea, and in hypothalamic and some pituitary tumors. Because prolactin secretion is normally inhibited in the nonpregnant woman, low levels in response to a prolactin-releasing hormone stimulation test indicate pituitary dysfunction.

Thyroid hormones. Hyposecretion of triiodothyronine and thyroxine is associated with a form of precocity involving an increased ovarian sensitivity to endogenous gonadotropins. In adults, hypothyroidism is usually associated with anovulation and dysfunctional bleeding. Elevated levels of thyroid hormones may indicate struma ovarii.

An elevated white blood cell count may indicate infection; a low hemoglobin and hematocrit may suggest dysfunctional uterine bleeding.

17-ketosteroids (17-KS). Urine levels of 17-KS measure the metabolic products of testosterone; elevated 17-KS levels indicate hypersecretion of androgens (as in polycystic ovaries and certain ovarian and adrenal tumors).

Other confirming tests
Several special tests help confirm the clinical evaluation. Radiographic studies include ultrasonography of the ovaries and adrenal glands to confirm diagnosis of a hormone-secreting tumor. A computerized tomography scan of the head can rule out pituitary or hypothalamic tumors. Mammography and thermography detect breast masses. (See *Breast mammography in fibrocystic disease,* page 166.) X-rays of the spine may show osteoporosis, which can occur in menopause. X-rays of the skull can rule out tumors and determine bone age. Other diagnostic tests include laparoscopy, laparotomy, and biopsy. (See *Laparoscopy: Visualizing abnormality,* page 167.) These tests detect tumors and help to diagnose true hermaphroditism. Buccal smears detect chromosomal abnormalities.

Treatment: Medical or surgical
Treatment depends on the type and severity of the patient's complaint, her age, and other significant factors, such as desire to achieve or avoid conception. Medical treatment includes hormone replacement and drug therapy

Wedge resection in polycystic ovaries

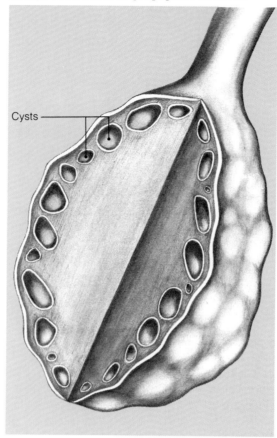

Bilaterally enlarged polycystic ovaries contain follicular cysts within a thickened capsule, which is due to excessive collagen deposits. Elevated luteinizing hormone levels cause thecal hypertrophy and hyperplasia.
Polycystic ovaries (Stein-Leventhal syndrome) may result in sterility, oligomenorrhea, or hirsutism.
Treatment includes drug therapy (such as with clomiphene citrate) to induce ovulation or surgical wedge resection of the ovary if drug treatment fails. Wedge resection removes diseased tissue and may allow greater responsiveness to gonadotropic stimulation, thus breaking the cycle of persistent anovulation.

to correct imbalance or relieve its symptoms. Surgery removes lesions and corrects abnormalities. Treatment may also include nutritional, psychological, and genetic counseling.

If the patient's symptoms result from ovarian hypofunction, treatment may include hormone replacement with estrogens (such as Premarin, Estinyl, and diethylstilbestrol) and progestogens (such as Provera and norgestrel). Estrogen-progesterone combinations are used to treat certain menstrual disorders (also used as oral contraceptives).

During menopause, estrogen suppresses hot flashes and may relieve dyspareunia and reduce the possibility of osteoporosis and fractures. However, these potential benefits must be weighed against the risks of side effects, possible breast or endometrial cancer,

Breast mammography in fibrocystic disease

Normal

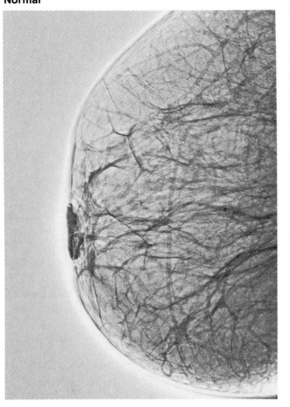

Abnormal

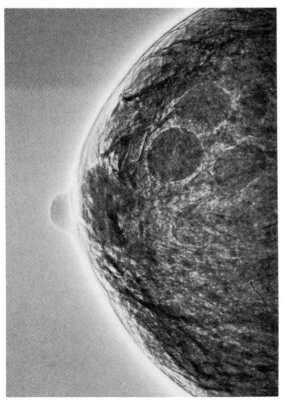

The lower mammogram reveals multiple benign cysts in fibrocystic disease. The upper mammogram shows a normal breast.

and thromboembolic disease. Progesterone controls bleeding in dysfunctional uterine bleeding and also induces decreased gonadotropin secretion in true precocious puberty.

Clomiphene citrate (Clomid), human menopausal gonadotropin (HMG), and HCG are used to treat ovulatory failure. Clomiphene stimulates and corrects abnormal patterns of gonadotropin secretion. HMG and HCG induce ovulation by replacing inadequate quantities of gonadotropins.

Thyroid hormone replacement reverses precocious puberty caused by ovarian sensitivity to gonadotropins in hypothyroidism. In galactorrhea associated with hypothyroidism, thyroid hormone replacement suppresses the release of prolactin, which is secreted in response to thyrotropin-releasing hormone.

Parlodel (bromocriptine mesylate), a dopamine receptor agonist, induces secretion of PIF to suppress prolactin in patients with galactorrhea. (Remember that central nervous system drugs such as tranquilizers inhibit PIF secretion, resulting in increased prolactin levels.) In mild galactorrhea, breast binders may decrease the nipple stimulation that can increase lactation.

Surgery is recommended for excision of feminizing or masculinizing ovarian tumors and of some pituitary tumors. It's also appropriate in patients with polycystic ovaries, which may be treated by wedge resection. This procedure may restore spontaneous ovulatory menstrual cycles and thus, fertility. (See *Wedge resection in polycystic ovaries,* page 165.) However, Clomid therapy is used more frequently. Surgical treatment is also effective for certain breast disorders; for example, aspiration or excision of benign cystic breast lesions (see *Aspiration: Two steps in one,* page 168); subcutaneous mastectomy and insertion of prosthetic implants in some patients with severe fibrocystic breast disease; and reduction mammoplasty in macromastia.

Supplemental doses of iron are used to treat anemia in dysfunctional uterine bleeding.

Nutritional counseling may be needed in hypothalamic amenorrhea resulting from poor nutrition (because of careless dieting or persistent anorexia). As the patient gains weight, gonadotropic responsiveness increases. Psychological counseling may be indicated for women unable to conceive, those with androgen-related disorders, and those unable to cope with menopause. Genetic counseling may be needed in families demonstrating chromosomal abnormalities.

Laparoscopy: Visualizing abnormality

With this invasive technique, a small fiberoptic telescope (laparoscope), inserted through the anterior abdominal wall, permits visualization of the peritoneal cavity. Laparoscopy can detect cysts, adhesions, fibroids, anatomical abnormalities, and infection. Laparoscopy also provides access for procedures such as lysis of adhesions, ovarian biopsy, tubal sterilization, removal of foreign bodies, and fulguration of endometrial implants.

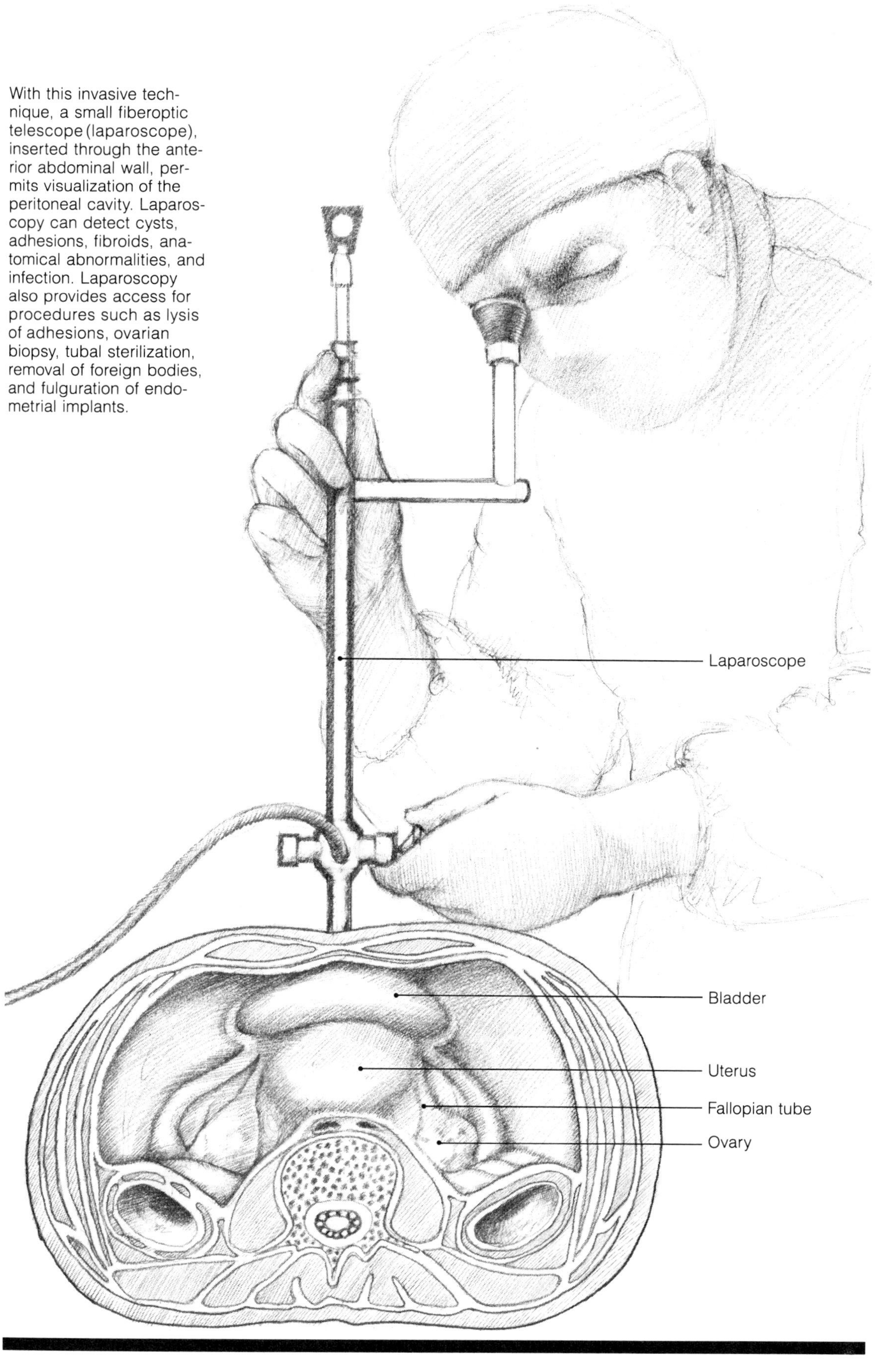

Laparoscope

Bladder

Uterus

Fallopian tube

Ovary

NURSING MANAGEMENT

As you help see the patient through clinical evaluation, diagnostic testing, and treatment, remember that thorough patient teaching and sensitive psychological support are critical to successful management of female gonadal disorders.

Begin a nursing history with a focus on patient concerns, including her perception of the disorder's effect on her life-style. Ask her to describe the onset of symptoms. Consider the patient's age and medical and family history, which may help you identify risk factors for certain disorders. Also note reproductive age to guide you in asking further questions.

Ask about menstrual history. What was the age of menarche? Was it preceded by breast development and pubic hair growth? Ask about the duration of the menstrual cycle, typical amount of bleeding, and any irregularities. Be sure to record the date of her last menstrual period. Assess the patient's nutri-

tional status; poor nutrition can cause amenorrhea. What are her exercise habits? Strenuous exercise, such as marathon running, can also affect the menses.

Ask about previous pregnancies, including spontaneous and induced abortions. Document any problems encountered during pregnancy and lactation.

Ask the patient about sexual habits and the use of contraceptives. Has she ever used oral contraceptives? If so, when? A patient with amenorrhea may be pregnant or could be suffering from postpill amenorrhea.

Ask if the patient has noticed breast changes. Question her about engorgement and when it occurs; often it's associated with the onset of menses. If a nonpregnant patient notices any secretion from the breasts, ask her to describe its color, consistency, amount, frequency, and duration. Ask if the patient performs monthly breast exams, and note any abnormal findings.

Ask about recent infection or surgery, such as dilatation and curettage.

Ask the patient with virilization to tell when it started and to describe its effects (such as abnormal hair growth and changes in voice and genitalia).

Has the patient experienced headaches, visual problems, or seizures? These could indicate a pituitary tumor and may be associated with precocious puberty.

In the patient with hot flashes or dyspareunia, are these symptoms associated with physiologic or premature menopause? Ask the menopausal patient about symptoms of depression and osteoporosis.

Physical examination

Gather the necessary equipment, including examination gloves, lubricant, and a light source. First, observe the patient. Is she adequately developed for her age? Remember that abnormally short stature is associated with gonadal dysgenesis. Also, excessive weight or thyroid hormone imbalance can cause menstrual dysfunction.

Assess the patient from head to toe. In postmenopausal women, check for a male balding pattern, which can follow increased androgen secretion. Excessive androgen production can cause excessive growth of facial and body hair at any age. Other symptoms include oily skin, acne, and voice changes.

Also perform a neurologic examination, which can suggest the presence of a pituitary tumor.

Aspiration: Two steps in one

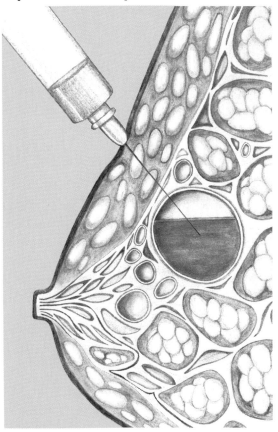

Needle aspiration combines diagnosis and treatment. This procedure allows cytologic evaluation of breast lesions, such as a single, palpable mass in fibrocystic disease. If laboratory evaluation is negative and a follow-up exam shows the mass has disappeared, treatment is considered adequate. Aspiration is also used to evaluate ovarian and cervical cysts.

Palpating the breast

During palpation, keep breast variations in mind. The young breast has a firm elasticity; the middle-aged breast may feel lobular; the older breast often feels stringy or granular. Other normal variations include premenstrual fullness, nodularity, and tenderness.

With the patient in a supine position, place a pillow under her shoulder on the side you are examining. This helps to spread the breast evenly and makes nodules easier to find.

Systematically examine the entire breast, including the periphery, tail, and areola. Use the pads of your three fingers in a rotating motion to gently compress breast tissue against the chest wall.

Use any of the palpation techniques illustrated below. Also, teach them to your patient so she can perform a breast self-examination at home. Encourage her to select one method and to use it routinely.

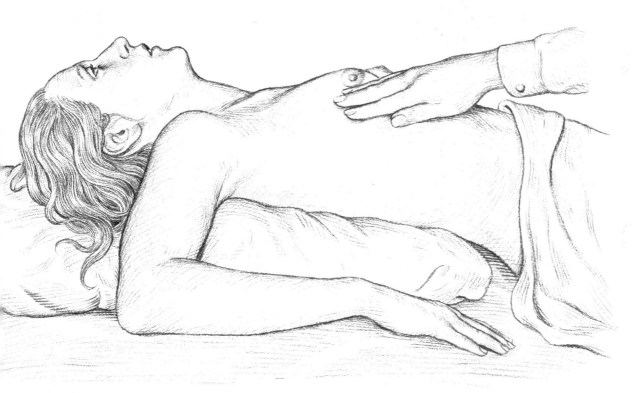

Spiral

Quadrant

Spokes/radial

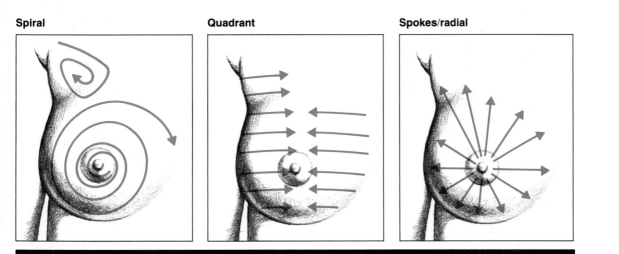

Palpating internal genitalia

With special training, you may be asked to perform internal examinations. Your caring attitude and careful explanation of each technique during the examination will help your patient relax.

To palpate your patient's vagina, insert your gloved and lubricated index and middle fingers. Use a palm-up position with the thumb abducted and the fourth and little finger folded on the palm of the hand, as illustrated here. The vagina is normally 3″ to 3½″ (7.5 to 9 cm) long and capable of expansion.

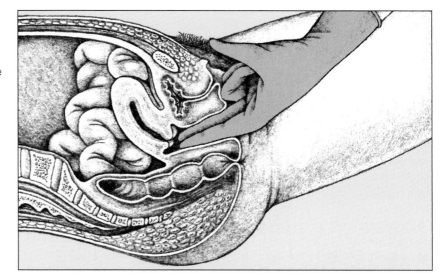

To palpate the cervix, sweep your fingers from side to side across the cervix and around the os. The cervix should feel moist, smooth, and firm but resilient, and should protrude ⅝″ to 1⅛″ (1.5 to 3 cm) into the vagina.

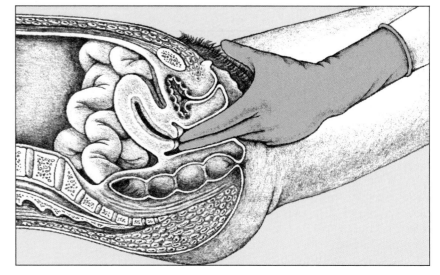

Next, observe the breasts. Note their size, symmetry, contour, and general appearance. While inspecting the nipples, note any discharge. Palpate the breasts with the patient in the supine position. If a breast disorder exists or if the patient is at risk for breast cancer, also palpate while the patient is seated. (See *Palpating the breast,* page 169.)

Palpate the abdomen. Document any tenderness or enlargement. Percuss the abdomen. Remember that dullness in the pelvic area may indicate an ovarian tumor. (See also Chapter 2.)

Next, a pelvic-rectal examination is required. With special training, you may be asked to perform this procedure, depending on hospital policy. Observe the genitalia (be sure the patient has emptied her bladder). Is development appropriate for the patient's age? Expect to see early excessive develop-ment with pubic hair in precocious puberty, clitoral enlargement in excessive androgen secretion, and sexual infantilism in ovarian hyposecretion.

With the patient in the lithotomy position, use a gloved hand to palpate the labia. They should have a soft, homogeneous texture. Palpate the internal genitalia to assess the patient for an abnormally short vagina and for cervical absence (in testicular feminization). Next, palpate the cervix, normally located on the anterior wall, with a sweeping motion. (See *Palpating internal genitalia.*)

Palpate for an ovarian tumor. Place your free hand on the patient's right lower quadrant and your gloved and lubricated fingers in the right lateral fornix. Maneuver your abdominal hand downward and, using your pelvic hand for palpation, identify the right ovary and any masses. Remember that in the postmenopausal patient, you may be unable to palpate the ovaries because of ovarian atrophy.

Focus on patient education

Teach the patient everything she needs to know about her disorder that will help her cope with its effects on her life. Use the information from your assessment to help you formulate nursing diagnoses and thereby plan appropriate nursing interventions. Some examples follow.

Inability to cope with precocious sexual development. Help the young patient understand her condition, feel good about herself, and interact positively with others. Provide a calm, supportive atmosphere, and encourage her and her family to express their feelings about these changes. The dramatic physical changes produced by precocious puberty can be upsetting, even alarming, for the child and her family. Reassure the child about her appearance; tell her that her peers will eventually catch up in their physical development.

Explain her condition to the child in terms she can understand to prevent feelings of shame and loss of self-esteem. Provide appropriate sex education, including information on menstruation and related hygiene.

Suggest that the parents continue to dress their daughter in clothes appropriate for her age that don't emphasize her premature physical development. Warn them against expecting more of her than they would expect of other children her age.

Evaluate your care. You'll know your teaching has been effective if the patient and her family ask appropriate questions about her condition, and if the child shows a positive interest in her appearance and interacts normally with her family and peers.

Disturbance in self-concept related to masculinizing effects of an ovarian tumor. To help the patient deal effectively with these changes, tell her that all females secrete androgens. Then explain the causes for increased androgen secretion and its effects. If appropriate, explain that surgery can correct this disorder. Suggest appropriate use of cosmetics and clothing to emphasize femininity. Encourage the patient to express her feelings. Provide reassurance and support.

You've managed this patient successfully if she understands and accepts the disorder and shows an interest in improving her appearance.

Knowledge deficit related to an inability to conceive. Help the patient understand her dis-

order. Review the normal menstrual cycle and the abnormality that is causing her infertility. Encourage her to ask questions and express her feelings. She may feel a loss of self-esteem, anger, guilt, or inadequacy. Give the patient information about diagnosis and treatment; also advise her of available options, such as adoption.

Consider your interventions successful if the patient asks appropriate questions and can describe the causes of her disorder and the options available.

Sexual dysfunction related to perceived decreased sexual desire during premature menopause. Help the patient understand menopause and her sexual desires. Explain the physiology of menopause and the effects of decreased hormone secretion. Provide an accepting, tolerant atmosphere; encourage the patient to express her feelings. Explain that she's not alone; many others also experience menopause at an early age and must deal with its effects. Discuss with the patient the effects her behavior has on her partner. Convey the importance of expressing acceptance, and explore ways of expressing love.

Evaluate your intervention by considering how well the patient understands menopause. Can she identify her feelings and their sexual implications? Can she identify the need and methods to express her love for her partner?

Discomfort related to breast tenderness from fluid accumulation in breast tissue. Reduce the patient's anxiety to help relieve her emotional and physical symptoms. Reassure the patient that this discomfort will subside. To help relieve breast discomfort, handle the patient gently during your examination and position her comfortably (off the tender area). Suggest that the patient wear a well-fitting bra and avoid constrictive clothing. To reduce discomfort, encourage the patient to take prescribed drugs as ordered.

When your intervention is successful, discomfort subsides and the patient follows prescribed treatment.

Your special role

Nurses are in a key position to help the patient with a female gonadal disorder. Your responsibilities include recognizing the disorder during the physical exam and teaching and supporting the patient throughout diagnostic testing and treatment. Your sympathetic psychological support in helping the patient cope with the impact on her self-image may be your most important contribution.

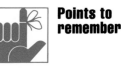

Points to remember

- Hypersecretion of ovarian hormones can result in precocious puberty, amenorrhea, or virilization.
- Hyposecretion of ovarian hormones can result in abnormal gonadal development and genital differentiation, amenorrhea or other menstrual abnormalities, or premature menopause.
- Abnormal ovarian hormone secretion can cause precocious breast development or breast hypoplasia.
- Psychological support and patient education are critical aspects of managing female gonadal disorders.
- Nurses should teach all female patients to perform monthly breast examination; early detection of lumps greatly improves prognosis.

13 GIVING SUPPORTIVE CARE IN MALE GONADAL DISORDERS

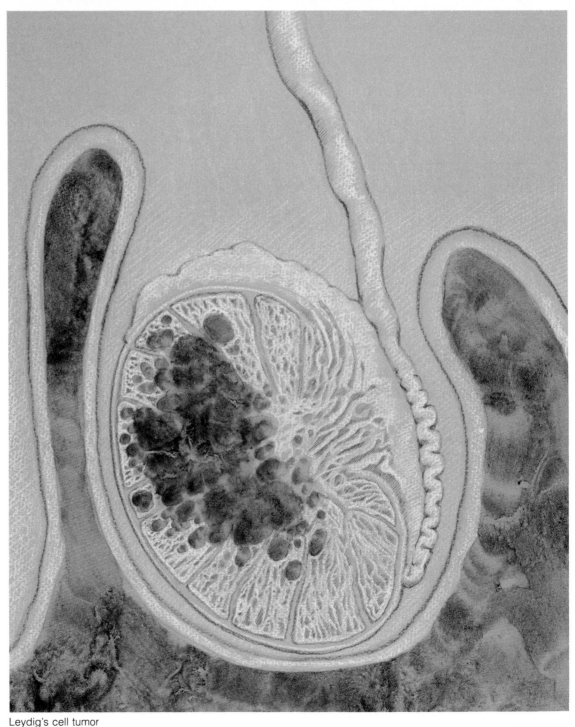

Leydig's cell tumor

Male gonadal disorders can strike at any time from conception to maturity, burdening the victim with retarded sexual development, infertility, potentially crippling psychological problems, and occasionally malignancy. Many of these disorders have genetic or idiopathic causes that often produce irreversible impairments and thus respond poorly to treatment. Even vigorous treatment, which can overcome the distressing effects of some gonadal disorders, may not restore normal sexual development.

Given the tremendous emphasis American society places on male sexuality, you can appreciate the potentially devastating psychological effects such disorders can have. Helping patients cope with these debilitating effects will challenge your counseling skills to the utmost. Indeed, you may find such counseling a greater challenge than any aspect of physical care. Prepare to meet it by learning to understand the physiologic mechanisms and overall management of this difficult group of disorders.

Male embryonic development
The developing embryo has the potential to become male or female. Without the influence of androgens, the fetus naturally develops into a female. Male differentiation requires, first, a testis-organizing factor, or H-Y antigen, which is present in the Y chromosome; and second, a functional testis, which is activated by expression of the H-Y antigen. The mechanism of translation of this sex factor into a functional testis is still poorly understood. Male internal and external genitalia, in turn, require the presence of two substances *in utero*: müllerian regression factor, which prevents the differentiation of fetal male ducts into female uterus and fallopian tubes; and testosterone, which initiates male external genitalia differentiation. Fetal testosterone secreted in response to stimulation by placental human chorionic gonadotropin (HCG) also stimulates differentiation of the internal male ducts: formation of the embryonic wolffian ducts into the vas deferens, seminal vesicles, and epididymis. (See *Structure of the testis,* page 174.) Dihydrotestosterone, a metabolite of testosterone produced in the peripheral tissues, stimulates development of external genitalia, urethra, and prostate.

Maturation of the testes and development of external sex characteristics (puberty) occur when pituitary gonadotropin secretion and gonadal sensitivity to the gonadotropin have reached balanced adult levels.

Androgen influence crucial
Male gonadal disorders are broadly divided into *hypergonadism* and *hypogonadism,* reflecting excessive or deficient androgen secretion. In hypergonadism, excessive prepubertal androgen secretion produces sexual precocity, usually in males younger than age 10.

In hypogonadism, low androgen secretion can cause many abnormalities, all resulting in impaired spermatogenesis and delayed development of secondary sex characteristics. (See *Male gonadal disorders,* page 175.)

Most hypogonadal men are infertile. However, infertility that's due to low testosterone secretion commonly responds to hormone replacement; idiopathic infertility usually does not. Male hypogonadism has no severe physical effects unless it is associated with malignant tumors or other debilitating causes.

PATHOPHYSIOLOGY
Several endocrine elements combine to develop and maintain male sex characteristics, sex drive, and production and delivery of viable sperm. This combination, dubbed the *hypothalamic-pituitary axis,* includes the hypothalamus, pituitary gland, testes, and end organs sensitive to gonadal hormones. Keep this in mind as you review gonadal disorders.

Many causes of hypergonadism
In *true* (or *primary*) *precocious puberty,* premature hypothalamic-pituitary axis maturation results from a variety of brain lesions, which in turn can result from tumors (usually nonpituitary), infection, or trauma. (See *How a tumor causes precocious puberty,* page 176.) The resultant increased pituitary gonadotropin and testosterone production stimulates premature Leydig's cell maturation, testicular enlargement, and spermatogenesis.

In *precocious pseudopuberty* (incomplete sexual precocity), gonadotropin levels do not rise; the testes tend toward immaturity, although external sexual organs are enlarged and secondary sex characteristics are developed. In this condition, excessive androgen levels come not from the gonads but from congenital adrenal hyperplasia or possibly a tumor in the adrenal cortex. Rarely, a malignant or benign interstitial testicular tumor may cause hypergonadism.

In *idiopathic precocious puberty,* no organic

cause for increased pituitary gonadotropin secretion can be found. This form of hypergonadism is present in about 50% of boys with premature sexual maturation and is often associated with mental deficiency.

Hypogonadism leads to infertility

Most hypogonadal disorders damage the seminiferous tubules. Whether they affect the tubules alone or also the androgen levels, their pathophysiologic effects are similar.

In *primary hypogonadism* (hypergonadotropic hypogonadism), both the seminiferous

Structure of the testis

Cross section of a testis

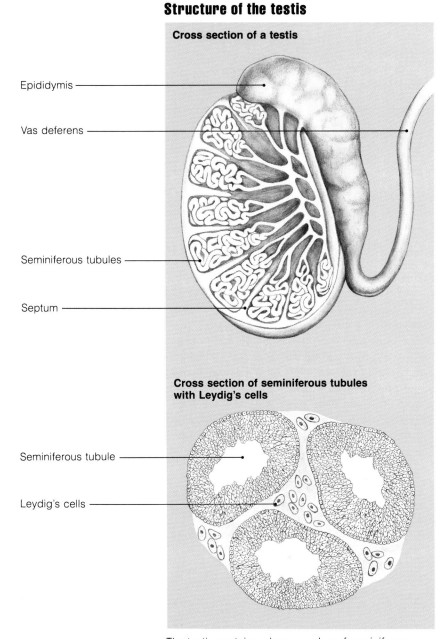

Epididymis

Vas deferens

Seminiferous tubules

Septum

Cross section of seminiferous tubules with Leydig's cells

Seminiferous tubule

Leydig's cells

The testis contains a large number of seminiferous tubules, where sperm are formed. Within the interstices between the tubules lie the Leydig's cells, which secrete testosterone, the most potent male sex hormone.

tubules and spermatogenesis are usually affected. Deficient gonadal hormone levels overstimulate the intact hypothalamus and pituitary gland to increase plasma levels of follicle-stimulating hormone (FSH) or luteinizing hormone (LH), or both. For this reason, primary hypogonadism is often called hypergonadotropic hypogonadism. Primary hypogonadism may also result from defective testosterone production, which may stem from hereditary enzymatic errors.

Testosterone resistance, caused by a lack of hormone receptors in target tissues, prevents hormone action, resulting in testicular feminization; genetic males with this condition appear female because of retarded virilization (male pseudohermaphroditism). The resulting feminization may be complete (no androgen response, phenotypic female) or incomplete.

In idiopathic gonadotropin deficiency, the lack of gonadotropin-releasing hormone (GnRH) leads to permanent LH and FSH deficiency.

Cryptorchidism (undescended testicles) results from testicular dysfunction and may lead to hypogonadism, even if only one testis is involved. (See *Cryptorchidism,* page 177.)

In *secondary hypogonadism* (hypogonadotropic hypogonadism), FSH and LH levels are abnormally low, possibly related to neoplasm, inflammation, trauma, vascular damage, or degenerative pituitary or hypothalamic lesions. It may occur alone or with other pituitary hormone deficiencies. Suppression of pituitary gonadotropins may also result from excessive levels of androgens or estrogens, as in adrenogenital syndrome.

Pituitary or testicular deficiency is sometimes linked to impotence, since testosterone is essential for normal libido and sexual function. Low testosterone levels may also result from chronic liver disease, metabolic disorders, uremia, and certain drugs, causing gonadal dysfunction that's not primarily related to the hypothalamic-pituitary axis. Hyperprolactinemic hypogonadism has also been reported; prolactin excess has an antigonadotropic effect and is usually associated with low testosterone levels.

Gynecomastia, a benign enlargement of the mammary glands, occurs transiently in many pubertal boys and may also be associated with hormonally active tumors, Klinefelter's syndrome, and metabolic disorders. Although its etiology is unclear, it may reflect a hormonal disturbance, such as an increase in the estrogen:androgen ratio.

MEDICAL MANAGEMENT

Diagnosing male gonadal disorders begins with a thorough patient history that includes medical, familial, and sexual evaluations to trace their often obscure sources. These evaluations require an array of special tests, including diagnostic hormone tests, biopsies, and chromosomal and radiographic studies.

Complex diagnostic tests

Male gonadal disorders may result from multiple genetic, anatomic, histologic, or hormonal factors. Hence, diagnostic testing involves evaluation of the hypothalamus, anterior pituitary gland, testes, and spermatic ducts, to measure levels of releasing hormones, gonadotropins, and androgens.

Hormonal studies. Serum levels of FSH and LH are most accurately determined by serial radioimmunoassays (RIA). Increased levels usually indicate primary testicular disease; decreased levels indicate a hypothalamic or pituitary defect.

Serum testosterone levels are also determined by RIA. Decreased levels may indicate primary or secondary hypogonadism.

To help differentiate hypothalamic from pituitary causes of hypogonadism, Gn-RH may be administered I.V. In patients with hypothalamic lesions, serum LH levels and, to a lesser extent, FSH levels rise in response to Gn-RH. In patients with pituitary lesions, the LH level does not rise. However, this test is not always reliable.

HCG challenge. The administration of human chorionic gonadotropin (HCG) specifically tests Leydig's cell function. This causes the testes to increase testosterone secretion if hypogonadism is due to hypothalamic or pituitary dysfunction. If it's due to testicular dysfunction, the HCG challenge doesn't increase testosterone secretion.

Clomiphene test. Clomiphene citrate, an estrogen antagonist, may be given to stimulate LH and FSH secretion by competing for receptor sites in the hypothalamus and pituitary. In postpubertal children, lack of LH response following administration of clomiphene citrate indicates either a hypothalamic or a pituitary disorder.

Sex chromatin evaluation. Evaluating sex chromatin patterns from buccal smears, skin biopsies, or blood samples provides quick and accurate screening for sex chromosome abnormalities. If such abnormalities are suspected, a full karyotype—involving systematic arrangement of chromosomes according to size and shape—is done. The presence of female-type (chromatin-positive) chromatin material in phenotypic males with bilateral small testes may indicate a congenital primary testosterone disorder, such as Klinefelter's syndrome.

Histocompatibility Y antigen (H-Y antigen) analysis, a recent development in evaluating

Male gonadal disorders

Hypergonadism

True precocious puberty: Early pituitary gonadotropin secretion related to central nervous system lesions, tumors, idiopathic causes, or heredity.
Precocious pseudopuberty: Early secretion of androgens from adrenal cortex or testes related to adrenal hyperplasia, virilizing adrenocortical tumors, interstitial cell tumors of the testes, or iatrogenic causes (for example, androgen therapy).

Primary hypogonadism
(Hypergonadotropic hypogonadism)

Gonadal dysfunction, causing androgen deficit due to numerous genetic, developmental, or acquired conditions despite feedback of increased gonadotropins.
Cryptorchidism: Failure of testes to descend into the scrotum. Mechanism is believed to be due to hormonal or anatomic factors. Also associated with numerous complex genetic syndromes.
Klinefelter's syndrome: Genetic defect; increased number of X chromosomes in at least one cell line.
Sertoli-cell–only syndrome: Genetic defect; no germinal cells present.
Noonan's syndrome (male Turner's syndrome): Genetic defect; often hereditary.
Myotonic muscular dystrophy: Hereditary genetic defect; usually appears in third or fourth decade of life.
Varicocele: Abnormal dilatation and tortuosity of veins of spermatic cord in scrotum.
Orchitis: Testicular infection caused by venereal disease, mumps, and other systemic conditions.
Exposure to ionizing radiation or toxic substances: Destruction of testicular tissue caused by ionizing radiation, chemotherapeutic agents, pesticides, or industrial chemicals.

Secondary hypogonadism
(Hypogonadotropic hypogonadism)

Faulty interaction within the hypothalamic-pituitary axis, resulting in failure to secrete normal levels of gonadotropins.
Hypopituitarism: Deficiency of gonadotropic hormone secreted by anterior pituitary gland; caused by a pituitary or hypothalamic lesion.
Kallmann's syndrome: Genetic defect of the hypothalamus, causing deficiency of gonadotropin-releasing hormone.
Isolated luteinizing hormone (LH) deficiency (fertile eunuch syndrome): Lesion in hypothalamus or pituitary gland, causing LH deficiency.
Gynecomastia: Excessive development of male breasts caused by increased prolactin, increased estrogen:androgen ratio, neoplasms, decreased androgen activity, or as a side effect of various drugs.

In normal males, sex hormone function is controlled by a negative feedback mechanism that stimulates the hypothalamus. Responding, the hypothalamus secretes gonadotropin-releasing hormone (Gn-RH) that stimulates the anterior pituitary, which releases luteinizing hormone (LH) and follicle-stimulating hormone (FSH).

Acting on the Leydig's cells in the testes, LH causes them to mature and secrete testosterone, which engenders normal growth and development of male sex organs and expression of secondary sex characteristics. FSH stimulates seminiferous tubule development. If a hypothalamic tumor causes hypersecretion of Gn-RH in the child, this eventually leads to oversecretion of testosterone and premature sexual development.

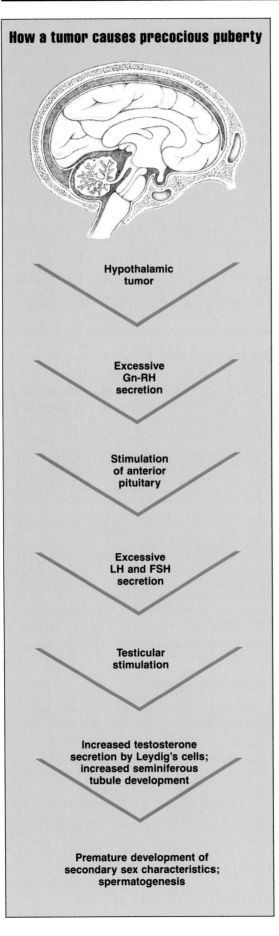

How a tumor causes precocious puberty

Hypothalamic tumor

Excessive Gn-RH secretion

Stimulation of anterior pituitary

Excessive LH and FSH secretion

Testicular stimulation

Increased testosterone secretion by Leydig's cells; increased seminiferous tubule development

Premature development of secondary sex characteristics; spermatogenesis

gonadal disorders of uncertain etiology, can determine the presence of the active male-determining gene of a Y chromosome. Amniocentesis reliably detects fetal chromosomal abnormalities through karyotyping.

Semen analysis. Semen analysis is usually the first test performed to evaluate male fertility. This test measures volume and assesses sperm count and motility through microscopic examination. Abnormal semen may require further testing, such as testicular biopsy; liver, thyroid, pituitary, and adrenal function tests; and screening for metabolic abnormalities.

Urine studies. Measuring urine testosterone levels can provide information on Leydig's cell function. Metabolic products of androgen secretion from the adrenal cortex and the testes (urinary 17-ketosteroids), which are also measured in urine, help screen for panhypopituitarism, congenital adrenal hyperplasia, and adrenal tumors.

Biopsy. Testicular biopsy provides morphologic information about the stage of spermatogenesis and tubule status. Biopsy can detect tubular disease, determine sperm maturation, and distinguish azoospermia due to obstruction from other causes.

X-ray studies. Skull films or computerized tomography scans may detect central nervous system (CNS) tumors invading the pituitary. Skull and hand films compare bone age with chronologic age in precocious puberty. Films of the seminal tract may show possible obstructions or developmental anomalies.

Treatment: Many options
Treatment of male gonadal disorders depends on their causes and severity; it may include surgery, radiation, hormone therapy, and psychotherapy.

Surgery. Surgical treatment may include excision of germinal cell tumors that cause hypergonadism, bilateral orchiectomy to remove highly malignant secreting tumors, or craniotomy to treat primary hypergonadal tumors. Seminal tract surgery removes ductile obstructions in some patients with azoospermia. Surgical reduction of breast tissue may be necessary to mitigate the psychological effects of gynecomastia. Orchiopexy may be necessary to repair cryptorchidism.

Radiation. Radiation is an adjunct to excision of testicular tumors or is the sole treatment of some tumors involving germinal or interstitial cells. It's also used to treat CNS tumors that cause hypergonadal disorders.

Hormones. Hormonal therapy is used widely

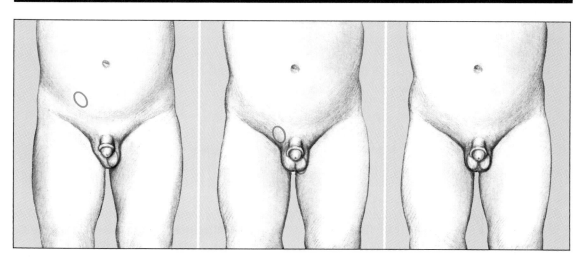

Cryptorchidism

Testosterone secreted by the fetal testes stimulates their descent from the abdomen to the scrotum, which usually occurs around the 8th month of gestation. In cryptorchidism, one or both testes fail to descend because of lack of testosterone or anatomic defects, such as an obstruction. If the testes do not descend by age 12 months, hormone therapy or surgery may be required to correct the defect. The illustrations depict the normal pathway of testicular descent.

in gonadal disorders. Medroxyprogesterone acetate (Depo-Provera) may be used to suppress testosterone secretion and thus inhibit further premature maturation in idiopathic precocious puberty. Bromocriptine, used in some centers, may suppress CNS tumors causing hyperprolactinemia and may correct impotence.

Testosterone replacement is often necessary in hypogonadal adolescents to mimic puberty. In primary testicular insufficiency, it maintains libido, potency, and hair and beard growth but will not restore spermatogenesis. Long-acting testosterone enanthate and cypionate, given I.M., appear to be the safest, most effective forms of androgen replacement.

When hypogonadal dysfunction results from decreased gonadotropins (hypogonadotropic hypogonadism), HCG produces all the effects of LH. Injections of HCG three times a week may stimulate the testes to normalize testosterone production. HCG is also used in cryptorchidism to induce testicular descent.

Psychotherapy. Most gonadal hyperfunction disorders occur during puberty, a traumatic time; supportive psychological care is particularly important and must take into account family dynamics and parental attitudes. Psychotherapy may also be valuable in treating patients who are infertile and impotent.

NURSING MANAGEMENT

Before you can provide skilled care for your male patient with a gonadal disorder, you should analyze your own feelings about it. Consider the inhibitions you might have about dealing with male sexuality; balance this against your knowledge and understanding of the disorder to be sure you can care for this type of patient comfortably and professionally—without letting your own feelings get in

the way of good treatment for him. Only then can you expect to offer the patient the reassurance and direction he needs.

The history: Draw out the anxious patient
The basis of good nursing care in patients with gonadal disorders, a thorough and well-focused history is essential but may be difficult to get; such patients are understandably anxious and sensitive about their privacy. Commonly, they are reluctant to volunteer the detailed information you need because of embarrassment, uneasiness with you, or fear of an unknown disease. So, to make this interview effective, make every effort to ensure privacy and try to put him at ease. As you begin, keep the patient's developmental stage in mind. Ask him about his chief complaint. He may mention only associated or vague symptoms at first, and you'll have to patiently draw him out.

Explore the history of his present illness. Ask whether he experiences pain or tenderness in the scrotum or penis; painful malignant testicular tumors and penile lesions may be the underlying cause of impotence.

Assess CNS symptoms. Has the patient experienced nausea and vomiting? Does he complain of headaches or visual disturbances? If so, determine their severity and pattern. Such symptoms may result from cerebral lesions causing precocious puberty.

Assess maturation of secondary sex characteristics by asking about the patient's shaving habits. The male who's hypogonadal before puberty develops only fine and sparse facial hair; the hypogonadal male who has previously reached sexual maturity has a slow, diminished rate of beard growth. Hypergonadal males may need to shave by age 10.

Impotence may mean different things to

different people, so if the patient uses this term be sure you find out what he means. Ask him about changes in his sex drive and frequency of erections and ejaculations.

If infertility is the complaint, ask how long he and his partner have been trying to achieve pregnancy. In hypogonadism, libido and potency may be diminished, depending on the degree and cause of testicular failure or hypothalamic-pituitary dysfunction.

Accurate history taking about infertility requires detailed questioning about environmental or iatrogenic causes. Ask about recent testicular injury, surgery, or infection, such as mumps or venereal disease. Febrile illness may cause a dramatic decline in sperm count and motility that can last as long as 3 to 4 months after the infection. Determine possible sources of environmental heat that may damage the spermatozoa. Does the patient wear tight underwear? Does he take saunas or frequent hot baths or steam baths? Does he spend long hours sitting (as in truck driving or long-distance biking)?

A past health history adds important information to the clinical profile. Ask about significant illnesses during the patient's growth and development. Find out and record the sequence of events during his puberty. Ask about his surgical history and whether he suffered any complications after surgery. Has he ever had an injury in the inguinal area? Ask about severe systemic allergic reactions and their effects and about exposure to radiation or toxic chemicals.

Does the patient have a history of metabolic, endocrine, or neurologic disorders? Such conditions as diabetes mellitus, panhypopituitarism, and multiple sclerosis can result in impotence and infertility. Include a good nutritional history because malnutrition can impair reproductive function.

Get a detailed medication history because many drugs can affect male gonadal function. For example, estrogens may cause gynecomastia, testicular atrophy, and impotence. Antihypertensives, cimetidine, tranquilizers, antineoplastic agents, and such cardiac drugs as propranolol and digitalis can produce hypogonadism or gynecomastia and can reduce libido and sperm count.

Get a family history. Many gonadal disorders are hereditary. Does evidence of gonadal dysfunction—genital abnormalities, cryptorchidism, testicular tumors, or other disorders—appear in family members? Remember that hypogonadism cannot be detected until the onset of puberty. What is the familial pattern for onset of puberty? This may serve as a baseline for evaluating the patient.

Finally, get a psychosocial history. Emotional well-being plays an important role in the patient's sexual functioning. Because stress and other psychosocial factors are often responsible for impotence and infertility, explore the patient's occupational, recreational, and domestic situations. Ask about use of alcohol or other CNS depressants; alcohol acts on the liver and, possibly, directly on the testes to alter normal testosterone production and spermatogenesis. Recent research indicates that prolonged use of marijuana may interfere with spermatogenesis and may cause gynecomastia.

The physical exam: Subtle clues

The physical examination is important despite significant variations in secondary sex characteristics among individuals and different racial groups.

Provide a private and comfortable environment for the patient. Before you begin, explain the procedures, letting the patient know you'll be using observation and palpation.

Since male gonadal disorders are seldom clinically obvious, look for subtle clues, such as the degree of virilization and its appropriateness for the patient's age, minor abnormalities of external genitalia, and testicular size.

Assess hair growth. To detect the subtle effects of gonadal dysfunction, note texture and distribution of body hair, keeping in mind the great variation among racial and ethnic groups. Orientals tend to have little body hair; Mediterraneans tend to have dark, profuse body hair. Many men of all races experience bitemporal or progressive baldness with aging. Pubic hair and beard growth are the most accurate areas in which to assess body hair. Male pubic hair normally is diamond-shaped, grows thickest over the symphysis pubis, and continues over the scrotum to the inner thighs. In severely hypogonadal adolescents, sparse pubic hair may be the only secondary sex characteristic to appear. Mild hypogonadism is marked by scant facial hair and feminine pubic hair distribution.

Assess body habitus. Prepubertal androgen deficiency causes disproportionately long bone growth and delayed epiphyseal closure. The most accurate body habitus measurement of androgen activity is height and span of the upper and lower body segments. In prepubertal eunuchoidism, the arm span exceeds height by 2″ (5 cm), and the upper:lower body segment ratio is also abnormal. In hypogonadism, the lower segment (symphysis pubis to soles) constitutes more than 55% of the patient's height. Tall stature, narrow shoulders, poor muscle development, and unusual fat distribution causing female contours are common. In sexual precocity, bone maturation accelerates but the epiphyses close prematurely; in later life, the patient appears stunted.

Assess the breasts for gynecomastia. Palpate to differentiate true gynecomastia from non-endocrine-related overgrowth of fatty tissue. If gynecomastia occurred with puberty, or if the patient is taking drugs that may cause gynecomastia, it is not pathologic. Otherwise, the patient should be tested for hypogonadism, testicular tumors, or other conditions.

Assess skin texture, voice timbre, and olfactory sense. If hypogonadism occurs after maturity, lack of testosterone causes pale yellow skin and fine wrinkles around the eyes. Hypogonadal men also have high-pitched, juvenile voices because normal laryngeal enlargement does not occur during puberty. Anosmia (absence of smell) is commonly associated with Kallmann's syndrome, in which the olfactory lobe of the cerebrum fails to develop.

Examine the testes. Note the size, position, and descent of the testes in the scrotum. Normally, the testis is about 1¾″ to 2⅛″ (4.4 to 5.4 cm) long and ⅞″ to 1¼″ (2.1 to 3.2 cm) wide; it weighs about ¾ oz (21 g). A length of less than 1⅝″ (4 cm) is considered abnormal. Palpate the scrotum to establish that the testes are present. Cryptorchidism or anorchia (complete absence of one or both testes) may exist. Palpation may reveal masses, cysts, hernias, or varicocele. Transillumination (shining a light through the scrotum to backlight the testes) differentiates hydrocele or spermatocele from solid masses. In most patients with hypogonadism, the testes are atrophied; in postpubertal hypogonadism, they may be soft and not as infantile. Small, hard testes are a mark of Klinefelter's syndrome. Testicular enlargement accompanies early development of other sex characteristics in precocious puberty, not in precocious pseudopuberty.

Formulate nursing diagnoses

Realize, as you form your nursing diagnoses, that much of your effort must be directed toward helping the patient and his family accept and cope with the patient's altered body image. This is not an easy task. You'll need all of your communication skills to provide important information about a body system that is so highly personal.

Altered body image related to precocious puberty. Your goals are to enable the patient and his family to accept the altered body image through recognition of the condition's possible causes and consequences and to help the patient learn to function near his chronologic age despite accelerated physical maturity.

Review with the patient and his family information about the causes of precocious puberty and the physical changes that have occurred or are expected, such as early skeletal and muscular development, appearance of secondary sex characteristics, possible spermatogenesis, and premature epiphyseal closure. Inform them of testing and treatment options. Remind parents that, although their child's sexual development is precocious, his psychological age parallels his chronologic age. Assure the child that other children experience the same changes. Guide the parents in teaching hygiene and sex education. Explain that sexual precocity from cerebral lesions may cause nausea, vomiting, headaches, visual disturbances, and hydrocephalus.

Provide emotional support through the diagnostic phase, and continue support if a CNS cause is determined. The prognosis may not be encouraging, and you should help the patient and his family express their concerns and feelings. Be sure to emphasize the normal aspects of the patient's development.

Your interventions are successful if the patient and his family ask questions about the causes and effects of his disorder, if they can identify the most likely changes, if they verbalize their feelings, and if the parents give the patient affection and support.

Social isolation related to hypergonadal or hypogonadal appearance. Your goal is to help the patient to accept himself through interaction with family, peer group, and society as appropriate to his age and mental development. Emphasize to the patient and, if necessary, his parents that he will probably develop mentally at the same rate as his peers. Of course, in some cases of primary hypogonadism mental deficiency coexists, and you may need to make appropriate referrals.

Counsel the patient to maintain good grooming and to choose clothing that minimizes his abnormal appearance. Help him to think about being in social situations.

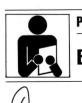

PATIENT-TEACHING AID

Examining your testes

Dear _____

To help detect abnormalities early, you should examine your testes once a month. Eventually, you'll become familiar with their configuration and will be able to recognize anything abnormal. The best time to examine them is right after a warm bath; the scrotum, which tends to contract when cold, will be relaxed, making the testes easier to examine.

With one hand, lift your penis and check the scrotum (the

than the right (see below, left).

Next, check the testes for lumps and masses. Locate the crescent-shaped structure at the back of each testis. This is the epididymis, which should feel soft.

Next, examine each testis (below). To examine your left testis, place your index and middle fingers on its underside and place your thumb on top. Roll the testis between your thumb and fingers. A normal testis is egg-shaped, rubbery-firm, and movable within the scrotum; it should feel smooth, with no lumps. Make sure you check the entire testis. In the same manner, use your right hand to examine your right tes-

Basic anatomy

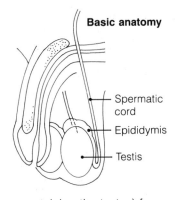

- Spermatic cord
- Epididymis
- Testis

sac containing the testes) for any change in shape, size, or color. The scrotum's left side normally hangs slightly lower

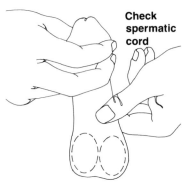

Check spermatic cord

The spermatic cord extends upward from the epididymis. Gently squeeze the spermatic cord, above your left testis, between the thumb and first two fingers of your left hand (above). Then repeat on the right side, using your right hand. Check for lumps and masses by palpating along the entire length of the cord.

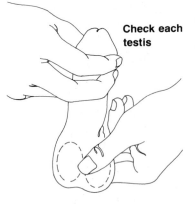

Check each testis

tis, which should be the same size as the left testis. If you notice any lumps, masses, or changes, notify your doctor.

Encourage him to find ways to interact with others, such as joining a club or group that he enjoys. Elicit support from his family and friends. Try to involve them in teaching other people about gonadal disorders. Understanding of these disorders by more and more people will help patients feel less isolated.

Your interventions are successful if the patient takes pride in his appearance with careful grooming and neat dressing, if he shows no signs of self-destructive behavior, if he begins or maintains contact with his peers and joins in their activities, and if he and his family readily discuss their concerns with each other and the nursing staff.

Knowledge deficit regarding effects of gonadal disorders. Your goals are to help the patient and his family understand the patient's physi-

cal changes and to encourage the patient to know about and take an interest in self-care. Explain the level of physical development he will attain, advising that, in most cases, sexual precocity will not be so threatening later in life when the patient's peers have also matured except that he may be short. If the patient lost total testicular androgenic function before puberty, advise him and his family to expect him to have eunuchoid proportions without secondary sex characteristics and with greatly reduced sexual function. Partial loss will cause a less striking decrease in sex characterization.

Men who develop hypogonadism after sexual maturity can expect reduced prostate size, slowly diminishing body hair growth, complexion changes, and, possibly, slightly reduced sexual function. Advise the patient that gynecomastia and acne may result from testosterone's action on the breasts and sebaceous glands.

If androgen therapy is warranted, instruct the patient and his family about the dosage schedule, route of administration, and side effects of the prescribed testosterone preparation. You may also have to show them how to give intramuscular injections. If therapy proves successful, teach the patient how to perform a monthly testicular self-examination. (See *Examining your testes*.)

Your interventions are successful if the patient is accurately informed about his disease and can adequately explain it to significant others, if he dresses neatly and appears well-groomed, if he takes his medications correctly and reports significant changes to the health-care team, and if he makes follow-up visits to the doctor or clinic.

Sexual dysfunction related to hypogonadism. Your goals are to help the patient demonstrate functionally adaptive behavior; to foster the development or continuation of productive interpersonal relationships; and to promote increased communication between the patient, the health-care staff, and significant others.

Depending on the patient's age, provide clear and accurate information about his sexual potential. If he is prepubertal, advise his family to expect that spermatogenesis and sex drive will be absent or greatly reduced. If he's postpubertal, explain that his sex drive will gradually diminish but won't disappear entirely. If a fertile male exhibits a genetic defect, provide genetic counseling. If hypogonadism was abrupt and led to infertility, as in iatrogenic causes, special support and counseling may be needed.

Explain that in primary (hypergonadotropic) hypogonadism, no treatment is effective; however, in secondary (hypogonadotropic) hypogonadism, replacement therapy with HCG may promote fertility.

Once the patient knows what to expect, explore with him the present and future impact of his infertility and diminished sexual function on his partner and his social life. Help him develop coping behavior that lets him function as normally as possible in interpersonal relationships.

Teach the patient to avoid habits that may interfere with normal spermatogenesis. Any activity that increases scrotal temperature, such as wearing tight underwear, taking hot baths, or habitual bike riding, may impair spermatogenesis. Instruct the patient to have regular physical exams and to protect his testes during athletic activity. Counsel him to receive prompt treatment for venereal disease and surgical correction of such anatomic defects as cryptorchidism.

If extensive evaluation and treatment suggest that infertility is idiopathic, additional teaching and support are necessary. Refer the patient and his partner for family counseling and, if warranted, to adoption agencies. Your interventions are successful if the patient realizes what to expect in his sexual function, if he and his partner can discuss it, and if they know where to find additional counseling.

Anxiety related to the need for surgical intervention. Your goals are to help the patient understand and accept curative or palliative surgery and, after surgery, to make him comfortable and to avoid complications.

Before surgery, teach the patient and his family about the surgery, according to hospital or doctor's guidelines. Before and after the operation, inform him about the type of incision and dressing, about I.V.s and drainage tubes, mobility restrictions, and prevention of postoperative complications. Be available to answer questions and to reinforce information given by other health-care team members.

Give extra support if the patient faces surgery for CNS causes of hypogonadism because the possibility of malignancy and the delicacy of the surgical area may exaggerate anxiety. Help the patient and his family realize that orchiopexy may not always result in fertility but that it's necessary to eliminate the risk of cancer in undescended testes.

Your interventions are successful if the patient understands the surgical procedure and its relevance to his gonadal disorder, if he and his family understand the prognosis of his disorder, and if he rests calmly and comfortably after the procedure.

A special challenge

Providing nursing care for the patient with a gonadal disorder may test your dedication and commitment more than most other diseases. The task demands more than making sure the patient takes his medication, is made comfortable, or understands his disease. It demands that you confront your own attitudes and concepts about human sexuality, a highly charged and intimate area of life. Only when you have your own attitudes firmly in control can you help the patient and his family adjust to abnormalities of sexual function.

Points to remember

• Besides retarding sexual development and causing infertility and possible malignancy, male gonadal disorders may impose a devastating psychological burden on the patient.
• Psychotherapy is an important adjunct to treatment because many male gonadal disorders become evident at puberty, an already emotionally charged period.
• True precocious puberty, a form of hypergonadism, can result from increased pituitary gonadotropin production or from tumors.
• Hypogonadal disorders may occur because of seminiferous tubule damage as well as from genetic or acquired conditions.
• The monthly testicular self-examination can play an important role in preventive health care.

APPENDICES

Endocrine drugs

Pituitary replacement hormones

Drug, dose, and route	Interactions	Side effects	Special considerations
desmopressin acetate 0.1 to 0.4 ml intranasally daily in 1 to 3 doses	None significant	Overhydration	Give only intranasally. Because patient may have difficulty measuring and inhaling drug, teach correct method of administration. Titrate dosage to avoid nocturia and allow the patient sufficient sleep. Adjust fluid intake to reduce risk of overhydration and sodium depletion, especially in very young or old patients.
lypressin 1 or 2 sprays in either or both nostrils q.i.d. Give additional dose at bedtime, if necessary, to prevent nocturia.	None significant	Overhydration	If dosage is inadequate, increase frequency rather than number of sprays. To administer uniform, well-diffused spray, hold bottle upright, with patient standing and holding his head upright. Inadvertent inhalation may cause chest tightness, coughing, and transient dyspnea. Instruct patient to carry drug with him at all times because of its fairly short duration.
vasopressin (aqueous) vasopressin tannate 5 to 10 units I.M. or S.C. (aqueous) b.i.d. to q.i.d.; for chronic therapy, 2.5 to 5 units (tannate) I.M. or S.C. every 2 to 3 days	*Lithium, demeclocycline:* reduced antidiuretic activity. Use together cautiously. *Chlorpropamide:* increased antidiuretic response. Use together cautiously.	Overhydration, hypersensitivity	Avoid I.V. administration of vasopressin tannate in oil. Place tannate in oil in warm water for 10 to 15 minutes. Then shake well before withdrawing I.M. dose. Overhydration occurs more frequently with long-acting tannate oil suspension than with aqueous solution. Use minimum effective dose to reduce risk of overhydration.

Thyroid replacement hormones

Drug, dose, and route	Interactions	Side effects	Special considerations
levothyroxine sodium (T₄ or L-thyroxine) Initially, 0.025 to 0.1 mg P.O. daily, increased by 0.05 to 0.1 mg q 1 to 4 weeks. Maintenance dose: 0.1 to 0.4 mg daily	*Cholestyramine:* impaired absorption of levothyroxine. Separate doses by 4 to 5 hours. *I.V. phenytoin:* free thyroid released. Monitor for tachycardia.	Nervousness, insomnia, tremors, tachycardia, angina pectoris	Because all brands aren't bioequivalent, warn patient stabilized on one brand to avoid switching to another brand or to generic levothyroxine. Levothyroxine has slow onset; prolonged duration. When changing from liothyronine to levothyroxine, start levothyroxine several days before withdrawing liothyronine, to avoid relapse.
liothyronine sodium (T₃) Initially, 25 mcg P.O. daily, increased by 12.5 to 25 mcg q 1 to 2 weeks. Maintenance dose: 25 to 75 mcg daily	*Cholestyramine:* impaired absorption of liothyronine. Separate doses by 4 to 5 hours. *I.V. phenytoin:* free thyroid released. Monitor for tachycardia.	Nervousness, insomnia, tremors, tachycardia, angina pectoris	Liothyronine has a prompt onset and a short duration of action. When changing from levothyroxine to liothyronine, stop levothyroxine and begin liothyronine. Increase in small increments after symptomatic effects of levothyroxine disappear.
liotrix Initially, 15 to 30 mg P.O. daily, increasing by 15 to 30 mg q 1 to 2 weeks. Maintenance dose: varies according to patient's response	*Cholestyramine:* impaired absorption of liotrix. Separate doses by 4 to 5 hours. *I.V. phenytoin:* free thyroid released. Monitor for tachycardia.	Nervousness, insomnia, tremors, tachycardia, angina pectoris	Commercially prepared forms of liotrix contain different amounts of each ingredient; do not change brands without considering differences in potency. Thyrolar-½ contains 25 mcg T₄ and 6.25 mcg T₃; Euthroid-½ contains 30 mcg T₄ and 7.5 mcg T₃. Give drug before breakfast to prevent insomnia.
thyroglobulin Initially, 15 to 30 mg P.O. daily, increased by 15 to 30 mg at 2-week intervals. Maintenance dose: 60 to 180 mg daily	*Cholestyramine:* impaired absorption of thyroglobulin. Separate doses by 4 to 5 hours. *I.V. phenytoin:* free thyroid released. Monitor for tachycardia.	Nervousness, insomnia, tremors, tachycardia, angina pectoris	Monitor pulse rate and blood pressure. Tell patient to immediately report chest pain (especially in elderly), palpitations, sweating, or nervousness. Give drug before breakfast to prevent insomnia.
thyroid USP (desiccated) Initially, 60 mg P.O. daily, increased by 60 mg q 30 days. Maintenance dose: 60 to 180 mg daily	*Cholestyramine:* impaired thyroid hormone absorption. Separate doses by 4 to 5 hours. *I.V. phenytoin:* free thyroid released. Monitor for tachycardia.	Nervousness, insomnia, tremors, tachycardia, angina pectoris	Monitor pulse rate and blood pressure. Tell patient to immediately report chest pain (especially in elderly), palpitations, sweating, or nervousness. Give drug before breakfast to prevent insomnia.

Thyroid hormone antagonists

Drug, dose, and route	Interactions	Side effects	Special considerations
methimazole Initially, 5 to 20 mg P.O. t.i.d. Maintenance dose: 5 mg daily to t.i.d.	None significant	Leukopenia, thrombocytopenia, agranulocytosis, diarrhea, nausea, vomiting	Periodically monitor CBC to detect impending blood dyscrasias. Doses exceeding 30 mg/day increase risk of agranulocytosis. Tell patient to report fever, sore throat, or mouth sores. Give drug with meals to reduce GI side effects.
propylthiouracil 100 mg P.O. t.i.d.	None significant	Leukopenia, thrombocytopenia, agranulocytosis, diarrhea, nausea, vomiting	Periodically monitor CBC to detect impending blood dyscrasias. Tell patient to report fever, sore throat, or mouth sores. Give drug with meals to reduce GI side effects.

Parathyroid drugs

Drug, dose, and route	Interactions	Side effects	Special considerations
calcitonin (Salmon) 100 to 400 MRC units I.M. once or twice daily	None significant	Transient nausea and vomiting, facial flushing, tetany, anaphylaxis	Keep epinephrine handy because of risk of anaphylaxis. Facial flushing and warmth occur in 20% to 30% of patients within minutes of injection and usually last 1 hour. Reassure patient that effect is transient. Observe patient for signs of hypocalcemic tetany (muscle twitching, tetanic spasms, and convulsions) during therapy.
calcium salts 500 mg to 1 g I.V. q 1 to 3 days (determined by serum calcium levels)	*Cardiotonic glycosides:* increased digitalis toxicity. Give calcium cautiously, if at all, to digitalized patients.	Vasodilation, bradycardia, tingling sensations, feeling of heat, local vein irritation; with rapid I.V. injection, syncope	If possible, administer I.V. into large vein and keep patient recumbent for 15 minutes. Severe necrosis and sloughing of tissues follow extravasation. Calcium gluconate causes less irritation to veins and tissue than calcium chloride.
furosemide 80 to 100 mg I.V. q 1 to 2 hours	*Aminoglycoside antibiotics:* potentiated ototoxicity. Use together cautiously. *Chloral hydrate:* sweating, flushing.	Volume depletion and dehydration, transient deafness with overly rapid I.V. injection, orthostatic hypotension, hypokalemia	Give I.V. doses over 1 to 2 minutes. Monitor blood pressure and pulse rate during rapid diuresis. Also monitor serum potassium levels and watch for signs of hypokalemia (muscle weakness, cramps). Patients also on digitalis are at increased risk of digitalis toxicity because of potassium-depleting effect of this diuretic.
mithramycin (plicamycin) 25 mcg/1 kg I.V. daily for 1 to 4 days	None significant	Thrombocytopenia; bleeding ranging from epistaxis to generalized hemorrhage; facial flushing; nausea; vomiting	Frequently check serum calcium levels, and watch for tetany, carpopedal spasm, Chvostek's sign, and muscle cramps. Therapeutic effect in hypercalcemia may not occur for 24 to 48 hours, but may last 3 to 15 days. Monitor platelet count and prothrombin time before and during therapy. Observe for signs of bleeding, especially facial flushing.
vitamin D₂ (ergocalciferol) 0.625 to 5 mg P.O. daily with calcium supplementation	*Mineral oil, cholestyramine resin:* inhibited GI absorption of oral vitamin D. Space doses. Use together cautiously.	Hypercalcemia, headache, dizziness	Monitor serum and urine calcium and phosphorus levels every 2 weeks. Give I.M. injection of vitamin D dispersed in oil to patients who cannot absorb oral vitamin D. Each mg of vitamin D equals 40,000 USP units.

Adrenomedullary drugs

Drug, dose, and route	Interactions	Side effects	Special considerations
metyrosine Initially, 250 mg P.O. q.i.d. May be increased up to 500 mg q day to a maximum of 4 g daily in divided doses	*Phenothiazines and haloperidol:* impaired catecholamine synthesis, causing extrapyramidal symptoms. Use cautiously.	Sedation, diarrhea, crystalluria, extrapyramidal symptoms	For optimal preoperative preparation, give for at least 5 to 7 days. Warn patient that sedation occurs initially but subsides after several days' treatment. Instruct patient to increase fluid intake to prevent crystalluria. Daily urine volume should be at least 2,000 ml.
phenoxybenzamine Initially, 10 mg P.O. daily. Increase daily dose by 10 mg q 4 days. Maintenance dose: 20 to 60 mg daily	None significant	Orthostatic hypotension, miosis, nasal stuffiness, dry mouth, impotence, tachycardia	Drug may take several weeks to achieve optimal effect. Nasal congestion, miosis, and impotence usually decrease with continued therapy. Monitor heart rate and blood pressure frequently. Tachycardia may require propranolol.
phentolamine 50 mg P.O. q.i.d. For diagnosis: 5 mg I.V. Before surgery: 2 to 5 mg I.M. or I.V.	None significant	Dizziness, weakness, flushing, hypotension, tachycardia, diarrhea, nausea, nasal stuffiness	When drug is given for diagnostic purpose, check blood pressure before and during administration. Don't give sedatives or narcotics 24 hours before diagnostic test. Administer norepinephrine to counteract severe hypotension, if necessary.

Adrenocortical drugs

Drug, dose, and route	Interactions	Side effects	Special considerations
aminoglutethimide 250 mg P.O. q.i.d. May be increased in increments of 25 mg daily q 1 to 2 weeks to maximum daily dose of 2 g	None significant	Severe pancytopenia, drowsiness, nausea, anorexia, morbilliform skin rash	Perform baseline hematologic studies and monitor CBC periodically. Monitor thyroid function studies since drug may decrease thyroid hormone production. Tell patient to report skin rash that persists for more than 8 days. Reassure him that drowsiness, nausea, and loss of appetite usually diminish after 2 weeks of therapy, but tell him to notify doctor if symptoms persist.

cortisone actetate
25 to 300 mg P.O. or I.M. daily or on alternate days
 	
dexamethasone
0.25 to 4 mg P.O. b.i.d., t.i.d., or q.i.d.
 	
prednisone
2.5 to 15 mg P.O. b.i.d., t.i.d., or q.i.d.
	Amphotericin B, diuretics: hypokalemia.
	Barbiturates, phenytoin, rifampin: decreased effect. Dose may need to be increased.
	Indomethacin, aspirin: increased risk of GI distress and bleeding. Give together cautiously.
		Euphoria, insomnia, hypokalemia, hyperglycemia, peptic ulcer and G.I. irritation, fluid retention with possible hypertension and congestive heart failure	Warn patient on long-term therapy about cushingoid symptoms. Teach patient early signs of adrenal insufficiency (fatigue, muscle weakness, joint pain, fever, anorexia, nausea, dyspnea, dizziness, fainting). Instruct patient to carry a card indicating need for supplemental systemic glucocorticoids during stress, especially as dose is decreased. Monitor weight, blood pressure, and serum electrolytes. Patients with diabetes may need increased insulin; monitor urine for sugar.
			   Give once-daily doses in the morning for better results and less toxicity. Give P.O. dose with food when possible. Unless contraindicated, give salt-restricted diet rich in potassium and protein. Potassium supplement may be needed.
			   Corticosteroid doses are highly individualized, depending on patient and his condition.

fludrocortisone 0.1 to 0.2 mg P.O. daily	None significant	Sodium and water retention, hypokalemia	Increase dietary intake of potassium, protein, and, if ordered, sodium. Provide a potassium supplement, if necessary. Warn patient that mild peripheral edema is common. Monitor blood pressure and serum electrolytes. Weigh patient daily and report sudden gain.
mitotane 9 to 10 g P.O. daily in divided doses	None significant	Depression, somnolence, vertigo, severe nausea, vomiting	Assess and record behavioral and neurologic signs daily for baseline data throughout therapy. To reduce nausea, give antiemetic before administering. Warn ambulatory patient of CNS side effects and advise him to avoid tasks requiring alertness or coordination.

Antidiabetic drugs

Drug, dose, and route	Interactions	Side effects	Special considerations
acetohexamide Initially, 250 mg P.O. daily; may increase dose q 5 to 7 days to maximum 1.5 g daily, divided b.i.d. or t.i.d. **chlorpropamide** Initially, 250 mg P.O. daily; may increase dose q 5 to 7 days to maximum 750 mg daily once in morning **tolazamide** Initially, 100 mg P.O. daily; may adjust at weekly intervals by 100 to 250 mg; maximum dose 500 mg b.i.d. **tolbutamide** Initially, 1 to 2 g P.O. daily as single dose or divided b.i.d. or t.i.d.; maximum dose 3 g daily	*Anabolic steroids, chloramphenicol, clofibrate, guanethidine, MAO inhibitors, oral anticoagulants, phenylbutazone, salicylates, sulfonamides:* increased hypoglycemic activity. Monitor blood glucose. *Beta blockers, clonidine:* prolonged hypoglycemic effect and masked symptoms of hypoglycemia. Use together cautiously. *Corticosteroids, glucagon, rifampin, thiazide diuretics:* decreased hypoglycemic response. Monitor blood glucose.	Bone marrow aplasia, nausea, vomiting, heartburn, rash, facial flushing, hypoglycemia	Teach patient about his disease. Stress importance of following therapeutic regimen; adhering to diet, weight reduction, exercise, personal hygiene; avoiding infection. Teach how and when to test for glycosuria and ketonuria and how to recognize and intervene for hypoglycemia. Patient may require hospitalization during transition from insulin therapy to oral antidiabetic. Monitor urine glucose and ketones at least t.i.d., before meals. Emphasize need for a double-voided specimen. During periods of increased stress, such as infection, fever, surgery, or trauma, patient may require insulin therapy. Monitor closely for hypoglycemia. Advise patient to avoid alcohol to reduce risk of facial flushing.
glipizide Initially, 2.5 to 25 mg daily; maximum dose 30 mg daily **glyburide** Initially, 2.5 to 20 mg daily; maximum dose 30 mg daily	*Beta blockers, clonidine:* prolonged hypoglycemic effect and masked symptoms of hypoglycemia. Use together cautiously. *Corticosteroids, glucagon, rifampin, thiazide diuretics:* decreased hypoglycemic response. Monitor blood glucose.	Bone marrow aplasia, nausea, vomiting, hypoglycemia (*frequency* of all side effects is lower than with acetohexamide, chlorpropamide, tolazamide, and tolbutamide)	Don't use drug in elderly and debilitated patients. Advise patient to take drug with meals and to avoid alcoholic beverages or to use them cautiously.

Antidiabetic drugs (continued)

Drug, dose, and route	Interactions	Side effects	Special considerations
regular insulin S.C. or I.V. dose varies according to patient's condition, diet, exercise program, and use of other therapeutic drugs **isophane insulin suspension (NPH)** Variable dose, S.C. only **prompt insulin zinc suspension (Semilente)** Variable dose, S.C. only **insulin zinc suspension (Lente)** Variable dose, S.C. only **protamine zinc insulin suspension (PZI)** Variable dose, S.C. only **extended insulin zinc suspension (Ultralente)** Variable dose, S.C. only	*Beta blockers, clonidine, guanethidine, MAO inhibitors:* prolonged hypoglycemic effect. Monitor blood glucose. *Corticosteroids, thiazide diuretics:* decreased insulin response. Monitor blood glucose.	Hypoglycemia, hyperglycemia (rebound, or Somogyi, effect), lipoatrophy, lipohypertrophy	Check expiration date on bottle before use. To mix insulin suspension, swirl vial gently or rotate between palm and thigh. Avoid vigorous shaking since this causes bubbles and air in syringe. Advise patient not to alter the order of mixing insulins or change the model or brand of syringe or needle. Remember that insulins vary in their onset, peak effect, and duration of action: *(see table below)*

Type	Onset (hr)	Peak (hr)	Duration (hr)
Regular insulin (S.C.)	½ to 1	2 to 5	6 to 8
Semilente	½ to 1½	5 to 10	12 to 16
NPH	1 to 1½	8 to 12	24
Lente	1 to 2½	7 to 15	24
PZI	4 to 8	14 to 20	36
Ultralente	4 to 8	10 to 30	>36

Miscellaneous drugs

Drug, dose, and route	Interactions	Side effects	Special considerations
bromocriptine mesylate 1.25 to 2.5 mg P.O. b.i.d. or t.i.d.	None significant	Dizziness, headache, orthostatic hypotension, nausea, abdominal cramps	First-dose phenomenon (orthostatic hypotension) occurs in 1% of patients. Affected patients may collapse for 15 to 60 minutes but usually can tolerate subsequent treatment without ill effects. Give drug with meals or snacks to decrease nausea and dizziness.
chlorotrianisene 12 to 25 mg P.O. daily or cyclically (3 weeks on, 1 week off) **diethylstilbestrol** 0.1 to 5 mg P.O. daily or cyclically	None significant	Thromboembolism, increased risk of stroke, pulmonary embolism, nausea, vomiting	Explain to patient on cyclic therapy for postmenopausal symptoms that, although withdrawal bleeding may occur during week off drug, fertility hasn't been restored. Tell diabetic patient to report positive urine tests so antidiabetic dose can be adjusted. Teach female patient how to self-examine breasts.
chorionic gonadotropin, human (HCG) 10,000 units I.M. 1 day after last dose of menotropins	None significant	Pain at injection site, headache, fatigue	In infertility, encourage daily intercourse from day before therapy begins until ovulation occurs. When used with menotropins to induce ovulation, advise patient of possible multiple births. Be alert for symptoms of ectopic pregnancy—usually evident between weeks 8 and 12 of gestation.
clomiphene citrate 50 to 100 mg P.O. for 5 days	None significant	Nausea, vomiting, hot flashes, breast discomfort, visual disturbances	Drug can be repeated until conception occurs or until three courses of therapy are completed. Tell patient to report visual disturbances immediately. Teach her to take basal body temperature and to record it on graph to determine when ovulation occurs.
medroxyprogesterone acetate 5 to 10 mg P.O. daily for 5 to 10 days	None significant	Breakthrough bleeding, edema, pulmonary embolism, breast tenderness	Tell patient to report vaginal bleeding. Teach her to self-examine breasts. Drug should be discontinued if thromboembolic disorder is suspected.
menotropins (HMG) 75 IU each of FSH and of LH I.M. daily for 9 to 12 days, followed by or administered with chorionic gonadotropin	None significant	Ovarian enlargement with pain and abdominal distention, nausea, vomiting	Reconstitute with 1 to 2 ml sterile saline injection and use immediately. In infertility, encourage daily intercourse from day before chorionic gonadotropin is given until ovulation occurs. Advise patient of possible multiple births.
testosterone cypionate **testosterone enanthate** 100 to 400 mg I.M. q 4 to 6 weeks.	*Oral anticoagulants:* reduced prothrombin time with possible bleeding. Use cautiously.	Acne, edema, weight gain, hirsutism, jaundice	Watch for ecchymoses and petechiae with concomitant anticoagulant therapy. Monitor prothrombin time. Inject deep into upper outer quadrant of gluteal muscle. Report soreness at site; possibility of postinjection furunculosis. Control edema with salt restriction or diuretics. Monitor weight routinely.

Rare endocrine syndromes

Syndrome and cause	Clinical features	Treatment
Achard-Thiers syndrome Results from adrenal hyperplasia with increased androgens and 11-oxysteroids	Obesity, diabetes mellitus, and hirsutism	Adrenal surgery, if possible
Anorchia (vanishing testes syndrome) Unknown cause. Destruction of testes occurs before 14th week of gestation	Vas deferens, with testicular vessels, end blindly or in a rudimentary epididymis. At pubertal age, eunuchoidism and absence of secondary sex characteristics	Long-acting testosterone for life
Bartter's syndrome Unknown cause, possibly congenital	Secondary aldosteronism characterized by hyperplasia of renal juxtaglomerular cells, hyperreninemia, hypokalemia, failure to thrive, and low or normal blood pressure	Partial adrenalectomy; aldosterone antagonists; indomethacin with spironolactone or triamterene
Beckwith-Wiedemann syndrome Unknown cause	Somatic gigantism at or shortly after birth with macroglossia, omphalocele, hypoglycemia, bilateral noncystic renal hyperplasia, and cryptorchidism	Glucagon, cortisone, diazoxide
Chiari-Frommel syndrome Unknown cause. May result from hypothalamic or pituitary dysfunction	Amenorrhea and lactation persist for longer than 6 months after discontinuing weaning. Accompanied by headache, backache, emotional instability, and abdominal pain	Surgery, radiation, bromocriptine
Diencephalic syndrome Results from neurogenic tumors	In infants and children, excessive GH secretion produces tumors in and around third ventricle. Affected patients appear alert and euphoric despite cachexia and emaciation	Surgery, if possible
DiGeorge's syndrome Unknown cause	Congenital absence of thymus and parathyroid glands causes tetany, dehydration, and severe infections.	Thymus transplant, calcium, antibiotics
Forbes-Albright syndrome Unknown cause. May result from pituitary tumor in 50% of patients	Amenorrhea, galactorrhea	Hypophysectomy, radiation, bromocriptine
Houssay syndrome Results from necrosis or infarction of pituitary in diabetic patients	Signs and symptoms of diabetes disappear, but those of hypopituitarism become suddenly or progressively evident.	ACTH and corticosteroids to correct hypoglycemia and other features of hypopituitarism
Kallmann's syndrome Unknown cause. May result from autosomal dominant trait	Olfactogenital dysplasia, causing anosmia, absence of secondary sex characteristics, hypertension, mental retardation, and occasionally, color blindness	Gonadotropin, testosterone, or estrogen
Laurence-Moon-Biedl syndrome Unknown cause	Primary and secondary hypogonadism, with retinitis pigmentosa, mental retardation, obesity, polydactyly	None
Leprechaunism (Donohue's syndrome) Unknown cause. May result from autosomal recessive trait	Intrauterine growth failure resulting in dwarfism with prominent eyes, thick lips, large ears and phallus, breast hyperplasia, hirsutism, and islet cell hyperplasia	None
MEN I (multiple endocrine neoplasia I or Wermer's syndrome) Unknown cause. May result from dominant autosomal trait	Pituitary, parathyroid, and pancreatic adenomas accompanied by peptic ulcer. Severity varies according to affected glands, but primary hyperparathyroidism and hypergastrinemia are most common.	Surgery, if possible; hormonal replacement
MEN II (multiple endocrine neoplasia II or Sipple's syndrome) Results from dominant autosomal trait	Medullary carcinoma of thyroid accompanied by pheochromocytoma and, at times, parathyroid tumors, neurofibromas, diabetes mellitus, and diarrhea.	Surgery, chemotherapy
MEN III (MEN II-b) Unknown cause	Resembles MEN II, except for low incidence of parathyroid tumors.	Surgery, if possible
Nelson's syndrome Results from an ACTH-secreting pituitary adenoma	Adenoma growth occurs in some patients with Cushing's disease after bilateral adrenalectomy, causing pigmentation of skin and mucosae and visual field defects	Radiation of hypophysis or hypophysectomy
Prader-Willi syndrome Unknown cause. Usually affects males	First months: areflexia, poor or absent response to pain, feeding difficulties. After 6 months: active reflexes, obesity, short stature, small penis, cryptorchidism. At pubertal age: lack of development of secondary sex characteristics.	Symptomatic: antidiabetics, amphetamine to control hyperphagia, testosterone replacement, low caloric intake
Soto's syndrome (cerebral gigantism) Unknown cause	Aberrant growth in children: large, elongated head, prominent forehead, large ears and jaw, antimongoloid slant to eyes, and elongated chin. Also, coarse facial features, subnormal intelligence, and impaired coordination	None
Verner-Morrison syndrome Results from neoplastic changes in islets of Langerhans or other body areas	Severe, watery diarrhea, hypokalemia, and achlorhydria	Surgical removal of tumor
Waterhouse-Friderichsen syndrome Usually occurs with meningococcemia, but also with other infections	Adrenal destruction, usually occurring in infants and children, producing adrenal crisis	Treatment of sepsis and adrenal crisis; adrenal hormone replacement
Wolman's syndrome Results from autosomal recessive trait	Congenital adrenal hypoplasia occurring in first weeks of life, with forceful vomiting, abdominal distention, watery diarrhea	None

Selected References and Acknowledgments

Selected References

Brunner, Lillian, and Suddarth, Doris. *Textbook of Medical-Surgical Nursing,* 5th ed. New York: J.B. Lippincott Co., 1984.

Brunner, Lillian, and Suddarth, Doris. *The Lippincott Manual of Nursing Practice,* 3rd ed. New York: J.B. Lippincott Co., 1982.

Campbell, Claire. *Nursing Diagnosis and Intervention in Nursing Practice.* New York: John Wiley & Sons, 1978.

Childs, Belinda P. "Insulin Infusion Pumps—New Solution to an Old Problem," *Nursing83* 13:54-57, November 1983.

Corbett, Jane V. *Laboratory Tests in Nursing Practice.* East Norwalk, Conn.: Appleton-Century-Crofts, 1982.

Cryer, Philip E. *Diagnostic Endocrinology,* 2nd ed. New York: Oxford University Press, 1979.

Dillon, Richard S. *Handbook of Endocrinology: Diagnosis and Management of Endocrine and Metabolic Disorders,* 2nd ed. Philadelphia: Lea & Febiger, 1980.

Evangelisti, J.T., and Thorpe, C.J. "Thyroid Storm—A Nursing Crisis," *Heart & Lung* 12:184-194, March 1983.

Guthrie, Diana W., and Guthrie, Richard A. *Nursing Management of Diabetes Mellitus,* 2nd ed. St. Louis: C.V. Mosby Co., 1982.

Halsted, Charles H., and Halsted, James A. *The Laboratory in Clinical Medicine.* Philadelphia: W.B. Saunders Co., 1981.

Hershman, Jerome, M., ed. *Endocrine Pathophysiology: A Patient-Oriented Approach,* 2nd ed. Philadelphia: Lea & Febiger, 1982.

Honigman, R.E. "Deciphering Diagnostic Tests: Thyroid Function Tests," *Nursing82* 12:68-71, April 1982.

Kee, Joyce L. *Laboratory and Diagnostic Tests with Nursing Implications.* East Norwalk, Conn.: Appleton-Century-Crofts, 1982.

Keller, Paul J. *Hormonal Disorders in Gynecology.* New York: Springer-Verlag, 1981.

Krieger, Dorothy T., and Bardin, C. Wayne, eds. *Current Therapy in Endocrinology 1983-84.* St. Louis: C.V. Mosby Co., 1983.

Laycock, John, and Lee, Julius. *Essential Endocrinology.* New York: Oxford University Press, 1983.

Muthe, Norma C. *Endocrinology: A Nursing Approach.* Boston: Little, Brown & Co., 1981.

Netter, Frank. *The CIBA Collection of Medical Illustrations.* West Caldwell, N.J.: CIBA Pharmaceutical Co., 1974.

Niedringhaus, L. "A Nursing Emergency: Acute Adrenal Crisis," *Focus on Critical Care* 10(1):30-36, February 1983.

Quinlan, M. "Solving the Mysteries of Calcium Imbalance: An Action Guide," *RN* 45(11):50-54, November 1982.

Robinson, Lisa. *Psychiatric Nursing as a Human Experience,* 3rd ed. Philadelphia: W.B. Saunders Co., 1983.

Sanford, S.J. "Symposium on Endocrine Disorders. Dysfunction of the Adrenal Gland: Physiologic Considerations and Nursing Problems," *Nursing Clinics of North America* 15:481-98, September 1980.

Skylar, D.L., et al. "Algorithms for Adjustment of Insulin Dosage by Patients Who Monitor Blood Glucose," *Diabetes Care* 4:311-18, March/April 1981.

Tepperman, Jay. *Metabolic and Endocrine Physiology,* 4th ed. Chicago: Year Book Medical Pubs., 1980.

Toft, A. D., et al. *The Diagnosis and Management of Endocrine Diseases.* St. Louis: C.V. Mosby Co., 1982.

Van Son, Allene. *Diabetes and Patient Education: A Daily Nursing Challenge.* East Norwalk, Conn.: Appleton-Century-Crofts, 1981.

Vaughan, Victor C., III, et al. *Nelson Textbook of Pediatrics,* 12th ed. Philadelphia: W.B. Saunders Co., 1983.

Wardell, Sandra. *Acute Intervention: Nursing Process Through the Life Span.* Reston, Va.: Reston Publishing Co., 1979.

Widmann, Frances K. *Clinical Interpretation of Laboratory Tests,* 9th ed. Philadelphia: F.A. Davis Co., 1983.

Williams, Robert H. *Textbook of Endocrinology,* 6th ed. Philadelphia: W.B. Saunders Co., 1981.

Wittkower, Eric D., and Warnes, Hector, eds. *Psychosomatic Medicine: Its Clinical Applications.* New York: J.B. Lippincott Co., 1982.

Acknowledgments

◆ p.16 Adapted from Saul M. Genuth, "General Principles of Endocrine Physiology," in R.M. Berne and M.N. Levy (eds.), *Physiology.* St. Louis: C.V. Mosby Co., 1983.
◆ p.34 Photo courtesy of Caroline Dolinskas, Department of Radiology, Pennsylvania Hospital, Philadelphia.
◆ p.54 Photo courtesy of Phillip Felig, John D. Baxter, Arthur E. Broadus, Lawrence A. Frohman, *Endocrinology and Metabolism.* New York: McGraw-Hill Book Co., 1981, p. 193.
◆ p.58 Photo courtesy of Robert Williams, *Textbook of Endocrinology,* 6th ed. Philadelphia: W.B. Saunders Co., 1981, Fig. 3-52, p. 98.
◆ p.66 Adapted from *Patient Care* magazine. Copyright © 1982 Patient Care Communications, Inc., Darien, Conn. All rights reserved.
◆ p.96 Photo courtesy of Morrie Kricun, Associate Professor, Hospital of the University of Pennsylvania.
◆ p.113 Photo courtesy of James W. Lecky, Department of Radiology, University of Pittsburgh School of Medicine, Pittsburgh, Pa.
◆ p.131 Adapted from *Diabetes Mellitus,* 7th ed. Indianapolis: Eli Lilly & Co., 1976.
◆ p.140 Chart adapted from Joan Luckmann and Karen C. Sorenson, *Medical-Surgical Nursing,* 2nd ed. Philadelphia: W.B. Saunders Co., 1980.
◆ p.152 Chart adapted from M. Davidson, *Diabetes Mellitus, Diagnosis and Treatment,* vol. 2, New York: Wiley Medical Pub., 1981, p. 427.
◆ p.156 Graph adapted from F.D. Hofeldt, E.G. Lufkin, L. Hagler, et al., *Diabetes* 23, 1974. Reproduced with permission from the American Diabetes Association, Inc.
◆ p. 166 Photo courtesy of Adele K. Friedman, Associate Professor of Radiology, Department of Radiology, Hospital of the University of Pennsylvania.

INDEX

i = illustration; t = table

i = illustration; t = table

i = illustration; t = table

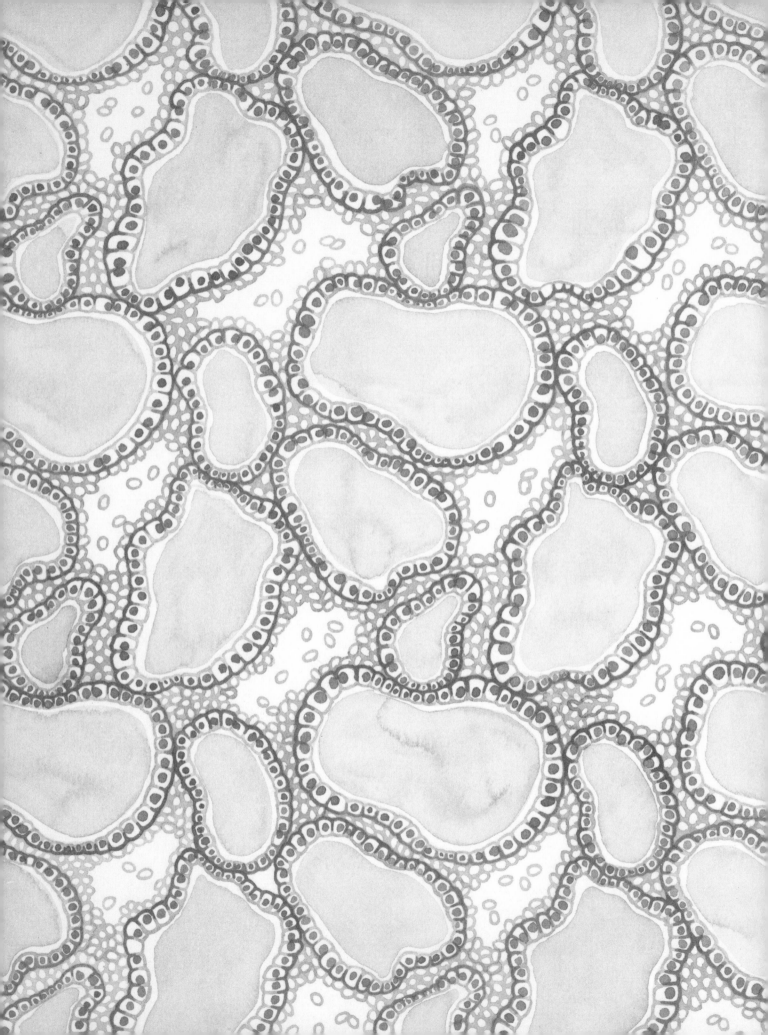